An Atlas of
REPRODUCTIVE
PHYSIOLOGY IN MEN

THE ENCYCLOPEDIA OF VISUAL MEDICINE SERIES

An Atlas of
REPRODUCTIVE
PHYSIOLOGY IN MEN

By

E. S. E. Hafez

with

B. Hafez and S. D. Hafez

Reproductive Health Center
Kiawah Island, SC, USA

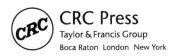

CRC Press
Taylor & Francis Group
Boca Raton London New York

CRC Press is an imprint of the
Taylor & Francis Group, an **informa** business

First published 2004 by The Parthenon Publishing Group

Published 2023 by CRC Press
Taylor & Francis Group
6000 Broken Sound Parkway NW, Suite 300
Boca Raton, FL 33487-2742

ISBN 13: 978-1-84214-235-6 (hbk)

Visit the Taylor & Francis Web site at
http://www.taylorandfrancis.com

and the CRC Press Web site at
http://www.crcpress.com

Library of Congress Cataloging-in-Publication Data
Hafez, E.S.E. (Elsayed Saad Eldin), 1922-
    An altas of reproductive physiology in men / E.S.E. Hafez, B. Hafez, and S.D. Hafez
        p.; cm – (The encyclopedia of visual medicine series)
    Includes bibliographical references and indexes.
    ISBN 1-84214-235–6 (alk paper)
        1. Andrology–Atlases. 2. Generative organs, Male–Atlases. I. Hafez, B. II. Hafez, S. D.
    III. Title. IV. Series.
        [DNLM: 1. Genitalia, Male–Atlases. 2. Reproduction–physiology–Atlases. WJ 17
    E138a 2003]
    QP253.H342003
    612.6′1–dc22   2003056536

British Library Cataloguing in Publication Data
    Hafez, E.S.E. (Elsayed Saad Eldin), 1922–
        An atlas of reproductive physiology in men. – (The encyclopedia of visual medicine series)
        1. Generative organs, Male – Atlases 2. Human reproduction – Atlases
        I. Title II. Hafez, B. III. Hafez, S.D.
        612.6′1

    ISBN 1842142356

Typeset by Siva Math Setters, Chennai, India

Note/Disclaimer:
This book is not a substitute for professional medical advice, diagnosis or treatment, nor is it an official endorsement of any product or procedure. Readers should consult their respective physician for medical advice.

Contents

Preface

It is hoped that this Atlas is both entertaining and useful, allowing the readers to enhance God's gifts to man in more ways than perhaps previously thought. It is estimated that some 40–50% of involuntary childlessness in couples is due to infertility in men. Andrology, the science of the male reproductive system, is a field not well established in medicine, in science or in the public consciousness. Only in the past 10–15 years have researchers begun to specialize in andrology. In the course of conversation, it seemed that, despite plenty of Viagra® hype, there were many questions and very few explanations. Unlike gynecology, the science of andrology is a young discipline and is currently generating some amazing new insights as well as many new puzzling questions.

This Atlas summarizes in simple tables and elaborate illustrations some of the latest research findings in the field: male endocrinology, neuroendocrinology, growth factors, wellness, sperm quality, fertility and male reproductive dysfunction, erectile dysfunction, genes, andrology, immuno- and molecular andrology, male contraception, and future research directions. A few groups of enthusiastic researchers have devoted special attention to human andrology and rapid development is anticipated owing to the application of modern technology, which has advanced so spectacularly in recent years.

Stress, an ill-defined term, is a phenomenon that has quite different meanings for the politician, social scientist, physician, nurse, psychotherapist, physiologist and molecular biologist. Stress, either endogenous or exogenous, is a real or perceived challenge that disturbs homeostasis. Stressors include violence, bereavement, redundancy or unemployment, and physical, chemical, biological or psychological insults. The ability to adapt to stress and cope depends on genetic, experiential, social, and environmental factors. The stress response reflects a set of integrated cascades in the nervous, endocrine and immune defense systems. Recent advances in molecular genetics have made a significant impact on the precision of assessing the physiopathological processes of the stress response.

The chapters of this Atlas are multidisciplinary in nature, and in their range and depth they reflect our intention to bridge the gap between basic and clinical science. There is a chapter devoted to laboratory techniques, morphological, anatomical, biochemical, immunological, hereditary and microbiological parameters and their clinical application. For the evaluation of important parameters, several methods have been included to enable the andrologist to select the most suitable method, depending on the available apparatus. A few specialized techniques such as GnRH and hCG tests, steroid metabolism *in vitro*, RNA extraction and RT-PCR, H-steroid receptor binding, flow cytometry, nucleus decondensation and chemotaxis assays have been included in the hope that they might be applied in certain clinical situations.

E. S. E. Hafez
Reproductive Health Center
Kiawah Island, SC, USA
2003

Dedication

This atlas is for all research workers in andrology dedicated to the improvement of quality of life

Acknowledgements

The senior author is grateful to his co-authors for their support, discussion and editorial skills and to Ms Cindy Lloyd for her elegant secretarial and clerical help. We are indebted to several academics who have allowed us to include their valuable illustrations and research results in the Atlas, particularly Professor Nabil K. Bissada (Medical University of South Carolina, USA), Professor Bruno Lunenfeld (Bar Illan University, Bar Ilan, Israel) and Professor Carl Pinkert (University of Alabama, Birmingham, Alabama, USA). We thank Parthenon Publishing for their enthusiasm, encouragement, and Herculean efforts, and for giving generously of their intellect, expertise, sound advice, and unstinting work. We are greatly indebted to friends and colleagues who made the writing of this Atlas such a satisfying experience. Special thanks are due to the Society for the Study of Reproduction and the American Society of Andrology for giving permission to use illustrations from their journals. Finally, we would also like to thank those who answered our questions on the phone, via e-mail or in personal conversation in a patient and honest fashion.

CHAPTER 1

Hormones, neurohormones and growth factors

HORMONES

Male reproduction is regulated and co-ordinated by an interaction of the endocrine glands and the central nervous system (CNS). Unlike the CNS, which controls body function through rapid, electric nerve impulses, the endocrine system uses chemical messengers or hormones to regulate slow body processes, e.g. growth and reproduction. The classic definition of a hormone is a physiological, organic, chemical substance (synthesized and secreted by a ductless endocrine gland), which passes into the circulatory system for transport. Hormones inhibit, stimulate, or regulate the functional activity of target organs or tissues. Growth factors are hormone-related substances controlling the growth and development of several organs, tissues and cultured cells. Unlike hormones, growth factors are produced and secreted by cells from different tissues to diffuse into target cells. This chapter deals with the biochemical structure, modes of communication and functional feedback of the major reproductive hormones as well as growth factors involved in male reproduction.

NEUROHYPOPHYSEAL HORMONES

The hormones of the posterior pituitary (neurohypophysis) differ from the other pituitary hormones in that they do not originate from the pituitary, but are only stored there until needed. The two hormones oxytocin ('milk letdown hormone') and vasopressin (antidiuretic hormone; ADH) are produced in the hypothalamus. These hormones are transferred from the hypothalamus to the posterior pituitary not through the vascular system, but along the axons of the nervous system.

The origin and function of neurohormones regulating male reproduction are summarized in Table 1.1. The decrease in membrane Na^+–k^+ ATPase activity in infertile men could be due to the fact that the hyperpolarizing neurotransmitters (dopamine, morphine and norepinephrine(noradrenaline)) are reduced and the depolarizing neuroactive compounds (serotonin, strychnine, nicotine and quinolinic acid) are increased. The schizoid neurotransmitter pattern of reduced dopamine, norepinephrine and morphine and increased serotonin, strychnine and nicotine is common to infertile men, and could predispose to the development of their infertility (Carpenter and Buchnan, 1994). The neurotransmitter patterns and upregulated isoprenoid pathway noted in infertile males are similar to those obtained in right hemispheric dominant individuals. In right hemispheric dominant individuals the isoprenoid pathway is upregulated with hyperdigoxinemia and increased tryptophan catabolism and reduced tyrosine catabolism. In left hemispheric dominant individuals the isoprenoid pathway is downregulated with hypodigoxinemia and reduced trytophan catabolism and increased tyrosine catabolism (Kurup and Kurup, 2003). Human male infertility therefore occurs in right hemispheric chemical dominance.

Table 1.1 Summary of origin and function of neurohormones regulating reproduction

Hormones	Origin	Neural pathways	Principal functions
Prolactin inhibiting hormone Prolactin releasing hormone	hypothalamus	neurons containing dopamine in the arcuate nucleus	Inhibits prolactin release stimulates prolactin release
Gonadotropin releasing hormone	ventromedial nucleus arcuate nucleus median eminence	negative feedback from gonads	stimulates tonic release of FSH and LH
	anterior hypothalamic area preoptic nuclei suprachiasmatic nucleus	hypothalamic cells sensitive to estrogen, touch receptors in skin and genitalia of reflex ovulating species	stimulates preovulatory surge of FSH and LH
Oxytocin	paraventricular nuclei supraoptic nuclei	tactile sensations from the mammary gland, uterus and cervix	induces uterine contractions and milk letdown, and facilitates gamete transport
Melatonin	pineal body	retina via retinohypothalamic fibers	inhibits gonadotropic activity in long-day breeders, e.g. hamster stimulates the onset of the breeding season in short-day breeders, e.g. sheep

FSH, follicle stimulating hormone; LH, luteinizing hormone

GROWTH FACTORS

There are three types of epithelial cell: secretory glandular cells, non-secretory basal cells and neuro-endocrine cells: The basal cells are stem cells for secretory epithelial cells and they are androgen-independent because they do not express androgen receptors (Ars). The neuroendocrine cells play a role in regulating the growth and function of the secretory cells. The mesenchyme comprises smooth muscle cells, fibroblasts, lymphocytes and neuromuscular tissue embedded in an extracellular matrix (Figure 1.1).

While mesenchymal–epithelial interactions play a fundamental role in male sex accessory organ development, the overall developmental process is triggered by androgens. Although the role of androgens is important, androgens alone are insufficient to maintain the normal homeostasis required for the proper function of the male sex accessory organs (Tanji et al. 2001). The mesenchyme of developing androgen target organs is the actual target and mediator of androgenic effects on the epithelium. Testosterone diffuses into the cell, where it is reduced by the enzyme 5α-reductase to the active androgen, 5α-dihydrotestosterone (DHT). DHT first binds to the AR of mesenchymal cells and this induces the transcription of stroma-derived growth factor, which will then interact with the AR-negative epithelial cells by a second-messenger system to culminate in the transcription of genes required for epithelial cell replication (Tenniswood, 1986).

Growth factors are potent mediators of cellular proliferation, differentiation and death (Steiner, 1993). Several growth factors either stimulate or inhibit growth in the male sex accessory organs: epidermal growth factor (EGF), transforming growth factor-α (TGF-α), transforming growth factor-β (TGF-β), insulin-like growth factor (IGF) I and II, hepatocyte growth factor (HGF) and others (Table 1.2).

HORMONE RECEPTORS

Hormone receptors belong to one of five superfamilies:

(1) Nuclear receptors are ligand-regulated transcription factors used by hydrophobic hormones;

(2) Some membrane receptors possess intrinsic enzymatic activity; examples are protein tyrosine kinase, serine-threonine kinase or guanylate cyclase;

(3) Cytokine receptors lack any intrinsic enzymatic activity but associate with soluble tyrosine kinases;

(4) Other receptors are primarily coupled to G proteins, which are effectors regulated by guanosine triphosphate (GTP);

(5) Ligand-gated ion channels use ions as second messengers (Bolander, 2000).

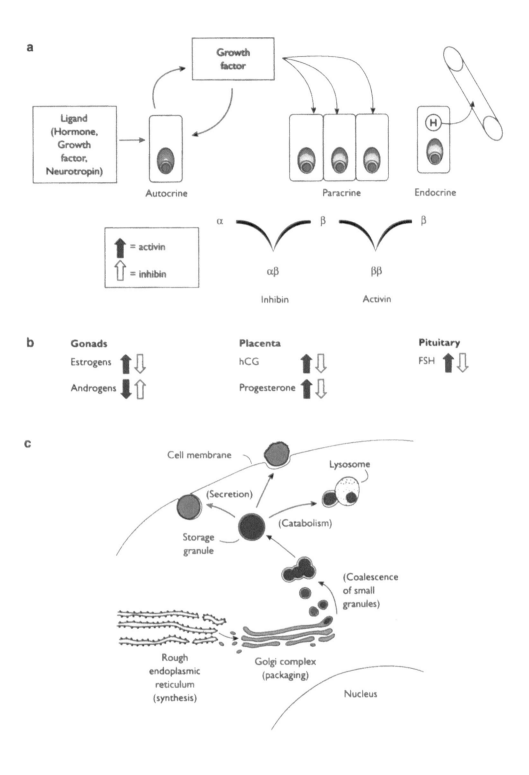

Figure 1.1 (a) Modes of intercellular communication. Locally produced growth factors acting in an autocrine/paracrine manner mediate endocrine action in target cells. (b) Summary of the physiological actions of inhibins and activins (adapted from Vale *et al*. 1994). (c) Synthesis, storage, secretion and catabolism of prolactin in a pituitary cell. The hormone is synthesized by rough endoplasmic reticulum, and packaged into granules by the Golgi complex. The granules coalesce to form mature storage granules and, upon appropriate stimulation, move to the cell surface for release by fusion of their membranes with the cell membrane. In the absence of continued stimulation for release, the granules, are incorporated into autophagic vacuoles where they are digested by lysosomal enzymes

Table 1.2 Putative autocrine/paracrine regulators and reproductive function

Putative regulator	Principal functions
ECF (epidermal growth factor)	May stimulate regrowth of epithelium following disruption of ovarian surface at ovulation
ECG-I-like peptides	Growth and development of neonatal uterus; relation of these peptides with estrogen action unknown
FGF (fibroblast growth factor)	18 000-Da protein stimulates proliferation of various cell types required for blastocyst implantation and embryonic development
GHRH (growth hormone releasing hormone)	Modulatory action of GHRH on gonadal function is dependent on follicle stimulating hormone (FSH) exerting synergistic action during ovarian follicle maturation
GM-CSF (granulocyte–macrophage colony-stimulating factor)	Secreted by placental cells; autocrine within certain cells of fetal placenta
	An important cytokine that serves as a basis for interaction between maternal immune system and reproductive tissues during mammalian pregnancy
IFN (interferon)	Cytokine with complex effects on cells of immune system in ovine and bovine studies. Conceptus produce IFN as major secretory factor before implantation
IGF (insulin-like growth factor)	Plays a role in early pregnancy in ruminants
	Endometrium synthesizes and secretes four IGF isoforms
	Testicular EGF plays a role in regulation of spermatogonial division and testicular IGF-I production stimulated by retinal, without cyclic changes in testicular IGF-I concentrations
Intrafollicular growth factor	Regulates steroidogenesis in granulosa cells in large ovarian follicles via aromatase activity
PAF (platelet-activating factor)	Phospholipid secreted by human blastocyst, an autocrine growth factor, needed for implantation
	PAF performs autiluteolytic and luteotropic function during pregnancy
PDGF (platelet-derived growth factor)	Promotes hatching and blastocyst outgrowth after *in vitro* microinjection of anti-PDGF antibodies into uterine lumen
Relaxin	Polypeptide, closely related structure to insulin and insulin-like growth factors, synthesized and secreted by corpus luteum
TNF (tumor necrosis factor)	Immunohistochemically localized in ovary: granulosa cells of antral follicle
	Increases thecal progesterone production and inhibits basal and FSH-stimulated progesterone in granulosa cells
	TNF and human chorionic gonadotropin (hCG) increase progesterone secretion above maximal dose of hCG

Nuclear receptors

Steroids and triiodothyronine are hydrophobic, readily pass through the plasma membrane, enter the nucleus and bind to transcription factors, whose activity they allosterically modulate. These ligand-regulated transcription factors are modular in structure. First, there is an amino-terminal transcription activation domain that recruits elements of the general transcriptional machinery, as well as proteins that nuclear alter chromatin structure. There is a DNA-binding domain, which targets the nuclear receptor to a specific group of genes, and a hinge region, which contains a nuclear translocation signal. The carboxy terminus harbors many functions. It possesses a second transcription activation domain, the ligand-binding site, a dimerization domain and receptor binding sites for molecular chaperones, called heat shock proteins (hsps), which stabilize the receptor. The last association does not occur in all nuclear receptor families (Bolander, 2000).

Although all nuclear receptors are homologous, they can be functionally divided into three families:

(1) The glucocorticoid family includes receptors for cortisol, aldosterone, androgens and progesterone. It is the most homogeneous group that requires hsps and forms homodimers that bind inverted repeats of the nucleotide sequence TGTTCT.

(2) The thyroid hormone family is the oldest and most diverse group, and includes receptors for triiodothyronine, retinoids, vitamin D, ecdysone and several eicosanoids and fatty acids. They usually form heterodimers with one of the retinoid receptors, serving as a common subunit. They do not require hsps and can bind either direct or inverted repeats of the sequence TGACC.

(3) The estrogen family includes only the estrogen receptor (ER), whose properties are intermediate to those of the other two families, like the

glucocorticoid family, it forms homodimers, requires hsps, and binds to inverted repeats; but these sequences resemble those recognized by the thyroid family (Bolander, 2000).

Estrogen receptor

Two ERs have been identified: ERα and ERβ. Phytoestrogens have a greater affinity for ERβ. ERα has 8 exons, on chromosome 6q. Its molecular weight is 66 000, it has 595 amino acid residues and a half-life of 4–7 h ERβ is localized to chromosome 14, q22-q24 and is in close proximity to Alzheimer's disease genes.

The ligand-binding domain of nuclear receptors is a three-tiered α-helical sandwich where the last helix projects away from the plane of the others and exposes the hydrophobic core. When the ligand binds, this terminal helix closes over it like a lid and creates a new surface for dimerization and transcriptional coactivator binding. In the glucocorticoid and estrogen families, this conformational change also induces hsp dissociation, which exposes the nuclear localization signal and leads to the nuclear accumulation of these receptors. The thyroid family lacks hsps and is constitutively located in the nucleus (Bolander, 2000). The structural alterations are associated with receptor phosphorylation (Bolander, 2000).

Falling hormone levels result in hormone-receptor dissociation and reversal of this process: the receptor is dephosphorylated; separates into monomers; and, for the glucocorticoid and estrogen families, exits the nucleus and reassociates with hsps.

Membrane receptors

Hydrophilic hormones, such as protein and peptide hormones, cannot penetrate the plasma membrane and, therefore, must interact with their receptors at the cell surface. These membrane receptors are integral membrane proteins; as such, they are restricted to the plasmalemma and must generate a second messenger to transmit the signal into the cell's interior. There are four major membrane receptor groups:

(1) Receptors with intrinsic enzymatic activity;

(2) Cytokine receptors;

(3) G protein-coupled receptors;

(4) Ligand-gated ion channels.

Steroids/receptors mediating their non-genomic effects

Steroids can act through the sex hormone binding globulin (SHBG). Because steroids are hydrohodic, they are transported in the blood bound to special transport proteins having hydrophobic pockets. However, SHBG is not just a transport protein; it has its own membrane receptor, which is coupled to cAMP synthesis. This production can be affected by the presence of sex steroids bound to the SHBG (Bolander, 1994, 2000; Nakhla *et al.* 1999).

These hormones are allosteric regulators of transcription factors; they could similarly be allosteric regulators of other molecules, such as enzymes or the cytoskeleton. For example, triiodothyronine directly binds and stabilizes the inactive monomer of pyruvate kinase; thyroxine binds microtubules and inhibits their polymerization (Davis and Davis, 1996; Giguere *et al.* 1996). Alternatively, these hormones may act allosterically on the membrane receptors of other hormones. For example, various sex steroids bind and potentiate the receptor for γ-aminobutyric acid (GABA), but inhibit the glutamate and oxytocin receptors (Grazzini *et al.* 1998; Rupprecht and Holsboer, 1999). Membrane receptors for some hydrophobic hormones are immunologically similar to the corresponding nuclear receptors. The transfection of the gene for the ER into cells lacking any such protein can generate both membrane and nuclear estrogen-binding sites (Razandi *et al.* 1999). The membrane receptor originates from the classic receptor either by alternate splicing of the mRNA or by post-translational modifications, such as the covalent addition of lipids (Bolander, 1994).

In some cases, the membrane receptor appears to be a unique protein distinct from the classic nuclear receptor. The membrane receptor for vitamin D displays a ligand specificity not shared by the classic receptor. The progesterone receptor in vascular smooth muscle is one of the few such receptors that have been sequenced and its primary structure is unique (Falkenstein *et al.* 1996; Bolander, 2000).

Cross-activation of tyrosine kinase receptor

Activation of the tyrosine kinase receptor (TKR) and cytokine receptors is simple and straight forward. A hormone binds to its specific receptor, and induces oligomerization and transphosphorylation of the intrinsic or associated tyrosine kinase. TKR dimerization is not a static event. For example, the EGF family binds to four different isoreceptors that can heterodimerize, depending upon the ligand. This dimerization leads to transphosphorylation, activation, dissociation of the dimer and reformation of the dimer with unmodified partners, which are subsequently phosphorylated (Bolander, 1994, 2000; Gamett *et al.* 1997).

TKRs from completely different families can cross-phosphorylate each other. For example, the activated EGF receptor dimer can phosphorylate and activate the unoccupied platelet-derived growth factor (PDGF) receptor and the IGF I receptor (Burgaud and Baserga, 1996; Habib *et al.* 1998). Such cross-activation can also occur between TKRs and cytokine receptors: the activated stem call factor receptor (aTKR) can phosphorylate the erythropoietin receptor (a cytokine receptor); and growth hormone (a cytokine) can phosphorylate the EGF receptor (Wu *et al.* 1997; Yamauchi *et al.* 1997; Bolander, 1994, 2000).

INHIBIN

Inhibin consist of two dissimilar disulfide-linked subunits. These heterodimers, termed A or B, inhibit pituitary gonadotropin production (Figure 1.1). These effects of inhibin on the pituitary depend on formation of the dimers, while circulating free forms of the α-subunit have no suppressive effect on pituitary follicle stimulating hormone (FSH) secretion. Recently developed assays can specifically measure the bioactive inhibin dimers, inhibin A and inhibin B, as well as the inhibin α-subunit precursor pro-αC, using antibodies against different regions of the inhibin molecule. The function of pro-αC has not yet been determined, but serum concentrations greatly exceed those of inhibins A and B (Burger and Igarashi, 1988; de Kretser *et al.* 1989; Illingworth *et al.* 1996).

A large amount of inhibin pro-αC is secreted from the testes, and this molecule is suspected of participating locally in the physiology of male reproduction as a paracrine and/or autocrine regulator. The α-inhibin precursor modulates binding of FSH to its receptor as well as its biological activity. In this manner, even small concentrations of inhibin precursor proteins could regulate FSH action at the gonadal FSH receptor. Such activity would permit both paracrine and autocrine modulation of a target cell response to FSH through

varied secretion of the free α-subunit precursor, as well as endocrine regulation of systemic FSH when the mature α-subunit is secreted in combination with its β-subunit to form dimeric inhibin (Sehneyer *et al.* 1991; Tuohimaa *et al.* 1993; Anawalt *et al.* 1996).

Pro-αC has been detected in all men studied to date, including orchiectomized patients. There is no significant difference in pro-αC levels between normal men and men with various testicular diseases, expect that orchiectomized men had significantly lower pro-αC concentrations than all other groups.

In oligozoospermic men, inhibin A levels are undetectable, whereas inhibin B concentrations correlate negatively with serum FSH and positively with sperm count and bilateral testicular volume ($p < 0.0001$). The concentration of pro-αC is 557 pg/ml and shows no correlation with serum FSH, LH, testosterone, sperm concentration or bilateral testicular volume. Inhibin pro-αC was not correlated with inhibin B. Pro-αC is unlikely to be a uesful marker for spermatogenesis in infertile men compared with inhibin B (Fujisawa *et al.* 2002).

HYPOTHALAMIC–HYPOPHYSEAL–TESTICULAR AXIS

The hypothalamic–hypophyseal–gonadal axis is evaluated by measuring the luteinzing hormone (LH) and the FSH responses after the administration of synthetic gonadotropin releasing hormone (GnRH) (Figure 1.2). The results from this test are expressed as the percentage increments of the LH and FSH gonadotropins 30, 60 and 90 min after GnRH stimulation, or in absolute values, comparing the responses from the patients against the values from a normal population. The LH and FSH responses to the GnRH stimulus are both related to sex, age and individual sexual maturation. The pubertal increased sensibility of the adenohypohysis to the synthetic decapeptide GnRH is an unequivocal sign of the maturation of the hypothalamic-adenohypohyseal–gonadal axis maturation. The maximum increment of LH is obtained 30 min after GnRH stimulation, and for FSH the maximum increase is obtained after some delay (Roth *et al.* 1972; Garnier *et al.* 1974; Sprat *et al.* 1985). With the human chorionic gonadotropin (hCG) stimulation test one can measure the increments of the gonadal sex steroids testosterone, estradiol and 17-hydroxyprogesterone (17-OHP) 2, 24, 48 and 72h post-hGC stimulation. It

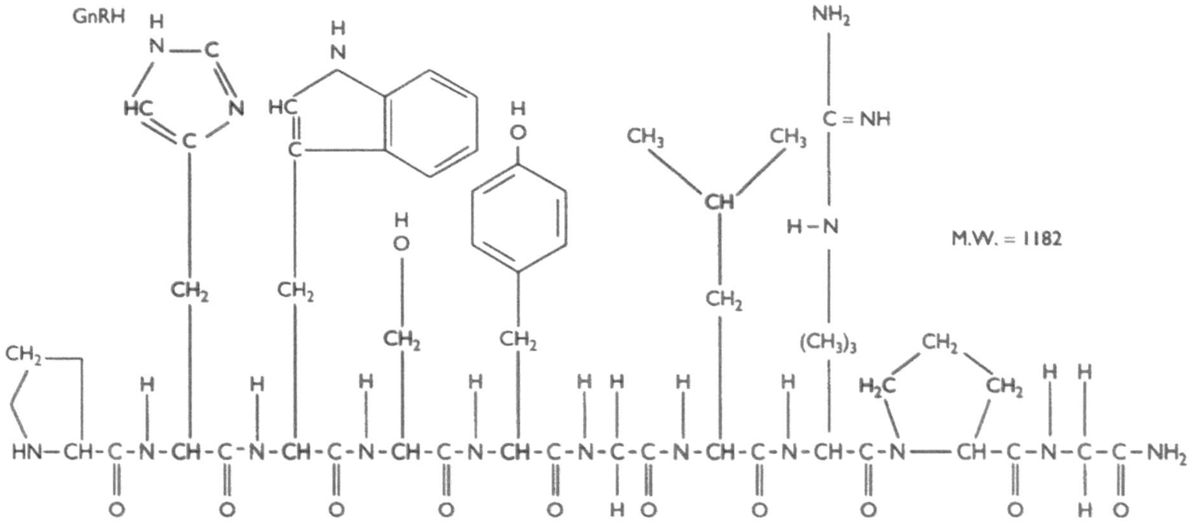

Figure 1.2 Amino acid sequence of gonadotropin releasing hormone (GnRH). (Reproduced with permission from Capen and Martin, 1989)

has been possible to identify gonadal steroid patterns, to differentiate a prepubertal from a postpubertal gonadal development (Martikainen *et al.* 1982).

Osuna *et al.* (2001) conducted an investigation in a Venezuelan population to evaluate the response of pituitary LH and FSH to the GnRH action in adolescents/adults. The gonadal steroid secretion 2, 24, 48 and 72h post-hCG administration was lower in the at stage adolescents Tanner 4. The gonadal steroid response post-hGC stimulation in the Tanner 5 adolescent group was similar to that obtained in adults. In late puberty the LH response to a GnRH stimulus is not related either to age or to sexual development, contrary to the FSH response obtained after GnRH and the gonadal steroid response after hCG stimulus, both of which are related to age and sexual development.

GONADOTROPIN RELEASING HORMONE ANALOG

Through the pioneer research of Lunenfeld and Gooren (2001), there are several GnRH agonists currently approved by the Food and Drug Administration (FDA). Application of a GnRH agoinst leads to a rapid increase of LH, FSH and sex steroids, such as testosterone in males (flare-up) followed by a downregulation of receptors, a desensitization and consequently a suppression of both FSH and LH, followed by suppression of sex steroids to castration levels (Figure 1.3). There are several short and long protocols that are effective for *in vitro* fertilization (IVF) and other similar procedures (Felberbaun *et al.* 2001). The long protocol is much more effective compared with stimulation without the administration of GnRH analogs, and is also more effective than other protocols for administration of GnRH agoinsts, like the short and ultra-short protocols.

PROLACTIN

Prolactin (PRL) exerts biphasic control of steroidogenesis in Leydig cells. That is, at a physiological concentration PRL enhances the stimulation of gonadotropin on Leydig cells and increases the production of progesterone or testosterone, and at a higher concentration PRL inhibits gonadotropin-induced steroidogenesis (Wesis-Messer *et al.* 1996). Several substances are known to regulate pituitary PRL secretion. Thyrotropin releasing hormone (TRH), vasopressin and vasoactive intestinal peptide secreted from the hypothalamus stimulate pituitary production of PRL, Whereas dopamine suppresses it (Behre *et al.* 1997). Plasma estradiol, testosterone or even physical or psychological stresses increase the plasma PRL level.

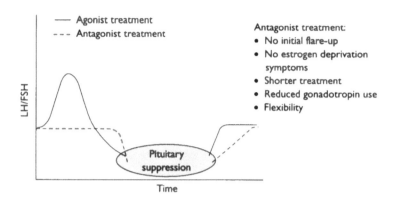

Figure 1.3 Effects of gonadotropin releasing hormone (GnRH) antagonist versus agonist treatment in levels of luteinizing hormone (LH) and follicle stimulating hormone (FSH). (Reproduced with permission from Lunenfeld, 2001)

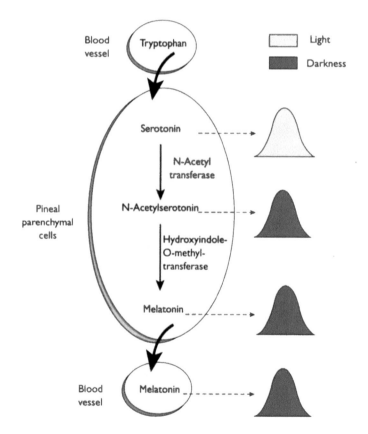

Figure 1.4 Formation of melatonin and diurnal rhythms in the pineal body and the blood

Table 1.3 Summary of physiological events during the reproductive cycle in men

Stages of life cycle	Age	Physioanatomical events
Fetal differentiation	5 (CRL 7)	gonadal primordia appear
(weeks of gestation)	6 (CRL 16)	seminiferous cords develop
	7 (CRL 29)	interstitial cells appear
	8 (CRL 40)	Müllerian ducts regress
	9 (CRL 50)	Wolffian ducts develop; urethral folds fuse into penis (first prostatic bud appears)
Adolescence (years)	12–17	extensive development of Leydig cells
	11–12	testicular spurt and fat spurt; seminiferous tubules differentiate (spermatogonia and primary spermatocyte);
	12–13	Straight public hair appears; Leydig cells differentiate; secondary spermatocytes appear; penis spurt and height spurt; kinky public hair appears;
	13–14	Voice deepening; first ejaculation; circumanal hair
	15–17	Spermatozoa appear; axillary hair; fat decreases; sweat and subaceous glands are large
Reproductive senescence	varies	testes size and firmness decrease; basement membrane and tunica propria of seminiferous tubules thicken; tubules decrease in diameter; degenerative changes in germinal epithelium; reduced sperm production; Sertoli cells obliterate, contain golden-brown pigment granules; progressive intertubular fibrosis causes separation of seminiferous tubules from blood supply; prostate gland enlarges, its contractions become weaker; number of coitus per year declines from 109 (35–44 years of age) to 81 (45–53 years) to 22 (65–74 years)

(Data from Charny et al. 1952; Tanner, 1965; Newman, 1970)

Table 1.4 Classification of 'androgenic' diseases in humans

High plasma androgen levels	Probably normal plasma androgen levels
Idiopathic precocious puberty in boys and girls	Hypersexuality and 'aggressive states' in adults males
Hirsutism in adult females	Acne and seborrhea in juveniles and young adults of both sexes
Male pattern baldness in adult females	Baldness in adult males in genetically susceptible individuals
All signs of virilization in females, e.g. those due to virilizing tumors or the administration of androgens	Benign prostatic hypertrophy; androgen-dependent cancer, e.g. prostatic carcinoma

MELATONIN

In humans melatonin may act at the testicular level by reducing sperm motility and concentration. However, long-term melatonin administration given to normal men had no effect on the secretory patterns of the reproductive hormones. It would appear that estrogen and possibly melatonin are required for human spermatogenesis to proceed normally, possibly by local production or action of these hormones (Figure 1.4). Both ERα and Erβ are demonstrated in human testes, and low concentrations of estradiol effectively inhibit germ cell apoptosis (Pentikainen et al. 2001). Also, aromatase was found within the Leydig cell cytoplasm of a normal adult human testis and in Sertoli cells (Inkster et al. 1995). The fact that ARs are expressed at the majority of sites at which ERs and aromatase are also expressed, suggests that the local balance between estrogen and androgen action is important (Swan et al. 2000).

HORMONAL DISTURBANCES

The physiological events during the reproductive cycle in men are summarized in Table 1.3. Androgenic diseases in men are classified into two major groups: those with a high plasma androgen level and those with a probably normal plasma androgen level (Table 1.4). Male hypogonadism and related phenomena during sexual maturity in boys are classified as: primary testicular failure; secondary testicular failure; and defective androgen action (Table 1.5).

DRUG DELIVERY SYSTEMS

Surfactant and polymer systems play an important role in durg delivery systems, where they contribute significantly to therapeutic efficiency. They allow control of the drug release rate, enhance effective drug solubility, minimize drug degradation, contribute to reduced drug toxicity and facilitate control of drug

Table 1.5 Causes of male hypogonadism and related phenomena during sexual maturity in boys

Syndrome	Etiology	Clinical manifestations	LH	FSH	Testosterone
Primary testicular failure					
Klinefelter's syndrome	chromosomal defect XXY or mosaic	variable; gynecomastia; small testes; eunuchoidism; sparse facial, axillary and pubic hair; azoospermia; occasional mental retardation	↑	↑	N or ↓
Noonan's syndrome (Ullrich–Turner syndrome)	unknown; occasionally abnormal sex chromosomes	variable; small testes; small penis; cryptorchidism; pulmonary valve stenosis; short stature; webbed neck; cubitus valgus; mental retardation	↑	↑	↓
Anorchia	congenital	no sexual maturation; complete lack of androgenization	↑	↑	↓
Seminiferous tubule failure	Sertoli cells only; orchitis (mumps; bacterial); irradiation; chemotherapy; idiopathic	normally androgenized testes may be normal or small; oligo-or azoospermia	N	N or ↑	N
Secondary testicular failure					
Hypothalamic–pituitary disease	tumor craniopharyngioma; granuloma; abscess	if acquired pre-puberty: lack of sexual maturation, no facial, axillary or pubic hair, high-pitched voice, poor strength, small penis and testis, azoospermia, impotence, fine skin, eunuchoidism if acquired post-puberty: loss of libido, impotence, azoospermia, decreased shaving, decreased testicular size, fine skin, decreased strength	↓	↓	↓
Hypogonadotropic hypogonadism		same as hypothalamic–pituitary disease acquired before puberty; variable anosmia or hyposmia (Kallmann's syndrome); color blindness; deafness; synkinesia	↓	↓	↓
Adrenogenital syndrome	enzyme deficiency in glucocorticoid synthesis by adrenal cortex, producing excess adrenal androgens with suppression of pituitary gonadotropins	pre-puberty: isosexual precocious sexual maturation, large penis, increased muscle bulk, acne, pubic and axillary hair Post-puberty: accentuated secondary sex characteristics, small testes, aggressive behavior, oligo-or azoospermia	N or ↓	N or ↓	↑
Drugs	androgens or estrogens—exogenously administered or sex steroid tumor	androgens—similar to description of adrenogenital syndrome	N or ↓	N or ↓	↑
		estrogens—pre-puberty: breast enlargement, failure of normal sexual maturation post-puberty: decreased facial hair, gynecomastia, female body contours, small testes, azoospermia	N or ↓	N or ↓	↓

(Continued)

Table 1.5 (Continued)

Syndrome	Etiology	Clinical manifestations	LH	FSH	Testosterone
Non-gonadal disease states	hyper- or hypothyroidism; systemic illness	sexual maturation usually normal but oligospermia may result	N	N	N
Defective androgen action					
Male pseudohermaphroditism (complete testicular feminization syndrome)	congenital total endorgan unresponsiveness to action of androgens	phenotypic XY female: no axillary or pubic hair; adequate breast development; immature testes either in abdomen, inguinal canal or labia majora; no internal female genitalia	↑	↑	↑
Incomplete (type I)	congenital partial endorgan responsiveness to action of androgens, X- linked recessive trait	ambiguous sex at birth: small phallus resembling a large clitoris; hypospadias; bifid scrotum; incomplete variable pubertal development; small penis and testes; gynecomastia; female pubic hair distribution; sparse facial hair; azoospermia; cryptorchidism; voice may fail to deepen	↑	N or ↑	↑
Incomplete (type II)	congenital inability to convert testosterone to dihydrotestosterone, autosomal recessive trait	identified as females at birth: severe hypospadias and underdevelopment of vagina; absent female internal genitalia; partial virilization at puberty with clitoromegaly	N	N	N

LH, luteinizing hormone; FSH follicle stimulating hormone; N, normal; ↑, increased; ↓, decreased.
Data from Chaves-Carballo and Hayles, 1966; Walsh *et al.* 1974; Wilson *et al.* 1974

uptake (Figure 1.5). Extensive investigations have been conducted on physicochemical characteristics of surfactants and polymers. However, these findings have not been fully implemented in drug delivery, as a result of lack of interdisciplinary communication. Scientists and engineers in both academia and industry are paying increasing attention to physicochemical aspects of surfactant and polymer systems and recognizing their importance for the design and controlled use of drug delivery formulations. Meanwhile there have been recent advances in biopharmaceuticals, genomics and proteomics. It is recognized that many new synthetic drugs are sparingly soluble, non-crystallizing compounds and are difficult to formulate by traditional means. Various types of surfactants and polymers are of significant in such cases. Of special interest are topics on micelles, liquid crystalline phases, liposomes, microemulsions, emulsions, gels and solid particles (Malmsten, 2002).

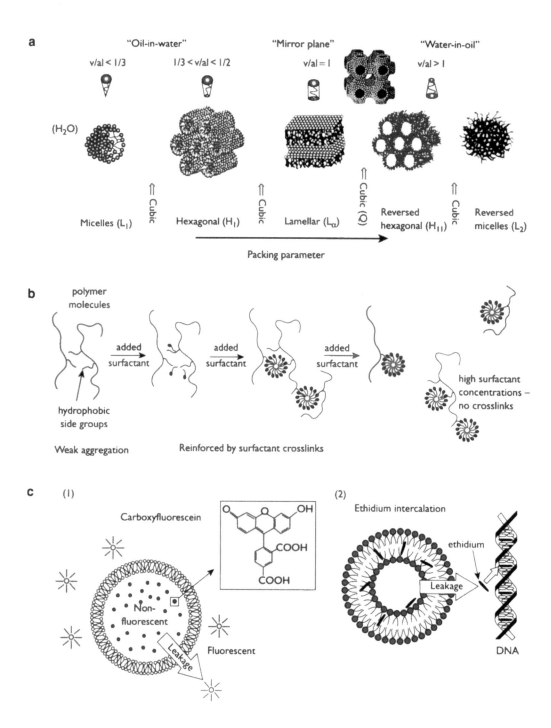

Figure 1.5 Diagrammatic illustrations of some surfactants/polymers in drug delivery systems.

(a) Association structures formed in surfactant and block copolymer systems, and the packing of surfactant molecules in different association structures. (Redrawn with permission from Jönsson et al. 1998).

(b) Effects of surfactant binding to hydrophobe-modified polymers. (Reproduced with permission from Jönsson et al. 1998).

(c) The use of (1) carboxyfluorescein and (2) ethidium for probing release from liposomes.

(d) Polymer-surfactant aggregates.

(e) The gradual progression of the microstructure with the system composition for a microemulsion prepared from non-ionic surfactants. (Redrawn with permission from Lindman et al., 2001).

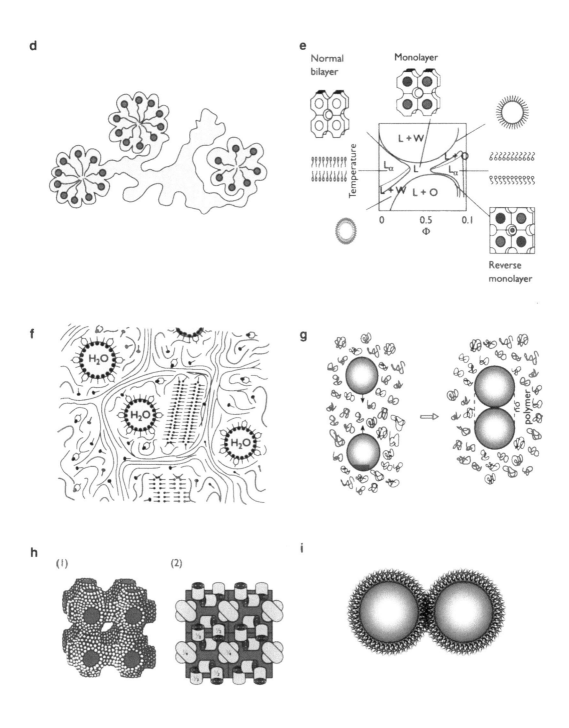

Figure 1.5 (Continued)

(f) The structure of a water/oil cream, consisting of both crystalline and amorphous domains, emulsion droplets, liquid crystalline phases and free emulsifiers. (Redrawn with permission from Junginger, 1994).

(g) Depletion flocculation.

(h) Two different possible cubic liquid crystalline structures: (1) bicontinuous and (2) close-packed slightly elongated micelles.

(i) Steric stabilization of polymer-coated particles

CHAPTER 2

Spermatogenesis/testicular tumors

The following topics will be discussed in this chapter:

(1) The testis;

(2) Spermatogenesis;

(3) Testicular tumors;

(4) Testicular torsion;

(5) Semen evaluation.

THE TESTIS

The testes develop in the abdomen, medial to the embryonic kidney (mesonephros). The plexus of ducts within the testis becomes connected to mesonephric tubules and so to the mesonephric duct, to form the epididymis, ductus deferens and vesicular gland. The prostate and bulbourethral glands form from the embryonic urogenital sinus and the penis forms by tubulation and elongation of a tubercle that develops at the orifice of the urogenital sinus. Male sexual differentiation, testicular descent and spermatogenesis require androgens, which are mediated through the androgen receptor (AR) that binds to the androgen-responsive element on DNA and regulates gene transcription.

During testicular descent, the gonad migrates caudally within the abdomen to the deep inguinal ring. It then traverses the abdominal wall to emerge at the superficial inguinal ring, which is, in fact, the much-enlarged foramen of the genitofemoral nerve. The testis completes its migration by passing fully into the scrotum. Descent is preceded by the formation of the vaginal process, a peritoneal sac extending through the abdominal wall and enclosing the inguinal ligament of the testis. For effective functioning, the testes must be maintained at a temperature lower than that of the body. Anatomic features of the testis and scrotum permit the regulation of testicular temperature. Temperature receptors in the scrotal skin can elicit responses that tend to lower the whole body temperature and provoke panting and sweating. The scrotal skin is noticeably lacking in subcutaneous fat. It is richly endowed with large adrenergic sweat glands, and its muscular (dartos) component enables it to alter the thickness and surface area of the scrotum and vary the closeness of the contact of the testes with the body wall.

Functional histology

The functional histology of the mammalian testis is shown in Table 2.1. The loops of the seminiferous tubules connect to the rete testis and the excurrent duct system. Each seminiferous tubule exhibits a wave of seminiferous epithelium represented along the length of the table (Figure 2.1). During embryonic differentiation of the male and female genital systems the undifferentiated system is composed of a large mesonephros, mesonephric duct, Müllerian duct and undifferentiated gonad.

The seminiferous tubules contain a complex series of developing germ cells that ultimately form the sperm, which are elongated cells consisting of a flattened head containing the nucleus and a tail containing the apparatus necessary for motility. The entire sperm is covered

Table 2.1 Functional histology of the testis

Segment

Tunica albuginea
A thick, white capsule of connective tissue surrounding the testis; made primarily of interlacing series of colleagenous fiber

Seminiferous tubules
Appear as large isolated structures, round or oblong in outline; varying appearance due to the complex coiling of the tubules at many different angles and levels. Between the tubules are masses of interstitial (Leydig) cells, which produce the male sex hormones

Spermatogonia
Lie in the outermost region of the tubule; round nuclei appear as an irregular layer within surrounding connective tissue. Nuclei are small and stain dark, owing to the presence of large numbers of chromatin granules

Primary spermatocytes
Located just inside an irregular layer of spermatogonia and Sertoli cells; nuclei are larger than those of the spermatogonia and stain lighter

Secondary spermatocytes
Maturation divisions and secondary spermatocytes are not seen in the average tubule, owing to the short duration of these stages

Spermatids
Located internally to primary spermatocytes. Layer of spermatids may be several cells thick. Sperm lie along the border of the lumen. The sperm heads are lodged in deep indentations of the surface of the Sertoli cell

Sertoli cells
Large and relatively clear, except for the prominent, dark-staining nucleolus. Cytoplasm is diffuse, and its limits are indefinite

by the plasmalemma or plasma membrane. The acrosome is a double-walled structure situated between the plasma membrane and the anterior portion of the sperm head.

In the seminiferous tubules the stem cells, called 'spermatogonia', divide several times before forming spermatocytes. The spermatocytes then undergo meiosis, thereby reducing the DNA content of the cells to one-half that of somatic cells. This series of cellular divisions, including the proliferation of the spermatogonia and the meiotic divisions, is known as spermatocytogenesis. The haploid cells resulting from this process are called spermatids, which undergo a progressive series of structural and developmental changes to form spermatozoa. These metamorphic changes are known as spermiogenesis. The developing germinal

cells are closely associated with the much larger Sertoli cells, which surround them during development.

The basement membrane or tunica propria that surrounds the seminiferous tubules contains a layer of contractile myoid cells. The principal permeability barrier between the blood and testis is thought to be the complexes at junctions between adjacent Sertoli cells. These Sertoli–Sertoli junctions, which are situated near the cellular base, contain multiple zones of adhesion (tight junctions) where the opposing membranes are fused. The occluding junctions divide the seminiferous tubules into two distinct compartments: a basal compartment containing spermatogonia and preleptotene spermatocytes; and an adluminal compartment, containing the more advanced stages of spermatocytes and spermatids, which freely communicates with the lumen of the tubule. The blood–testis barrier not only excludes entry of certain substances but also appears to function in retaining specific levels of other substances, such as androgen binding protein (ABP), inhibin and enzyme inhibitors, within the luminal compartments of the tubules.

Leydig cells

The interstital (Leydig) cells, which lie between the seminiferous tubules, secrete male hormones into the testicular veins and lymphatic vessels. Leydig cells play multiple and central roles in testicular development and sperm maturation. Several hormones control the functions and development of Leydig cells: luteinizing hormone (LH), chorionic gonadotropin and local factors, including insulin-like growth factor I and stem cell factor (Dafan, 1998; Yan *et al.* 2000; Mendis-Handagama and Ariyaratne, 2001). Just before puberty, the sustentacular (Sertoli) cells of the tubule form a barrier (Vazama *et al.* 1988), which isolates the differentiating germ cells from the general circulation. These sustentacular cells contribute to fluid production by the tubule and may produce the Müllerian-inhibiting factor found in the rete fluid of adult males (Vigier *et al.* 1983).

Besides central control by gonadotropins, testicular cells exchange numerous messages (steroids, growth factors, cytokines, etc.) that modulate Leydig cell function and especially testosterone synthesis (Lejeune *et al.* 1996; Saez, 1994). Testosterone, together with follicle stimulating hormone (FSH), plays a crucial role in the

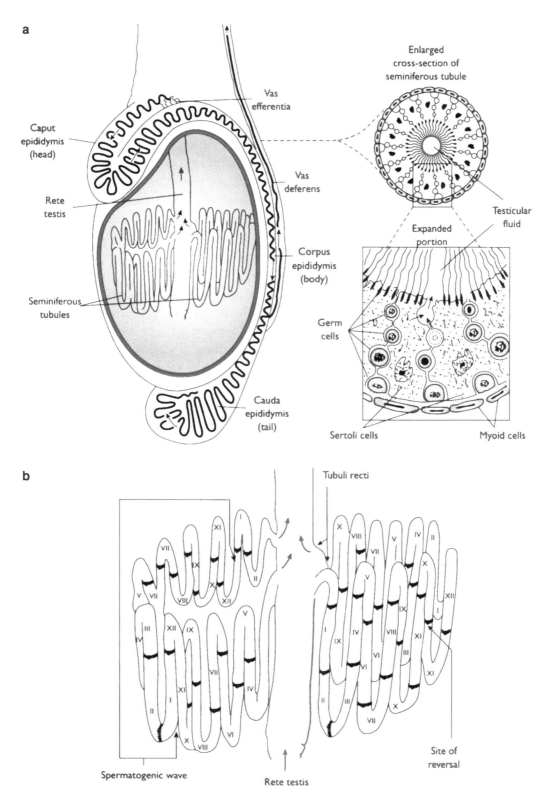

Figure 2.1 (a) Loops of the seminiferous tubules, the rete testis and the excurrent duct system. The pathway by which spermatozoa are transported to the exterior is indicated by arrows. (Modified from Setchell, 1977). (b) A seminiferous tubule in which the wave of the seminiferous epithelium is schematically represented along the length of the tubule. The succession of stages I to XII, the site of reversal in the middle of the tubule and the relationship of the wave to the rete testis are shown. The more advanced stages of each wave are located nearer the rete testis. An actual seminiferous tubule may contain 15 or more complete spermatogenic waves. (Adapted with permission from Perey *et al.* 1961)

development and maintenance of spermatogenesis (Sharpe, 1994; McLachlan *et al.* 1995). FSH modulates Sertoli cell function (Carreau *et al.* 1994).

Endocrine control

Normal testicular function requires hormonal stimulation by pituitary gonadotropins, which are in turn controlled by pulsatile secretion of gonadotropin-releasing hormone (GnRH) from the hypothalamus.

The testes produce not only the major androgen, testosterone, but also a series of related steroid hormones. The major action of androgens is on the Sertoli cells rather than directly on the germ cells. The myoid cells also appear to be androgen dependent. This steroid dependency is met by pulsatile production of androgens by the interstitial Leydig cells, which are adjacent to the seminiferous tubules (Figure 2.2). Leydig cells are stimulated to secrete androgens by pulses of pituitary LH. The androgens produced by the Leydig cells not only diffuse into the adjacent Sertoli cells but are secreted into the blood, where they feed back both at the hypothalamus and at the pituitary to block release of additional LH. Activin and inhibin, which are secreted by the Sertoli cells, have remarkable abilities to generate a diverse series of signals. Activins, potent FSH-releasing dimers (dimers of inhibin β-subunits), have paracrine (inhibiting growth hormone and adrenocorticotropin secretion), and autocrine (stimulating FSH secretion) mechanisms. Activin and inhibin also act within the gonads as autocrine and paracrine modulators of the production of steroids, other hormones and growth factors. Transforming growth factor (TGF), a multifunctional peptide induced in response to steroids, may be involved with the regulation of testicular function. Two groups of compounds are involved in regulation of the hypothalamic–pituitary– gonadal axis. These include neurotransmitters, dopamine, serotonin and norepinephrine (noradrenaline) and brain opioids and other peptides.

Sperm chromatin

Regular condensation of sperm chromatin occurs during spermatogenesis. A sequence of events ending ultimately in the decondensation of the sperm chromatin after penetration or injection into the oocyte is the prerequisite for successful fertilization. A complete failure of sperm head decondensation occurs in 10–38% of the unfertilized metaphase oocyte, whereas 76% of the penetrated oocytes that failed to progress to the pronuclear stage contained sperm nuclei (Selva *et al.* 1993; Dozortsev *et al.* 1994).

The failure of sperm decondensation in the oocytes may be due to a subtle sperm abnormality unrecognizable by conventional analysis, e.g. a structural or biochemical defect associated with chromatin packaging or organization during spermatogenesis (Aitken, 1994; Zamboni, 1994). Intrinsic abnormalities in membrane structure or chromatin organization are associated with the failure of the male pronucleus to develop (Urner *et al.* 1993). Nevertheless, development in pronuclear decondensation and centrosome reconcentration *in vitro* suggests a novel diagnosis assay for these previously undetectable types of male infertility (Stearns and Kirschner, 1994).

There is no correlation between chromatin decondensation and sperm counts in the ejaculate, morphology or the percentage of condensed chromatin. Therefore, chromatin decondensation *in vitro* is not recommended for predicting the fertilization potential of sperm and pregnancy rates in intracytoplasmic sperm injection (ICSI) (Hammadeh *et al.* 2002).

SPERMATOGENESIS

Flow cytometric analysis of spermatogenesis

Flow cytometric separation of testis cells into haploid, diploid and tetraploid fractions is performed as follows. Single-cell suspensions are thawed, centrifuged for 10 min at 500 g and the pellet resuspended in TNE buffer (0.2 ml). A 0.5-ml volume of propidium iodide (PI) (12 μg/ml final concentration) (Sigma, St Louis, MO, USA) is mixed with 0.1 ml of cell suspension. The stained suspension is held in ice for 3–30 min before being aspirated into a Becton Dickinson FAC-Sort Flow Cytometer (Becton Dickinson Corp., San Jose, CA, USA). Red fluorescence (BP650 LP filter) emitted from individual cells is recorded from approximately 10 000 cells per sample after excitation with a 488-nm argon laser.

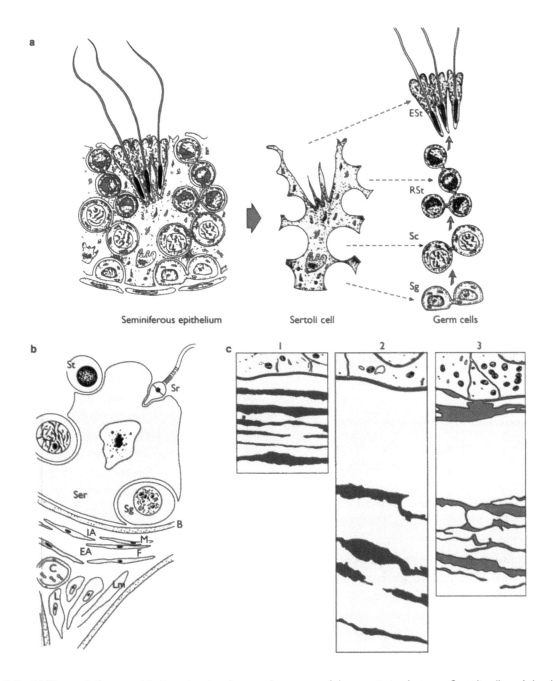

Figure 2.2 (a) The seminiferous epithelium showing the complex nature of the association between Sertoli cells and the developing germ cells, along with an illustration depicting dissociation of this cellular complex. The developing germ cells occupy intracellular spaces between adjacent Sertoli cells and move from the basement membrane towards the lumen during the spermatogenic process. The germ cells begin their developmental process as spermatogonia (Sg), become spermatocytes (Sc), then round spermatids (RSt) and finally elongated spermatids (ESt). Schematic dissociation of the seminiferous epithelium shows how the germ cells occupy the expanded intercellular spaces between adjacent Sertoli cells. (Adapted with permission from Fawcett, 1974.)

(b) Illustration showing the tubular and peritubular anatomy of the testes. B, basement membrane; C, blood capillary; EA, external acellular layer; F, fibroblast; IA, internal acellular layer; L, Leydig cell; Lm, lymph; M, myoid cell capable of contraction; Ser, Sertoli cell; St, spermatid; Sg, spermatogonium; Sr, spermatozoan.

(c) 1: Schematic representation of the normal relationship between the seminiferous epithelium (top) and the boundary tissue of the seminiferous tubules. The contractile cells are shown as dark areas and the intercellular spaces as light zones between them. 2: Thickened lamina propria of the seminiferous tubule, where the basement membrane (dark line on top) is far removed from the first layer of contractile cells. 3: A second mode of thickening of the boundary tissue; the intercellular space that is widened is not in direct contact with the basement membrane of the epithelium. Note some areolar areas between the contractile cells, where collagen bundles can be found. (Figure courtesy of Professor Bustos-Obregon, Santiago, Chile)

Flow cytometric analysis of haploid cells

Cell suspensions are stained with acridine orange by the one-step procedure: the thawed, filtered cell suspension as described above is adjusted with TNE buffer to a concentration of 10^6 cells/ml and held in ice until staining. An aliquot of the suspension (0.1 ml) is mixed with 0.8 ml consisting of 0.6 ml acridine orange (Fluka A.G., Switzerland) solution (6 μg/ml) in citric acid buffer (citric acid 0.1 mol/l, Na_2HPO_4 0.2 mol/l ethylenediaminetetra-acetic acid (EDTA) 1 mmol/l, NaCl 0.15 mol/l, pH 6) and 0.2 ml of lysis solution (Triton X 100 0.1%, NaCl 0.15 mol/l, and HCl 0.08 mol/l). After 3 min the chilled sample is aspirated into a flow cytometer (described above) gated to measure only haploid cells. Green flourescence (BP 530/30 filter) and red flourescence (BP 650 LP filter) were measured for 10 000 cells/sample after excitation with a 488 nm argon laser, and data were displayed as red/green dot-plot diagrams and analyzed using the WINMDI data processing program (Weissenberg et al. 2001).

Flow cytometry/spermiogenesis

Flow cytometry is a powerful method for evaluating any adverse effects upon spermatogenesis because, compared to conventional histological studies, one can examine many cells in a shorter time, providing statistically significant data based on a sample size of 10 000 cells per experimental run.

Flow cytometric examination of the haploid cell fraction reveals any defects in spermatogenesis at the level of maturation of the spermatids (spermiogenesis). When stained with propidium iodide and the histograms are examined, the haploid peak is shifted to the right, compared to that in control cell suspensions, suggesting an abnormal chromatin structure that allowed more dye to enter or to bind to the nucleic acid. Additional study using acridine orange confirms any changes on the maturation of the spermatid chromatin, which normally occurs during spermiogenesis. Flow cytometry is a valuable technique to evaluate any damage caused by chemotherapeutic drugs and/or toxicants in reproductive biology (Weissenberg et al. 2002).

Leydig cells

Testosterone biosynthesis in Leydig cells is dependent on endocrine stimulation by human chorionic gonadotropin (hCG), LH, or their intracellular second messenger, cyclic adenosine 3′, 5′-monophosphate (cAMP) (Nishimura et al. 2001). Such hormonal stimulation increases the amount of intracellular cholesterol associated with side-chain cleavage enzyme (P-450$_{scc}$), which results in accelerated testosterone production. In this steroidogenic pathway, reactive oxygen species (ROS) such as superoxide anion and other free radicals can be produced as a result of electron leakage either in the main reactions or as a result of interaction of steroid products or other pseudosubstrates with the enzyme. Excessive ROS are a major cause of male infertility (Roveri et al. 1992; Sikka et al. 1995).

Selenium, an essential micronutrient, has profound effects on several important biological functions. In the male reproductive system, this element is necessary for normal development of sperm (Ursini et al. 1999). Selenium concentration in semen is associated with sperm motility, with alterations affecting the incidence of asthenospermia. Decreased selenium content in the testis after hypophysectomy and a rise after administration of testosterone indicate that hormones responsible for spermatogenesis are involved in the maintenance of the testicular selenium concentration.

Selenoprotein is quantitatively important because it accounts for over 60% of plasma selenium in rats with normal selenium status. Expression of selenoprotein P messenger ribonucleic acid (mRNA) is ubiquitous in all rat and human tissues, having the highest abundance in kidney, testis, liver and lung. Selenoprotein P probably functions in selenium transport and as an antioxidant (Wu et al. 1973; Ramauge et al. 1996; Majorino et al. 1998; Nishimura et al. 2001). Selenoprotein P mRNA in the testis is expressed predominantly in interstitial Leydig cells, and involved in testosterone production by these cells (Iglesias et al. 1994). Selenoprotein P in Leydig cells might act to reduce oxidant stress associated with testosterone production.

Nishimura et al. (2001) examined the changes in selenoprotein P mRNA expression and testosterone production following stimulation by a stable analog cAMP in cultured Leydig cells (MLTC-1 cells) under normal oxygen concentrations. Selenoprotein P mRNA was analyzed by Northern blotting, while testosterone concentration in culture medium was measured by radioimmunoassay (RIA). When cAMP was added

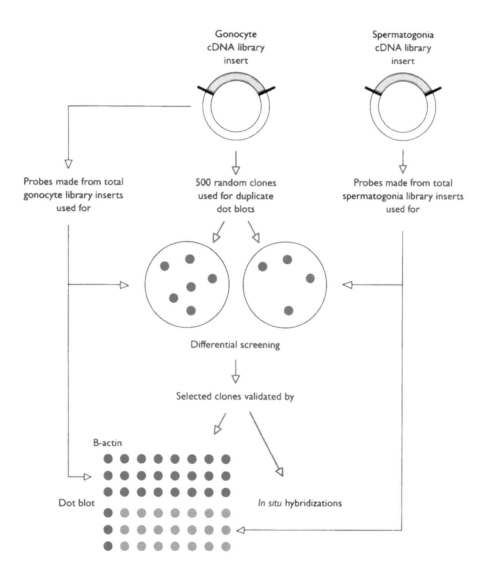

Figure 2.3 Scheme of the protocol used to select the differentially expressed genes in gonocytes compared to their expression in A$_s$, A$_{pr}$, and A$_{al}$ spermatogonia. (Reproduced with permission from Van Den Ham *et al*. 2002)

to cultures at 0, 0.01, 0.1, or 1 mmol/l, selenoprotein P mRNA expression showed does-dependent stimulation. cAMP was added at 0.1 mmol/l to cultures, and the selenoprotein P mRNA expression and testosterone concentration were evaluated after several incubation times. Selenoprotein P mRNA expression was maximal at 9 h. Testosterone concentration in the medium also increased, becoming maximal at 15 h. Selenoprotein P

induced in Leydig cells following cAMP stimulation may counteract oxygen toxicity from cAMP-mediated increases in testosterone production.

Somatic cell lines (Leydig cells)

There is a unique interaction between different types of somatic cell (such as Leydig, Sertoli and peritubular

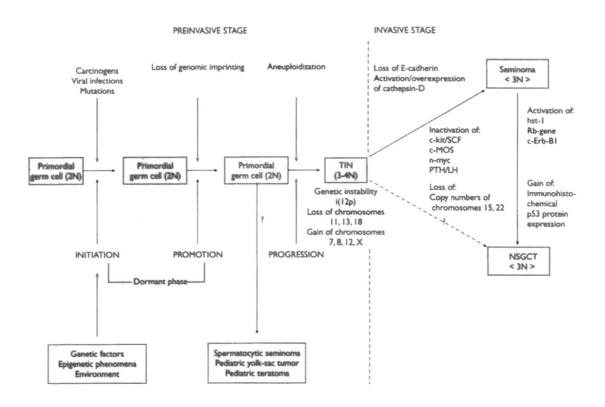

Figure 2.4 Molecular pathogenesis of testicular germ-cell tumors, as summarized from literature data. TIN, testicular intraepithelial neoplasia; PTH/LH, parathyroid hormone/luteinizing hormone; NSGCT, non-seminomatous germ-cell tumor. (From Heidenreich and Olbert, personal communication)

cells) on the one hand and germ cells on the other. Leydig cells synthesize testosterone and play multiple and central roles in testicular development and sperm maturation. Although several cell lines are derived from Leydig cell tumors, only a few of these retain any of the properties of the Leydig cells (Nagy *et al.* 1990; Musa *et al.* 2000). Transgenic mice that harbor the temperature-sensitive SV40 (tsSV40) large T-antigen gene are useful for establishing cell lines from tissues difficult to culture *in vitro* (Obinata, 1997).

Various cell lines with specific functions have been established from different organs by using transgenic mice, e.g. hepatocyte cells, gastric surface mucous cells, colonic epithelial cells and testicular Sertoli cells (Walther *et al.* 1996). Ohta *et al.* (2002a, b) established a Leydig cell line, TTE1, from the temperature-sensitive simian virus 40 large T-antigen transgenic mice. The cells show temperature-sensitive growth characteristics

and a differentiated phenotype at a non-permissive temperature. This was the first attempt in differentiating broad-scale gene expression in Leydig cells using the microarray technology. The ability to analyze broad-scale gene expression in this fashion (Figure 2.3) provides a powerful tool for investigating the molecular mechanisms of Leydig cell functions.

Nitrite production for nitric oxide in Leydig cells

Nitric Oxide (NO) production in Leydig cells is measured as the amount of nitrite in the culture medium (Green *et al.* 1982). Briefly, the Leydig cell culture medium is added to an equal volume of Griess reagent (one part 0.1% naphthylethylenediamine dihydrochloride to one part 1% sulfanilamide in 5% phosphoric acid). Absorbance at 550 nm is measured, and nitrite concentration is determined from comparison

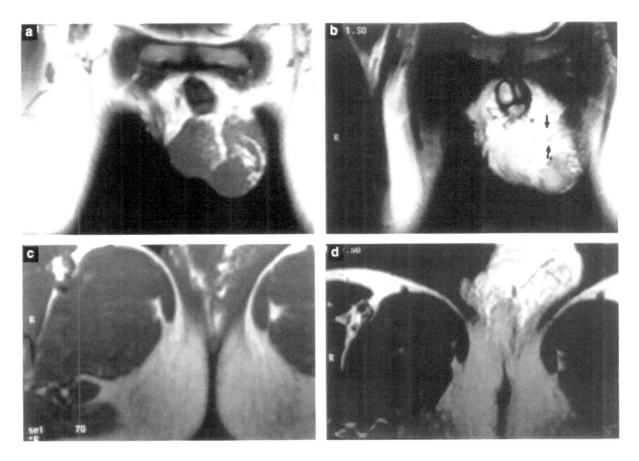

Figure 2.5 Coronal T1-weighted image demonstrating a lobulated lesion involving the upper aspect of the left hemiscrotum. The lesion shows intermediate T1 signal (a) and marked hyperintensity on T2 images (b) relative to muscle. Note several signal void (arrows) in several small focal areas, which possibly represent thrombus. On sagittal views, the mass had lower T1 signal (c) and intermediate T2 signal (d) relative to the testes. (Reproduced with permission from Lin *et al.* 2002, *Arch Androl*, 48:259–65. www.tandf.co.uk/journals)

with a calibration curve of known sodium nitrite standards.

Measurement of testosterone in Leydig cells

Testosterone concentration in Leydig cell culture medium is measured by an enzyme immunoassay (EIA) using a testosterone EIA kit (Cayman Chemical, Ann Arbor, MI, USA). Absorbance at 495 nm is measured, and testosterone is determined from a calibration curve of known testosterone standards.

Reactive oxygen species

Aerobic metabolism of human sperm produces different ROS (H_2O_2, O_2 and $-OHO$), which are potentially harmful to the sperm plasma membrane with its high content of polyunsaturated fatty acids. Seminal plasma contains high- and low-molecular weight factors that protect sperm against free radical toxicity. They include enzymatic ROS scavengers such as CuZn superoxide dismutase and catalase and the chain-breaking antioxidants ascorbate, urate, albumin, glutathione and taurine.

TESTICULAR TUMORS

Extensive investigations have been conducted on the incidence of testicular cancer, and gonadal function with testicular tumors after orchiectomy and/or chemotherapy (Berthehen and Skakkeboek, 1983; Carroll *et al.* 1987; Adami *et al.* 1994; de Wit *et al.* 1995; Brennemann *et al.* 1997; DeSantis *et al.* 1999) (Figures 2.4, 2.5). Testicular tumors are associated with congenital anomalies such as hypospadias

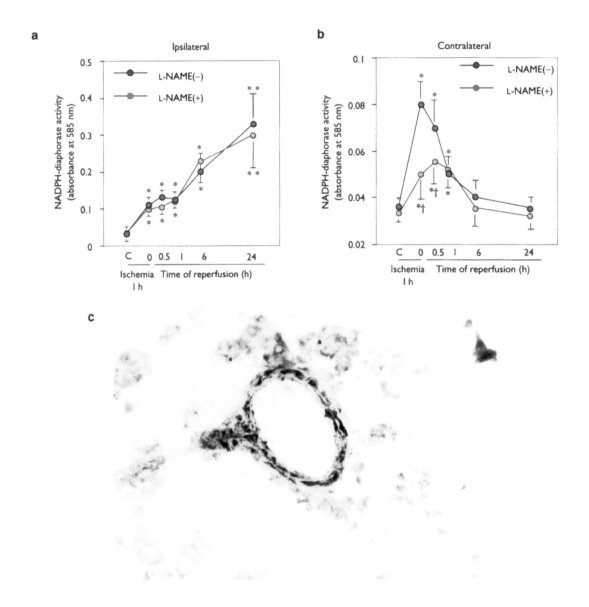

Figure 2.6 Time course and effect of L-NAME on reduced nicotinamide-adenine dinucleotide phosphate (NADPH)-diaphorase activity of ipsilateral (a) and contralateral testes (b). The activity after 1 h of ischemia followed by 0–24 h of reperfusion in the presence (closed circles, *n* = 8 per point) or absence (open circles, *n* = 6 per point) of L-NAME injected during the pre-ischemic period. Data are expressed as mean ± SEM. *$p < 0.05$; **$p < 0.01$ vs. control; †$p < 0.05$ between the two groups. (c) Cytochemical representation of NADPH-diaphorase activity in the contralateral testis during unilateral testicular torsion (× 400). (Reproduced with permission from Shiraishi *et al.* 2003, *Arch Androl*, 49:179–90. www.tandf.co.uk/journals)

or undescended testes (Petersen *et al.* 1998). This is particularly due to a pre-existing abnormality in the contralateral testis, high scrotal temperature due to a tumor-bearing testis, hormonal abnormality and the generation of anti-sperm antibodies. Another important issue is the effect of treatments including orchiectomy, radiotherapy, chemotherapy and retroperitoneal lymphadenectomy, which causes ejaculatory

disturbance. Although the introduction of a surveillance policy for stage I testicular germ cell tumors provides better long-term fertility outcome, some stage I patients still need prophylactic chemotherapy because of the high probability of recurrence (Figure 2.6).

Tomomasa *et al.* (2002) evaluated gonadal function in patients with testicular germ cell tumors, after two or

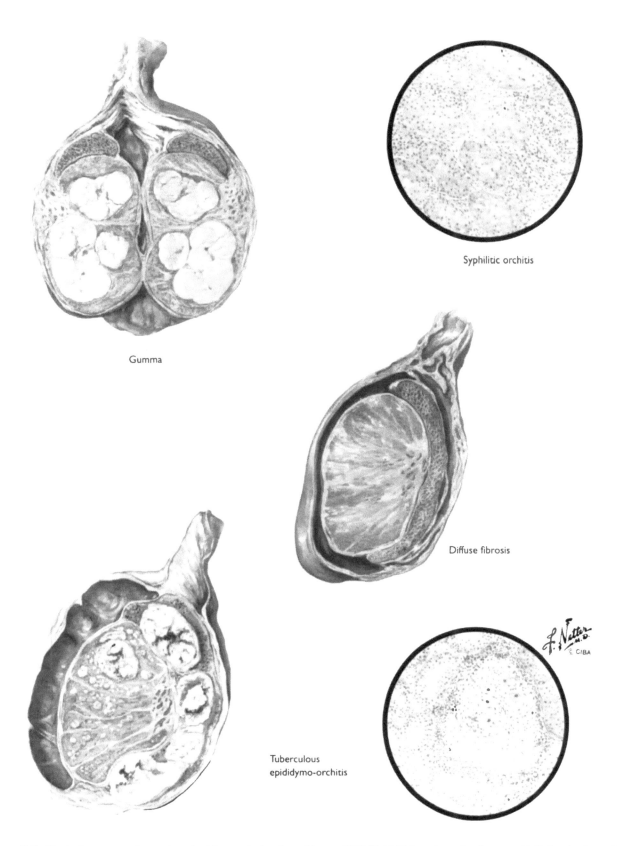

Gumma

Syphilitic orchitis

Diffuse fibrosis

Tuberculous
epididymo-orchitis

Figure 2.7 Testicular tumors (reproduced with permission from Netter, 1992 © 1965, Icon Learning Systems, LLC. A subsidary of MediMedia, USA, Inc. All rights reserved)

Table 2.2 Guidelines for tumor enucleation in testicular germ cell tumors

Tumor diameter less than 20 mm
Tumor must be organ confined
Multiple biopsies from the tumor bed to prove tumor-free resection rims
Normal preoperative testosterone and luteinizing hormone serum levels
Close follow-up, high compliance of patient and physician
Treatment in centers experienced in the management of testicular cancer

Table 2.3 Clinical staging of testicular germ-cell tumors (Lugano classification)

Clinical stage	Description
I	no evidence of metastases
IA	tumor limited to testis and epididymis
IB	infiltration of spermatic cord or tumor in cryptorchid testicle
IC	infiltration of the scrotum, trans-scrotal surgery, tumor developing after trans-scrotal or inguinal surgery
IX	extent of primary tumor cannot be evaluated
II	retroperitoneal lymph-node metastases
IIA	all lymph nodes ≤ 2 cm
IIB	more than one lymph node 2–5 cm
IIC	lymph nodes > 5 cm
IID	abdominal tumor palpable, fixed inguinal tumor
III	mediastinal and supraclavicular lymph-node metastases, visceral metastases
IIIA	mediastinal and supraclavicular lymph-node metastases only
IIIB	pulmonary metastases only
IIIC	hematogenous metastases outside the lung
IIID	persistent elevated markers without evidence of metastases

three courses of adjuvant chemotherapy, before and after orchiectomy. Sperm concentration gradually improved after chemotherapy following orchiectomy in 83% of patients. Serum levels of FSH, LH and pro-lactin (PRL) increased after orchiectomy. Serum levels of testosterone increased in four patients, but decreased in two after orchiectomy. Several factors including pre-existing intrinsic defect and disturbance of the hypothalamus–pituitary–gonadal axis are involved in the deterioration of gonadal function in patients with testicular germ cell tumors.

Although hemangiomas are the most common benign tumors in infancy, scrotal hemangiomas are extremely rare and comprise less than 1% of all hemangiomas. Scrotal hemangiomas that extend into adjacent areas of the perineum, thigh or anterior abdominal wall are common (Figure 2.7). Ultrasound is recommended as part of the preoperative assessment delineating the extent of a scrotal hemangioma. Since an absence of flow on Doppler studies does not exclude the dignosis of hemangioma magnetic resonance imaging (MRI) may provide more useful information for differentia-tion. In cases of cutaneous scrotal hemangiomas, con-servative treatment that waits for involution is widely accepted. In patients with scrotal masses, exploration with excision is the treatment of choice, even if a hema-gioma is likely. Lin *et al.* (2002) reported an intrascrotal tumor diagnosed preoperatively by color duplex ultrasonography and MRI in a 19-year-old male who subsequently underwent *en bloc* excision. Pathological examination identified a cavernous hemangioma.

Guidelines for tumor enucleation in testicular germ cell tumors are outlined by the German Testicular Can-cer Group, based on 72 cases (Table 2.2). Clinical stag-ing of testicular germ cell tumors is outlined according to the Lugano classification (Table 2.3).

Macrophages

The testes contain abundant macrophages and leuko-cytes. Circulating monocytes reach the gonad during fetal life and are a major source of testicular macrophages. The number of macrophages and their functions are largely determined by the local environ-ment. Macrophages undergo proliferation inside the testis during sexual development, as well as in adult-hood, in certain cases.

These cells are involved in immunological surveil-lance, immunoregulation and tissue remodeling. The phagocytic capacity of testicular macrophages became evident after the administration of the specific Leydig cell cytotoxin, ethylene dimethane sulfonate (EDS). Macrophages show an astonishing ability to secrete bio-logically active molecules. More than 100 macrophage secretory products have been identified. The secretory capacity of testicular macrophages implies a potential role in paracrine interactions with other gonadal cell types. Testicular macrophage products such as cytokines and 25-hydroxycholesterol have specific effects on Leydig cell steroidogenesis, Sertoli cells and spermatogenic cells (Frungieri *et al.* 2002).

TESTICULAR TORSION

Testicular torsion is a form of ischemia–reperfusion injury, which requires early diagnosis and surgical intervention. Testicular torsion causes testicular injury and subfertility. The pathophysiology of testicular torsion is associated with two types of cell death: necrosis and apoptosis. Possible involvement of autoimmunity has been observed in delayed injury of the contralateral testis. Unilateral testicular torsion (UTT) increases the biochemical changes due to tissue hypoxia and the level of norepinephrine (noradrenaline) (Shiriashi *et al.* 2003). Chemical sympathectomy prevents the hypoxic changes after UTT in the contralateral testis and to hypoxia due to reduced blood flow through an autonomic nerve reflex (Figure 2.6).

NO, derived from vascular endothelium, relaxes vascular smooth muscle. A basal NO release regulates vasodilatation and focal blood flow. On the other hand, NO plays an important role in the induction of apoptosis. Whereas NO protects the heart during ischemia–reperfusion through protein kinase C activation, Shiriashi *et al.* (2003) found the involvement of inducible NO synthase in the delayed injury after testicular torsion.

SEMEN EVALUATION

The World Health Organization established strict criteria for sperm normality, terminology for semen parameters and normal values of semen variables (see Chapter 3).

Sperm/seminal plasma

Semen analysis reference values are summarized in Table 3.1. Semen coagulation occurs in some mammalian species (humans, non-human primates and South American camelids). Various enzyme interactions regulate the process of coagulation and subsequent liquefaction of semen in llamas and alpacas – the semen is milky or translucent and may be viscous or semi-viscous. The ejaculated volume increases with time of copulation. Motility and especially sperm concentration vary the most during the copulatory period, with viable sperm varying the least (Bravo *et al.* 1997a,b, 2002).

Inflammation of the male genital tract is a potential cause of male infertility and is associated with increased numbers of leukocytes in seminal plasma (Yanushpolsky *et al.* 1996). Immature germ cells, but not leukocytes, in semen are negatively correlated with poor pregnancy outcome in *in vitro* fertilization (IVF). Leukocyte numbers in semen have been overestimated, owing to the inclusion of immature germ cells, because monoclonal immunocytochemical staining was not used in earlier studies (Tomlinson *et al.* 1993; Aitken *et al.* 1994; Aitken and Baker, 1995; Yanushpolsky *et al.* 1996). Granulocyte elastase in seminal plasma is a marker for leukocytospermia. Since semen leukocytes, but not immature germ cells, secrete granulocyte elastase, the measurement of granulocyte elastase by enzyme-linked immunosorbent assay (ELISA) is a convenient method for estimating the concentration of semen leukocytes. *In vivo* endogenous inhibitors, including secretory leukocyte protease inhibitor (SLPI) and α 1-protease inhibitor (α 1-PI), in seminal plasma are thought to protect spermatozoa from attachment by elastase (Moriyama *et al.* 1998).

Table 3.1 Semen analysis reference values. (Reproduced with permission from Sharlip, 2002)

On at least two occasions:
   Ejaculate volume of 1.5–5.0 ml
   pH of > 7.2
   Sperm concentration of > 20 million/ml
   Total sperm count of > 40 million/ejaculate
   Motility of > 50%
   Forward progression > 2 (scale of 0–4)
   Normal morphology > 50% of normal*, > 30% of normal[†], or > 14% of normal[‡]

And:
   Sperm agglutination < 2 (scale of 0–3)
   Viscosity < 3 (scale of 0–4)

*World Health Organization, 1987
[†]World Health Organization, 1992
[‡]Kruger (Tygerberg) Strict Criteria; World Health Organization, 1999

SPERM

Functional ultrastructure

The sperm has a flattened nucleus containing highly compact chromatin. The condensed chromatin is composed of deoxyribonucleic acid (DNA) complexed to a class of basic proteins, 'sperm protamines'. The chromosome number and hence the DNA content of the sperm nucleus is haploid (half the DNA of somatic cells of the same species). The haploid sperm cell results from the meiotic cell divisions that occur during sperm formation.

The acrosome – a thin, double-layered membranous sac layered over the nucleus during the last stages of sperm formation – contains acrosin, hyaluronidase and other hydrolytic enzymes, and is involved in the fertilization process. The equatorial segment of the acrosome is important because it is this part of the spermatozoon, along with the anterior portion of the postacrosomal region, which initially fuses with the oocyte membrane during fertilization.

Type B spermatogonia divide at lease once and probably twice to form the primary spermatocytes. The primary spermatocytes duplicate their DNA and undergo progressive nuclear changes of meiotic prophase known as preleptotene, leptotene, zygotene, pachytene and diplotene, before dividing to form secondary spermatocytes. Without further DNA sythesis, the resultant secondary spermatocytes divide again to form the haploid cells known as spermatids. The round spermatids are transformed into spermatozoa by a series of progressive morphological changes collectively known as spermiogenesis, which include condensation of the nuclear chromatin, formation of the sperm tail (flagellar apparatus) and development of the acrosomal cap.

The structure of the sperm shows the acrosome over the head and the central axonemal core and microtubules of the tail (Figure 3.1), the relationship of the sperm with the medium (Figure 3.2) and the functional ultrastructure of the sperm membrane (Figure 3.3).

The sperm is surrounded by a limiting plasma membrane that mediates many of the early events during fertilization. The membrane is derived originally from the plasmalemma of spermatogonia/spermatocytes in the testis, but is then modified considerably during spermiogenesis, epididymal maturation and capacitation (Jones, 1998).

Sperm nuclear decondensation

Reduced glutathione (GSH) plays an important role in protecting the cell from oxidative damage and might play a role in sperm nuclear decondensation. There is increased synthesis and levels of GSH during oocyte maturation.

Sperm membrane and reactive oxygen species

Membrane permeabilization seems to be a necessary condition for the internalization of key compounds that might induce sperm nucleus decondensation (Dozortzev et al. 1995; Ahmadi and Ng, 1999). Heparin–GSH acts as the physiological decondensing agent that induces the decondensation of mammalian

spermatozoon nuclei (Reyes, 1989). Heparin binds to the sperm plasma membrane in a process that seem to be analogous to the interaction between hormones and cell surface receptors (Delgado et al. 1982; Handrow et al. 1984). The mechanism that has been suggested to occur in rat liver cells may be explained by the fact that, when sperm cells are treated with heparin, it might release phospholipase A1 and heparin binds at the site of phospholipase A1 (Glimelius et al. 1978; Sanchez-Vazquez et al. 1996). Binding to the membrane and nuclear decondensation might be interrelated, with heparin first binding and then exerting a destabilization effect on the cell membrane. Another possibility is the action that heparin and/or GSH might have on reactive oxygen species (ROS).

Sperm chromatin anomalies affecting male fertility

During spermatogenesis, histones are replaced by small proteins of highly basic character – known as protamines – that are rich in cysteine residues. During spermatogenesis and epididymal maturation, disulfide bridges form between these residues, providing the chromatin with the added stability that is necessary to ensure the transport and integrity of the male genetic material. This state of chromatin condensation may be altered by various factors, such as a shortage of zinc from the prostate, or alterations in protamines, which affects the fertilizing capacity of the spermatozoon. The assessment of chromatin status is very important when evaluating the ability of spermatozoa to fertilize. Many techniques have been described for the evaluation of chromatin status, such as optical microscopy, electron microscopy and flow cytometry. Sperm chromatin defects have been correlated with the reduced ability of spermatozoa to fertilize, in the context of both assisted reproduction techniques and the general population. Patients with fertility problems are characterized by an increased frequency of spermatozoa with abnormal chromatin. Therefore, individuals who are infertile, owing to male factor, and those presenting varicocele have sperm with less condensed chromatin; this might, in part, explain their sterility (Feng, 2002).

Sperm motility

Motility assessment involves subjective estimation of the viability of spermatozoa and the quality of the

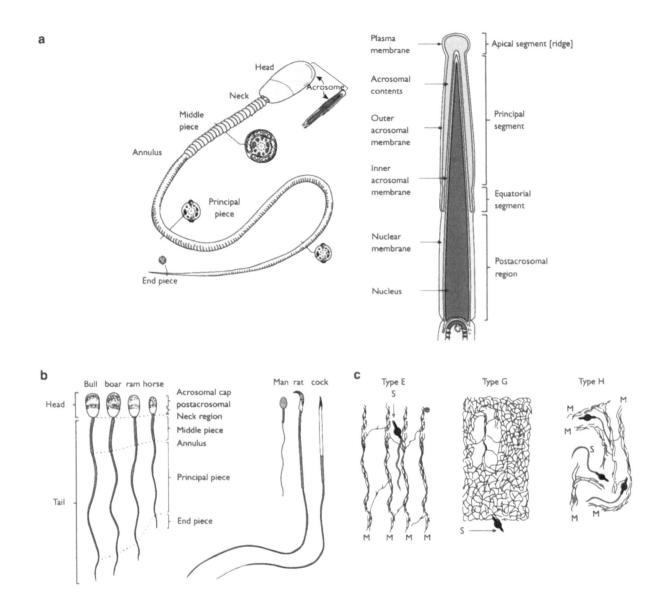

Figure 3.1 (a) Left: features of sperm without the overlying plasma membrane. The head with its acrosomal cap and the tail with its four anatomical divisions are shown. Cross-sections of the middle piece, principal piece, (2) and tail piece show the central axonemal core of 9 + 12 microtubules, the nine coarse outer fibers, the mitochondrial sheath, the dorsal and ventral longitudinal columns and the circumferential ribs. Right: a sagittal section of a sperm head showing the various anatomical subdivisions. The acrosome includes the apical (apical ridge), the principal and the equatorial segments. The outer membranes of the apical and principal segments make up what is called the acrosomal cap. The relationship of the acrosome, with its inner and outer membranes, to the nuclear and plasma membranes is also shown. (b) Comparison of the sperm of mammals and other vertebrates. The major structural features are given. Note the differences in the relative sizes and shapes. (c) Model of cervical mucus based on nuclear magnetic resonance (*NMR*) studies showing ovulatory or estrogenic (*E*), and luteal type (*G*) secretions. The estrogenic model illustrates the micelles (*M*) and intermicellar spaces open to sperm penetration. The progestational model (Type G) shows a dense network without a micellar structure, which acts as a barrier to spermatozoa. In type H, micells are probably broken and arranged in an irregular fashion, causing a disordered sperm migration pattern. *S*, sperm. (Reproduced with permission from Odeblad, 1969)

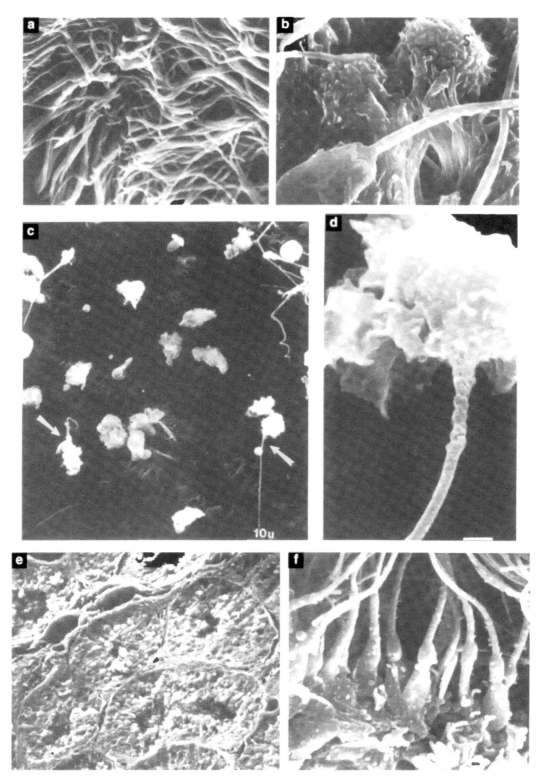

Figure 3.2 Scanning electron micrographs of sperm. (a) Sperm on the cervical epithelium 1 h postcoitus. Note the arrangement of sperm tails in a parallel formation (Reproduced with permission from Hafez, 1973). (b) Cervical epithelium showing non-ciliated secretory cells (S) with microvilli and ciliated cells. (c) Human ejaculate from a patient with unexplained infertility showing massive infiltration of leukocytes. Few 'free' sperm are present; not associated with the ruffled white cells. The smooth-contoured cells may be immature forms of each spermatid. (d) Ruffled leukocyte with a sperm during spermaphagy. (Reproduced with permission from Koehler *et al.* 1982). (e) Scanning electron micrograph of equine testis. Note the irregular shape of the seminiferous tubules and tails of spermatozoa protruding into the lumen (× 440). (f) Spermiation. Spermatozoa with cytoplasmic droplets are released from Sertoli cells (× 5280). (Reproduced with permission from Johnson, 1978)

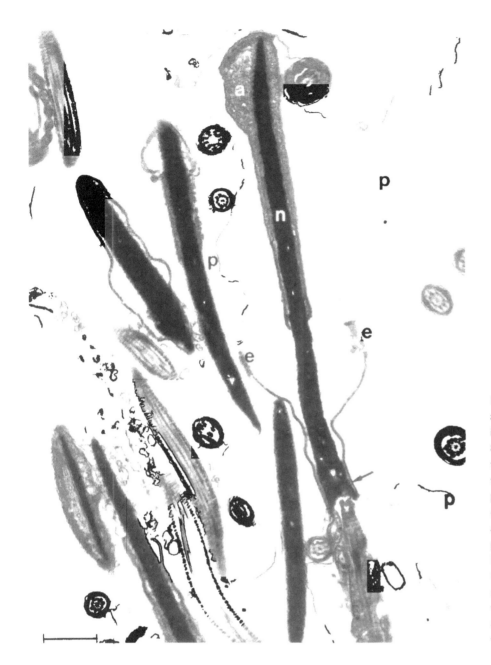

Figure 3.3 Electron micrograph of a thin section of sperm after being incubated for 26 h in the presence of 80 μmol/l heparin. It is also possible to observe the insertion point of the plasma membrane at the basal plate level in the implantation fossa (arrow). The sperm nucleus (n) appears highly condensed and the plasma membrane (p) completely loose, as well as the post-acrosomal membrane system (e) and the acrosome (a). Bar = 1μm. (Reproduced with permission from Reyes et al. 2002, Arch Androl, 48:209–19. www.tandf.co.uk/journals)

motility. Light microscopic analysis of sperm is most commonly used. Evaluation of sperm motility is conducted with fresh untreated and extended semen (Tables 3.2 and 3.3). Parameters of motility include:

(1) Percentage of sperm that are motile (normal is 70–90% motile);
(2) Percentage of sperm that are progressively motile;
(3) Sperm velocity (based on an arbitrary scale of 0 (stationary to 4 (fast));
(4) Longevity of sperm motility in raw semen (at room temperature: 20–25°C) and in extended

semen (at room temperature, or refrigerated temperature: 4–6°C).

Various patterns of motility are visualized. General patterns of sperm motility in diluted semen appear in a long semiarc pattern. The degree of vigor is used to score a sample. Many factors influence sperm motility (Figure 3.4). The extender may slightly alter motility, usually by increasing velocity measures. After initial extension, a high percentage of sperm may exhibit a circular motility pattern, which usually resolves after 5–10 min in the extender. If there is excessive fluid

Table 3.2 Motility pattern of human spermatozoa from fertile men and those with suspected infertility

Motility pattern	Tail	Head	Sperm movements and progression
Vibratory, circular	(a) slow or rapid quivering from side to side (b) vibrations of various types and frequency; bent in a curved shape (c) immotile	immotile or vibrating in one plane	motility without progression; perpendicular, oblique or horizontal clockwise or counter-clockwise
Darting	vibration with high velocity	irregular; propelling; no rotation	minimal and erratic or wandering path
Rotating	undulations of small amplitude pass down the tail	whole sperm rotates around its axis; periodic 'flashing' effect	rapid forward progress in a straight line
Asymmetric head and/or flagella	amplitude of tail wave is asymmetric at both sides	irregular propelling; usually no rotation	circular orbits if rotation is absent
Sperm with cytoplasmic droplet	amplitude of tail waves is unequal, or there are rapid vibrations	irregular; often rocking; seldom rotational	perpendicular, oblique; seldom progressive
Agglutinated sperm	(a) decreasing, vibrating motion (b) slow, vibrating motion	slow, irregular, propelling, rocking	depends on type of agglutination

Table 3.3 Sperm motility-evaluating procedures

Procedure	Comments
Progressive motility and quality of movement	rapid; easy; subjective; dependent on skilled person; probably statistically adaptable with non-parametric techniques; analyzes populations
Analysis of photographically produced sperm tracts	time-consuming but could become acceptable with newer computer-linked cameras; objective; permanent record for future clinical comparisons; analyzes populations
Sperm velocity test	rapid; objective; statistically adaptable; validity of nomogram has to be established for each laboratory; analyzes populations
Gravity	rapid; objective; statistically adaptable; requires treatment group to obtain sperm motility value other than unity; analyzes populations
Optical anisotropy	rapid; objective; statistically and computer adaptable; analyzes populations
Laser and nuclear magnetic resonance	rapid; objective; quantitative; statistically adaptable; analyzes populations; use limited unless future developments are productive
Single cell analysis	objective; time-consuming; because only a few cells can be analyzed, value to pathological conditions is limited; of considerable research value to study the mechanisms of motility

between the slide and the coverslip, it will appear that the sperm cells are reflecting light as they spiral (roll over), moving forward. In the case of less fluid the cells may appear to move in a two-dimensional pattern. Sperm with hyperactivated motility make an X-pattern.

Sperm motility can be evaluated by measuring the following parameters (Figure 3.4):

(1) ALH: amplitude of lateral head displacement (μm). Magnitude of lateral displacement of sperm head about its spatial average trajectory.

(2) LN: linearity. Curvilinear trajectory, VSL/VCL.

(3) WOB: wobble. Oscillation of actual trajectory about its spatial average path, VAP/VCL.

(4) VSL: straight line velocity.

(5) VCL: curvilinear velocity.

(6) VAP: average path velocity.

(7) AHL: beat cross frequency.

(8) O: angle of deviation.

(9) STR: straightness. Linearity of spatial average path, VSL/VAP.

(10) BCF: beat/cross frequency. Time-averaged rate at curvilinear sperm trajectory crosses its average path trajectory.

(11) MAD: mean angular displacement (degrees). Time average of absolute values of instantaneous turning angle of sperm head along its curvilinear trajectory.

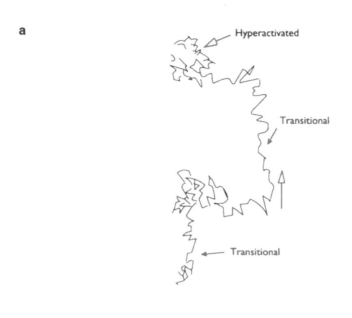

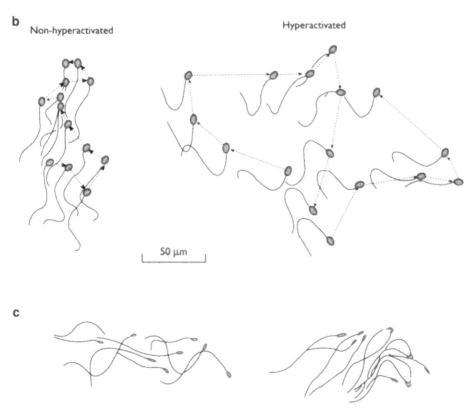

Figure 3.4 Sperm tail beating and head–centroid trajectory pattern for mammalian sperm. (a) Hyperactivated/transitional motility pattern; (b) sperm motility before/after hyperactivation; (c) various sperm motility *in vitro*. (Adapted from the literature)

Table 3.4 Stimulation of sperm motility and/or forward progression

Sugar and electrolyte solutions*

(1) Equal volumes of semen are mixed with one of the following solutions: (a) Baker's solution; (b) Joel's solution; or (c) Locke's solution.
(2) The mixtures are incubated at 37 °C and sperm motility and forward progression are observed every hour for 4 h.
(3) Comparisons are made with semen to which equal volumes of physiological saline are added.

Caffeine†

(1) 0.1 ml of modified Ringer's buffer solution containing 36 mmol/l caffeine is added to 0.5 ml semen. (The final concentration of caffeine is always 6 mmol/l).
(2) The mixture is incubated at 37°C and the sperm motility and forward progression are tested each hour for 5 h.
(3) Comparisons are made with semen to which only modified Ringer's buffer (in the absence of caffeine) is added.

Kallikrein‡

(1) 0.25 ml of semen is mixed with 0.25 ml of physiological saline containing 3×10^{-8} mol/l kallikrein.
(2) The mixture is incubated at 37 °C and sperm motility and forward progression are observed every hour for 4 h.
(3) The results are compared with semen incubated with physiological saline only.

L-Arginine**

(1) A standard sperm count is performed.
(2) The semen is diluted to a concentration of 20×10^6 spermatozoa/ml with physiological saline or modified Baker's solution.
(3) Equal volumes of semen are mixed with 8 mmol/l L-arginine (in physiological saline or Baker's solution), the final concentration of L-arginine always being 4 mmol/l.
(4) The mixture is incubated for 1 h at 37 °C.
(5) The sperm motility and forward progression are compared with semen incubated with physiological saline or Baker's solution in the absence of L-arginine.

*Schirren, personal communication
‡Schill, personal communication
**Keller and Polakoski, personal communication

Mitochondrial dysfunction-related free radical generation has been implicated in the pathogenesis of human male infertility. Mitochondrial dysfunction can lead to defective sperm motility. Increased free radical generation within the sperm cell can lead to cytotoxicity and sperm destruction (Kurup and Kurup, 2002). Various methods are used for *in vitro* stimulation of sperm motility (Table 3.4).

Molecular parameters of sperm motility

Hyaluronic acid increases human sperm motility and intracellular Ca^{2+} concentration, possibly via CD44 receptors. The activation of hyaluronic acid enhances phosphorylation of intracellular proteins, tyrosine-specific phosphorylation, autophosphorylation of receptors and production of inositol triphosphate. Other binding proteins for hyaluronic acid have been identified on the cell membrane of human sperm. Binding of hyaluronic acid to another receptor, PH-20, induced a rapid increase in intracellular calcium ions in macaque sperm, measured using the fluorescent Flur-3 indicator (Bains *et al.* 2002). An increase in intracellular calcium is associated with an increase in the motility of human sperm.

Molecular parameters of sperm membrane

Bains *et al.* (2002) confirmed, by three independent methods, the expression of CD44 on the surface of human sperm membranes. Frungieri *et al.* (2002) evaluated ,macrophage morphology, number and location as well as the expression of macrophage secretory products in testes employing immunohistochemistry and reverse transcriptase polymerase chain reaction (RT-PCR) analysis from paraffin-embedded material scratched from the slides or collected by laser capture microdissection (LCM) and laser pressure catapulting (LPC) of immunostained cells. The increased numbers of CD68-positive macrophages directly (via phagocytosis) or indirectly (via paracrine actions exerted through their secretory products) are involved in the regulation of steroidogenesis, Sertoli cell activity, germ cell survival and, in consequence, the pathogensis or maintenance of infertility states in the human testes.

Sperm transport in the female reproductive tract

The rate of sperm transport in the female reproductive tract is affected by various endocrine factors, viscosity of the cervical mucus and any microbiological contaminants (Figures 3.5 and 3.6).

In vitro manipulation of sperm

Several methods are applied for *in vitro* manipulation of sperm (Table 3.5).

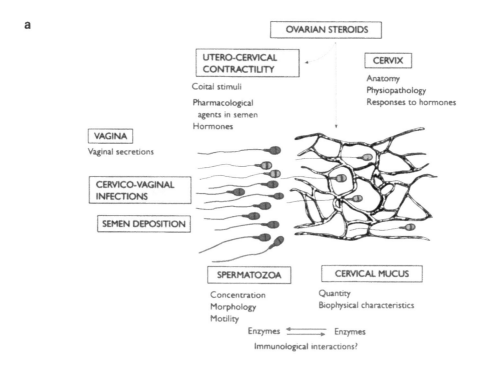

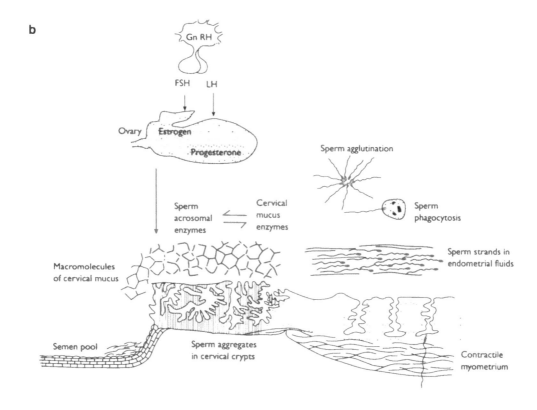

Figure 3.5 The biophysical, physiological, biochemical and immunological interactions among sperm, cervical mucus and various segments of the female reproductive tract. (b) Sperm transport through the cervix to the uterine lumen involves biochemical mechanisms as well as biophysical/physiological changes in cervical mucus, which in turn are controlled by endocrine factors. GnRH, gonadotropin releasing hormone; FSH, follicle stimulating hormone; LH, luteinzing hormone

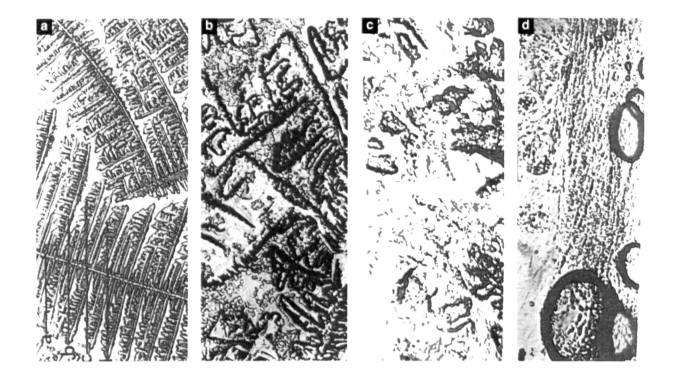

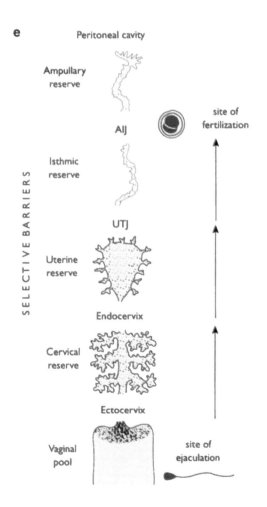

Figure 3.6 Ferning cervical mucus score. (a) Primary, secondary and tertiary stems, 3. (b) >> Stems, 2. (c) A typical fern crystallization, 1. (d) No crystallization, 0. (e) Diagram illustrating selective barriers and reservoirs of spermatozoa in the female reproductive tract

Table 3.5 *In vitro* manipulation of sperm

Techinique	Procedure	Rationale
Sperm washing	Percoll®, Sperm Isolate®, Modified Ham's F-10 medium, Tyrodes salt solution, or other isotonic media, prewarmed and filtered before use	retrograde ejaculation cryopreserved semen oligozoospermia, low sperm motility eliminate antisperm antibodies intrauterine insemination preparation
Sperm swim up	selection of sperm increase sperm quality	decreased motility, eliminate potential pathogens, eliminate leukocytes
Swim down	increase sperm quality	oligospermia
Semen manipulation for *in vitro* fertilization	swim up and swim down *in vitro* capacitation	eliminate cryopreservation media constituents
Semen and oocyte manipulation for enhancing fertilization	microfertilization	sperm transfer using zona drilling to enhance sperm access to the oocyte
Micromanipulation of sperm	intracytoplasmic sperm injection	micromanipulators used to introduce a sperm into a mature oocyte
Semen sexing	flow cytometric sorting	live sorting of X and Y sperm

Table 3.6 Morphology, count, motility and chromatin condensation of sperm of fertile and infertile men (reproduced with permission from Hammadeh *et al.* 2001, *Arch Androl*, 46:99–104. www.tandf.co.uk/journals)

	Patient group % (n = 90)	Control group % (n = 75)
Normal morphology ≥ 14%	12.1	23
Sperm count ≥ 20 × 10⁶/ml	55	100
Linear progressive motility	40	70
Nuclear maturity (chromatin condensation)	55	78

Chromatin condensation of sperm

Chromatin condensation of sperm is an important function during capacitation and fertilization. There are significant differences in nuclear maturity/chromatin condensation between fertile and infertile men (Table 3.6).

Nucleons

DNA in the nuclei of mature sperm is highly structured and exceptionally stable, and has a high degree of condensation (Hernandez *et al.* 1977). DNA in this state is entirely repressed with respect to synthesis at the time of its entry into the ovum. This may be due to the restructuring of sperm nuclei that begins in the testes during spermiogenesis and consists of the exchange of chromatin histones by more basic, arginine-rich protamines (nucleoprotamine complex). This displacement is complete, but in humans approximately 15% of the histones remain associated with sperm DNA (nucleohistone complex). The nucleohistone could designate initiation sites for chromatin decondensation, thus serving a structural role (Gatewood *et al.* 1987). The time course of sperm nucleus decondensation varies considerably among species (Delgado *et al.* 1980, 1982, 1999; Carranco *et al.* 1983).

Human, mouse, chinchilla and hamster sperm nuclei decondensed within 30–60 min after microinjection into hamster oocytes, whereas bull sperm nuclei decondensed only after a considerable time lag in the presence of high concentrations of dithiothreitol (DTT) and a detergent, and seemed to be completely resistant to the decondensing activity of glycosaminoglycans. Sperm chromatin has been distinguished into two classes according to the types of protamines present in the sperm nucleus. Bull sperm nuclei contain only protamine P1, which, being richer in cysteinyl residues, is supposed to be maximally cross-linked by disulfide bridges; therefore these nuclei are probably highly stable (Sanchez-Vazquez *et al.* 1996). The nucleon chromatin decondensation takes place by the action of heparin–GSH, under *in vitro* swelling conditions, displaying the same classic organization into 'hub-like' nuclear bodies joined by a network of chromatin fibers ranging in thickness from 25 to 1.5 nm. The mechanism takes place without the participation of sperm membranes, subcellular organelles, or other protein foreign to the sperm nuclei (Delgado *et al.* 1999).

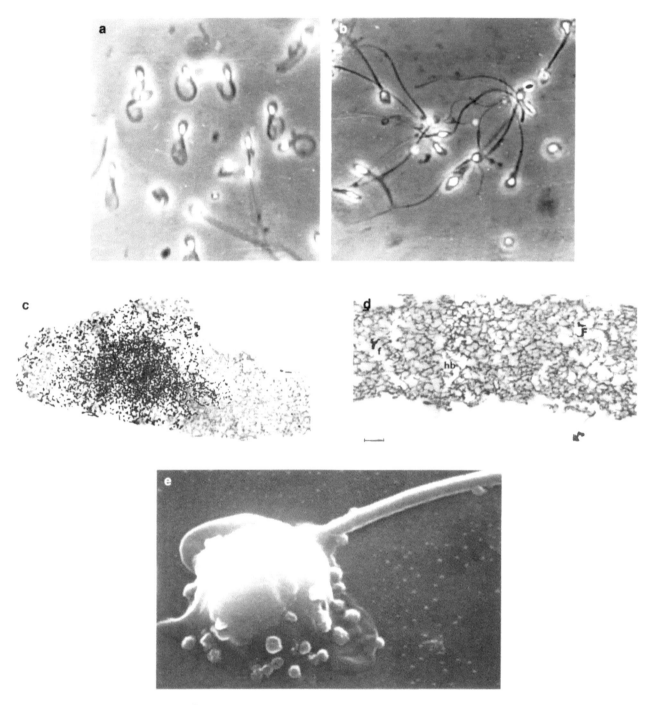

Figure 3.7 Hypo-osmotic swelling of treated human sperm. (a) Control: sperm treated with peanut oil showing coiled tails. (b) Sperm treated with pongam oil showing no coiling of the tails ($\times$ 500). (Reproduced with permission from Bandivdekar and Moodbidri, 2002, *Arch Androl*, 48:9–13. www.tandf.co.uk/journals). (c, d) Electron micrographs of thin sections of swelled nucleons after incubation in heparin-reduced glutathione. In both cases the chromatin is organized into 'hub-like' nuclear bodies (hb), joined by a network of chromatin fibers. (c) Nucleon middle decodensation stage. Nuclear chromatin initiates its decompaction at the periphery of the nuclear structure. (d) High-resolution electron microscopy of the bull decondensed spermatozoa nuclei. Chromatin fibers ranging in thickness from 25 (F) to 1.5 nm (f). Bar = 200 nm. (Reproduced with permission from Delgado *et al.* 2001, *Arch Androl*, 47:47–58. www.tandf.co.uk/journals). (e) Scanning electron micrograph of a spermatozoon during phagocytosis by leukocytes ($\times$ 11 000)

The nucleons reach 95% of chromatin decondensation in the presence of heparin plus GSH or heparin alone. The fact that the correlation between heparin and GSH concentrations needed to induce sperm nucleus decondensation was three-to-four-fold greater than in nucleons might be due to the complete lack of nucleon membranes. Heparin–GSH seems to induce nucleus decondensation by an ionic chromatin charge neutralization mechanism (Delgado *et al.* 2001) (Figure 3.7).

Nucleons have a useful tool in assisted fertilization. Human nucleons exhibit a metabolic activity represented by oxygen uptake, which increases ATP levels, suggesting the presence of aerobic synthesis of ATP (Sosa *et al.* 1974). Both mechanisms take place without the participation of the sperm membranes (plasmatic, acrosomal, nuclear), subcellular organelles or other forms of protein foreign to sperm nuclei. Cryopreservation is deleterious to sperm function, killing more than 50% of the spermatozoa during the process. Therefore, the implementation of a simple cryopreservation technique with the use of nucleons seems to be necessary to avoid all the basic steps required in a normal successful fertilization (capacitation, acrosome reaction, membrane integrity, excellent motility, cryoprotective medium, liquid nitrogen, etc.).

Sperm membrane integrity

Sperm used for artificial insemination (AI) depend mainly on the conservation of their fertilizing ability. Several methods have been used to evaluate this ability, based on several distinctive features, ranging from simple morphology (as the well-formed, tail-less or cytoplasm-containing sperm ratio) to highly computerized sperm motion analysis or the evaluation of intracellular calcium concentrations. One of the methods, evaluate specifically the activity of the trypsin-like acrosin release after its liberation from the acrosome, is a clear indicator of the loss of plasma membrane integrity. Other assays evaluate the kinematic characteristics of the sperm sample: head lateral displacement, straight motility, sperm flagella beating and wave amplitude. All these parameters evaluate the capacity of the sperm to penetrate through the egg vestments. Other techniques evaluate the perioxidative capacity on the sperm membrane lipids, as a membrane fluidity evaluation parameter or as membrane damage. Others

focus on the zona pellucida receptor aggregation capacity, a prerequisite for the acrosomal reaction, or the well-established transduction signaling aspects due to the correct establishment of the tyrosine kinase activity in the sperm receptor (Leyton and Saling, 1989; Ward and Kopf, 1993). Another target to evaluate is the total membrane function, as in the case of the chlortetracycline triple stain (Talbot and Chacon, 1980).

The methodologies have been looking for specific molecules using monoclonal or highly specific polyclonal antibodies or by looking at carbohydrate-containing proteins using sugar-specific lectins. Sperm membrane mapping has been performed with several lectins in several species. The peanut agglutinin is used since it recognizes terminal *N*-acetylgalactose or lactose residues. Serrano *et al.* (2001) developed an elegant technique using fluorescent-labeled peanut agglutinin plus a fluorescein extender that permits an easy evaluation for pig spermatozoon membrane integrity. Sperm integrity was evaluated before and after a zona pellucida-induced acrosome reaction in capacitated sperm. The sperm acrosome reaction was affected when the zona pellucida was reduced.

Enyzmes

Sperm are able to produce ROS (Aitken/Clarkson, 1987; Aitken *et al.* 1989; Iwasaki and Cagnon, 1992; Zini *et al.* 1993; Griveau *et al.* 1995); e.g. hydrogen peroxide (H_2O_2), hydroxyl radicals ($\bullet OH$) and superoxide anion ($\bullet O_2$). Several enyzmes are involved in their neutralization: superoxide dismutase, glutathione peroxidase/reductase system, catalase. ROS induce lipid peroxidation of the sperm membrane, which results in sperm dysfunction and subsequent infertility, or death of the sperm. ROS also induce ATP depletion, inhibit mitochondrial functions and inhibit sperm–oocyte fusion (Comporti, 1989; Aitken *et al.* 1991; Lamirande and Gagnon, 1992).

Tyrosine phosphorylation and motility parameters in human sperm

Initiation of sperm motility has been associated with protein phosphorylation as well as changes in intracellular calcium and pH. Several proteins become phosphorylated at the time sperm start moving actively. The majority of these proteins are phosphorylated on serine

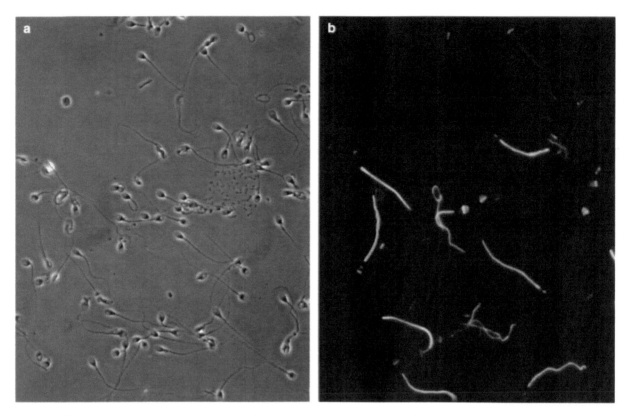

Figure 3.8 Photomicrographs showing immunolocalization of tyrosine phosphorylated proteins in human spermatozoa. Sperm were fixed and permeabilized with methanol and immunolabeled with a phophotyrosine antibody (4G10) and FITC-conjugated anti-mouse IgG, shown by (a) phase contrast and (b) fluorescent microscopy × 600. (Reproduced with permission from Bajpai *et al.* 2003, *Arch Androl*, 49:229–46. www.tandf.co.uk/journals)

or threonine residues and their phosphorylation is cAMP-dependent. Most of these studies have focused on the initiation/activation of sperm motility; therefore, much less is known about what modulates sperm movement after motility has commenced. Hyperactivated motility, characterized by vigorous, large-amplitude, whiplash-like flagellar beats with the sperm heads tracing erratic trajectories and considered to be critical for fertilization, is also poorly understood. Although calcium and cAMP are known to be required for its expression, the mechanisms controlling this type of motility in capacitated spermatozoa are a matter of speculation. Tyrosine phosphorylation has recently been associated with sperm capacitation. However, its involvement in sperm motion regulation remains to be clearly elucidated (Bajpai *et al.* 2003).

Bajpai *et al.* (2003) conducted extensive studies to verify whether tyrosine phosphorylation of human sperm proteins was essentially required for the maintenance of motility as well as the development of hyperactivation. Washed spermatozoa were incubated for 6 h

in Ham's F10 medium + 0.35% human serum albumin at 37 °C in 5% CO_2, with and without the following tyrosine kinase inhibitors: genistein, tyrphostin, erbstatin or herbimycin A, and the wide-spectrum kinase inhibitor, staurosporin. The concentrations of the inhibitors used in the experiments did not induce sperm toxicity, as measured by membrane integrity and mitochondrial function assays. Samples incubated without the inhibitors (control), increased their tyrosine kinase activity (by ELISA), the number and intensity of tyrosine phosphorylated (PY) protein bands (by Western blot), the incidence of PY-immunoreactive sperm (by immunofluorescence) and some of the sperm motion characteristics (computerized assisted semen analysis: CASA) such as velocity, amplitude of lateral head displacement (ALH) and hyperactivation. Among the selective protein tyrosine kinase inhibitors, genistein was the most active and consistent, inhibiting sperm tyrosine kinase activity, PY-proteins, incidence of PY-sperm and sperm motility and motion parameters such as velocity, ALH and hyperactivation. The rest of

a

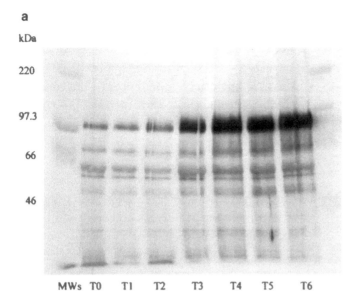

b

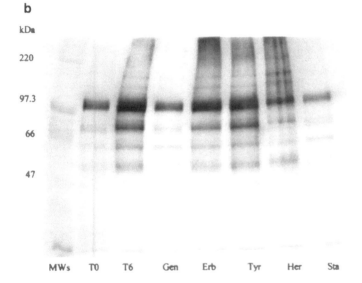

c

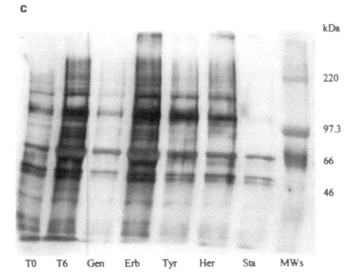

Figure 3.9 (a) Time-dependent increase in tyrosine phosphorylation of human sperm proteins during a capacitating incubation. Seminal plasma was washed off and spermatozoa were incubated for 6 h in Ham's F10 medium + 0.35% human serum albumin at 37 °C in 5% CO_2. Aliquots were taken every hour and solubilized in sodium dodecyl sulfate (SDS) buffer. Protein extracts from 1 million sperm per lane were separated by polyacrylamide gel electrophoresis, transferred to Immobilon P and immunolabeled with phosphotyrosine antibody (4G10) ($n = 5$). (b) Effect of kinase inhibitors on sperm protein tyrosine phosphorylation after a 6-h incubation in Ham's F10/HSA at 37 °C, in 5% CO_2. Proteins were extracted from washed sperm in an SDS buffer, loaded onto a 7.5% polyacrylamide gel (1 million cells/lane), separated by electrophoresis, transferred to Immobilon P sheets and immunolabeled with phosphotyrosine antibody (4G10). Molecular weight of bands was determined using a Kodak digital imaging system (v 2.1) ($n = 12$). (c) Effect of kinase inhibitors on tyrosine phosphorylation of soluble (Triton X-100) sperm proteins after a 6-h incubation in Ham's F10 HSA at 37 °C in 5% CO_2. Proteins were extracted from washed spermatozoa in an SDS buffer, solubilized with 0.05% Triton X-100, loaded onto a 7.5% polyacrylamide gel (1 million cells/lane), separated by electrophoresis, transferred to Immobilon P sheets and immunolabeled with phosphotyrosine antibody (4G10). Molecular weight of bands was determined using a Kodak digital imaging system (v 2.1) ($n = 5$). (Reproduced with permission from Bajpai et al. 2003, Arch Androl, 49:229–46. ww.tandf.co.uk/journals)

Table 3.7 Concentration of interleukin 6, interleukin 10 and prostaglandin E₂ (PGE₂) in seminal plasma of fertile and infertile men (Reproduced with permission from Camejo, 2003, *Arch Androl*, 49:111–16. www.tandf.co.uk/journals)

	Infertile (n = 45)	Fertile (n = 25)	p Value
Interleukin 6 (pg/ml)	47 ± 6.9	23 ± 4.8	p < 0.04
Interleukin 10 (pg/ml)	1.3 ± 0.3	4.9 ± 0.9	p < 0.04
PGE₂(µg/ml)	25 ± 3.9	30 ± 8.2	p = NS

Values are medians ± SE

the kinase inhibitors decreased motion characteristics to a varied extent and had different effects on phosphorylation parameters. In general, they decreased PY-phosphorylation of two proteins (of 83 and 54 kDa) present in whole sperm extracts, and two sets of proteins of low (39–49 kDa) and medium (55–87 kDa) molecular weight present in the Triton X-100-solubilized sperm protein fraction. This inhibition was evident regardless of the total tyrosine kinase activity of the samples or the incidence of PY-immunoreactive spermatozoa. These findings further support the association between motility and protein tyrosine phosphorylation in human sperm and point to certain proteins as the main linkers (Figures 3.8 and 3.9).

SEMINAL PLASMA

Seminal plasma is a composite secretion arising from a number of sources including the testes, epididymides and accessory glands of men. The chemical composition of seminal plasma is different from that of other body fluids. Seminal plasma contains unusually high levels of citric acid, ergothioneine, fructose, glycerylphosphorylcholine and sorbitol. Appreciable quantities of ascorbic acid, amino acids, peptides, proteins, lipids, fatty acids and numerous enzymes are also present. Antimicrobial constituents including immunoglobulins of the IgA class are constituents of seminal plasma. In addition, a variety of hormonal substances, including androgens, estrogens, prostagladins, follicle stimulating hormone, luteinizing hormone, chorionic gonadotrophin-like material, growth hormone, insulin, glucagon, prolactin, relaxin, thyroid releasing hormone and enkephalins are detected in seminal plasma.

At or immediately after ejaculation, seminal plasma is in a coagulated form. Proteolytic enzymes (mainly

originating from the prostate) normally cause liquefaction within 20 min. Presence of non-liquefied material after 1 h is regarded as pathological and indicative of defect in prostate function, usually due to infection.

There are significant differences in the concentrations of interleukin (IL)-6 and IL-10 and prostaglandin (PG) E² in seminal plasma of fertile and infertile men (Table 3.7).

Blood melatonin and testosterone levels are significantly higher than the comparable seminal plasma levels. Seminal plasma estradiol levels are significantly higher than the blood levels. There is no correlation between sperm concentration, motility or morphology and blood or seminal plasma hormone levels. Also, blood and seminal plasma hormone levels are not correlated. In normospermic men, seminal plasma estradiol levels are higher than blood hormone levels, suggesting local production of estradiol. This may imply that estrogen and/or the balance of androgen/estrogen is important in normal human spermatogenesis.

Functions

Four main functions of human seminal plasma are established: a vehicle for sperm transport; a coagulating system; an energy source; and a highly buffered medium to overcome the hostile acid pH of the vagina (Kelly and Critchley, 1997). Another possible contribution of human seminal plasma is the immunosuppressive activity that has been proposed to play a role in the prevention of lymphocyte responses against sperm autoantigens in the male and female reproductive tracts (Alexander and Anderson, 1987). Seminal plasma is a potent inhibitor of many immune functions, including inhibition of lymphocyte activation of delayed hypersensitivity reactions, complement activation and natural killer cell activity (Lord *et al.* 1977). The immunosuppressive effects of human seminal plasma are due to several components. However, PGE, specially PGE₂, plays a major suppressive role. Studies utilizing cultures of peripheral blood mononuclear leukocytes reported that PGE₂ and seminal plasma led to a marked increase in the IL-10/IL-12 ratio. PGE and IL-10 are implicated in inducing non-responsiveness in T cells (Groux *et al.* 1996). This might have been sufficient to ensure that no major response to spermatozoa was evoked in the male and female tracts. However, infections of the male reproductive tract can be a signal for an inflammatory response that alters the composition of seminal plasma and influences sperm quality (Purvis and Christensen, 1996). Reports have described variations in the concentrations of seminal cytokines (IL-1, IL-2, IL-12, IL-6, IL-8, tumor necrosis factor-α) between fertile and infertile men (Rajasekaran et al. 1995; Gruschwitz et al. 1996; Naz and Evans, 1998). IL-6 is a good marker of genital inflammation and infection.

Increased IL-6 concentration is observed in seminal fluid of patients with accessory gland inflammation as well as with accessory gland infection. Moreover, significant positive correlation was found between IL-6 levels in seminal plasma and sperm membrane lipid peroxidation (Camejo et al. 2001; Camejo, 2002). In vitro studies have reported that the seminal plasma of fertile men has more inhibitory mitogenic activity than that in oligoteratoasthenospermic men (Huleskel et al. 1997), and that seminal plasma from couples with unexplained infertility showed significantly lower suppressive activity on antibody-dependent cellular cytotoxicity than seminal plasma from fertile males (Sakin-Kaindl et al. 2001). It would appear that the decrease in suppressive activity might be due to a decrease of immunosuppressive molecules or increase of proinflammatory molecules. Camejo (2002) conducted extensive investigations to evaluate the relation between immunosuppressive PGE_2 and IL-10 to proinflammatory IL-6 in seminal plasma of infertile and fertile men.

The IL-6 concentration in seminal plasma of infertile men was significantly higher than that of fertile men ($p < 0.04$). However, levels of IL-10 were higher in the semen of infertile men than that of fertile men. Increase in proinflammatory cytokines, such IL-6, and decrease in immunosuppressive cytokines, such as IL-10, could alter the tolerance to sperm cells in the male and female tracts and reduce the favorable conditions to reach fertilization and implantation.

Phospholipid-binding proteins

Manjunah et al. (2002) studied phospholipid-binding proteins in the seminal plasma of various animals. Bovine seminal plasma contains major proteins designated BSP-A1, BSP-A2, BSP-A3 and BSP-30 (collectively called BSP proteins). BSP-A1 and -A2 have the identical amino acid sequence but they differ in the extent of glycosylation, and are considered to be the same chemical entity. BSP-A3 is not glycosylated and BSP-30 is highly glycosylated. All these proteins contain two similar domains (type-II structures) that appear to be responsible for binding properties of gelatin/collagen, physphorylcholine, heparin, high-density lipoprotein and low-density lipoprotein exhibited by BSP proteins. The BSP protein analogs have been purified and sequenced from boar (pB1) and stallion (HSP-1 and HSP-2) seminal plasma. The stallion seminal plasma also contains another form designated HSP-12. They isolated five forms (RSP-15-kDa, RSP-16-kDa, RSP-21-kDa, RSP-24-kDa, RSP-28-kDa) from the seminal plasma of the ram, and two forms (WBSP-17-kDa, WBSP-18-kDa) from the water buffalo.

Antioxidant enzyme activity

Owing to their high polyunsaturated fatty acid content, human sperm plasma membranes are highly sensitive to ROS-induced lipid peroxidation, decreasing membrane fluidity and sperm fertilizing capability. Human seminal plasma and sperm possess antioxidant systems to scavenge ROS and prevent ROS-related cellular damage. Investigations have been conducted on superoxide dismutase (SOD), catalase and GSH in human sperm and seminal plasma (Juelin et al. 1989). Varicocele was accused of causing infertility in approximately 19–41% of male patients attending an infertility clinic (Pryor and Howards, 1987). The relationship between varicocele and male infertility is well documented. Ozbek et al. (2001) examined the seminal plasma antioxidant activity of patients with GII–GIII varicocele and compared the results with healthy volunteer controls. Twenty infertile varicocele patients and 15 fertile controls were included in the study. After separation of sperm, SOD, catalase and glutathione peroxidase (GSH-Px) activity were assessed by enzymatic methods. The concentrations were significantly lower in the varicocele group compared to controls. It would appear that reduced ROS-scavenging enzyme activity in the seminal plasma of patients with varicocele is associated with impaired sperm function. Antioxidant enzyme supplementation may be helpful in this pathology.

CHAPTER 4

The epididymis

The caput epididymidis (head), in which a variable number of efferent ductules (13–20) join the duct of the epididymis, forms a flattened structure applied to one pole of the testis. It continues as the narrow corpus epididymidis (body), which terminates at the opposite pole in the expanded cauda epididymidis (tail). The wall of the duct of the epididymis has a prominent layer of circular muscle fibers and a pseudostratified epithelium of columnar cells. Three segments of the duct of the epididymis can be distinguished histologically; these do not coincide with the gross anatomic regions. There is a progressive decrease in the height of the epithelium and stereocilia and widening of the lumen throughout the three segments (Figure 4.1). The first two segments are concerned with sperm maturation, whereas the terminal segment is for sperm storage. The epithelial lining of the epididymis consists of different kinds of cells: principal columnar cells; small basal cells on the basal membrane; and some lymphocytes.

The lumen of the epididymal tubules is lined with epithelium made of a basal layer of small cells and a surface layer of tall columnar ciliated cells. Masses of sperm are often found in the lumen. Spaces between the tubules are filled with loose connective tissue. The ductus deferens leaves the cauda epidymidis and is supported in a separate fold of peritoneum; it is readily separable from the rest of the spermatic cord. The mucosa of the ductus deferens is thrown into longitudinal folds. Near the epididymal end, the epithelium resembles that of the epididymis: The non-ciliated cells have little secretory activity. The lumen is lined with pseudostratified epithelium. Large volumes of fluid leave the testis daily, and most of this is absorbed in the caput epididymidis by the initial segment of the duct of the epididymis. Transport of sperm through the epididymis takes several days. It is accomplished by the flow of rete fluid, the activity of the ciliated epithelium of the efferent ductules and contractions of the muscular wall of the duct of the epididymis. Maturation of sperm occurs during transit through the epididymis; motility increases as sperm enter the corpus epididymidis. The environment of the sperm in the cauda epididymidis provides factors that enhance fertilizing ability; sperm from this region give a higher fertility than those from the corpus epididymidis.

Sperm stored in the epididymis retain fertilizing capacity for several weeks; the cauda epididymidis is the principal storage organ, and it contains about 75% of the total epididymal sperm. The special ability of the cauda epididymidis to store sperm depends on low scrotal temperatures and on the action of male sex hormones. Sperm stored in the ampullae constitute only a small part of the total extragonadal sperm reserves. Small numbers of non-motile sperm appear in ejaculates collected weeks or even months after castration; these are mainly derived from the ampullae.

The blood supply and microvasculature of the epididymis are shown in Figure 4.2.

EMBRYOLOGY

The various embryological events that take place are crucial to the proper development of the epididymis. The sequence of events in the embryological development of the epididymis in man as compared to that in the mouse is shown in Figure 4.3. Sex determination is the process

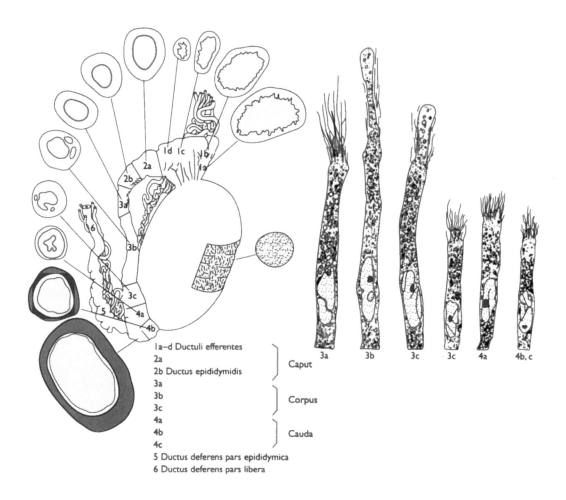

1a–d Ductuli efferentes
2a
2b Ductus epididymidis   } Caput
3a
3b   } Corpus
3c
4a
4b   } Cauda
4c
5 Ductus deferens pars epididymica
6 Ductus deferens pars libera

Figure 4.1 Left diagrammatic illustration of the human testis and epididymis. The epididymis is dissected free from adjacent connective tissue and divided into different sections according to cytological characteristics of the epithelium. Transverse sections of the excretory duct system in different segments of the epididymis show regional differences in the width of the lumen, and the characteristics of the epithelium. The black contour reflects the thickness of the smooth muscle layer. (Figure courtesy of Professor Holstein.) Right: common types of cells of the epithelium from different segments of the ductus epididymidis

by which genetic information dictates the formation of either a testis or an ovary. There are situations of sex reversal in which the genetic sex and the phenotypic sex do not match. These cases have been the basis for the identification of several genes involved in sex determination.

Gene expression/epididymal function

The epididymal epithelium secretes proteins in a highly regulated and regionalized manner, so that sperm encounter luminal fluid proteins in a specific sequence. Each segment of the epididymis has its won microenvironment uniquely controlled by the cells' differential response to extracellular signals and mediated by specific signaling molecules and DNA binding proteins, ultimately resulting in region-specific gene expression and secretion of proteins. Future research is required to identify the secretory proteins that interact with sperm, and the specific signals/transduction pathways and regulatory proteins involved in this highly orchestrated sequence of

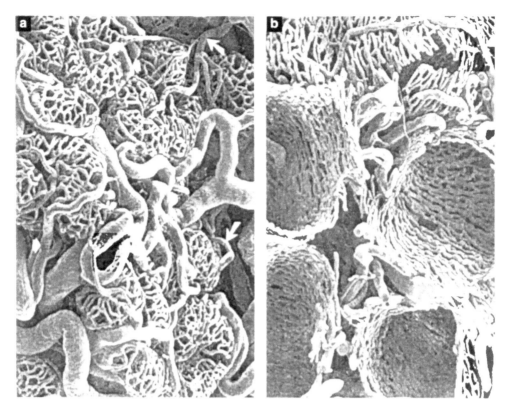

Figure 4.2 (a) Microvasculature of the efferent ductules of a pig showing the polygonal capillary architecture, the ramification of feeding vessels (long arrows) and the confluence of capillaries into draining vessels (arrowheads). (b) Microvasculature of the epididymal duct in the caput region in a pig epididymis. Note the circular arrangement of the capillaries and the longitudinal course of an arteriole (long arrow) feeding the capillaries through circular ramifications (from Setchell, personal communication)

molecular events. Such advanced research requires the application of transgenic technology and gene activation.

FUNCTIONS/STRUCTURE/ ULTRASTRUCTURE

Functional histology

The mucosa is unciliated and composed of principal, apical, narrow, mitochondria-rich, light (clear) basal cells, and intraepithelial leukocytes (halo cells). Depending on the species, the epididymis can be subdivided into several distinct regions: initial segment, intermediate zone, caput, corpus and cauda. The initial segment is wide with a few sperm in the lumen, and it is lined by a tall, actively secretory epithelium with characteristic cytology that resembles the proximal tubules of the kidney, which also reflects its major function: reabsorption of nearly 90% of the luminal fluid.

Neural control

The neutral control of the epididymis is important of sperm transport, especially during ejaculation, and normal function of these tissues, as with other tissues of the body, is possible only with a normal blood supply and lymph drainage. The nerve supply to the epididymis is derived from the inferior (caudal) mesenteric ganglion (IMG) or plexus, which lies near the caudal mesenteric artery, and the pelvic plexus, found on the lateral aspect of the pelvic viscera. The hypogastric nerves receive sympathetic fibers from the IMG, and contribute branches to the middle spermatic nerves, which run along the ductus deferens to the epididymis.

The hypogastric nerves also supply fibers to the inferior spermatic nerves, through the pelvic plexus. The hypogastric nerves arise from the intermesenteric plexus or the superior hypogastric plexus, and

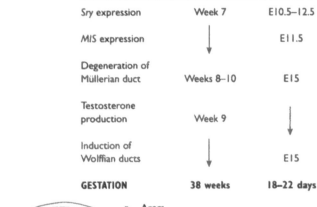

	Human	Mouse
Germ cell migration	Week 5	E7–E12.5
Formation of sex cords	Week 6	E12
Development of Müllerian ducts		E14

END OF INDIFFERENT STAGE

Sry expression	Week 7	E10.5–12.5
MIS expression		E11.5
Degeneration of Müllerian duct	Weeks 8–10	E15
Testosterone production	Week 9	
Induction of Wolffian ducts		E15
GESTATION	**38 weeks**	**18–22 days**

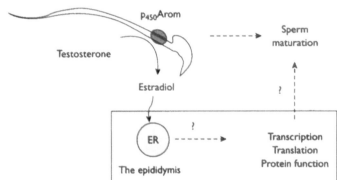

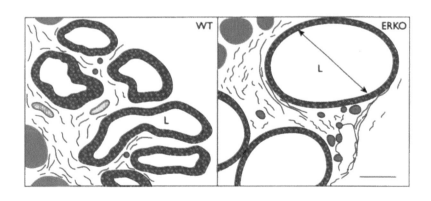

Figure 4.3 Top: timetable of important events during the embryological development of the human and mouse epididymis. Development in the rat follows approximately the same timetable as the mouse. Note that classic human embryology tests define the end of the indifferent stage as the time when *Sry* is expressed; however, studies in the mouse have shown that *Sry*-induced mesonephric cell migration into the developing gonad is necessary for testis cord formation. Center: sperm carry P450 aromatase, which converts androgens to estrogens in the lumen of the efferent ductules and epididymis. This luminal estrogen will enter the epithelial cells and target estrogen receptors (ER), where as yet unidentified genes are transcribed to produce proteins having the potential to regulate sperm maturation in the head of the epididymis. Bottom: schematic illustration of proximal efferent ductules in wild-type (WT) and α-ERKO mice. The lumen (L) is small in WT but greatly dilated in the α-ERKO male. Bar = 100 μm. (Adapted with permission from Hess *et al.* 2002, *Arch Androl*, 48:32–41. www.tandf.co.uk/journals)

contribute fibers mainly through the pelvic plexus to the inferior spermatic nerves. Fibers from the hypogastric nerves may also join the middle spermatic nerves, which pass along the spermatic artery to the caput epididymidis (Setchell, personal communication).

Structural/ultrastructural changes during aging

There are several structural changes in the epididymal epithelium during aging: occasional intraepithelial cysts/hyperplasia of the epithelium, eosinophilic to amphophilic round cytoplasmic bodies in interstitial cells, proteinaceous luminal debris and a decrease in the diameter of the cauda epididymidis. Ultrastructural changes include damaged mitochondria and bundles of filaments. Several theories have been proposed to explain the mechanisms of aging on the epididymis: the specific gene theory. e.g. the *klotho* gene; the telomere theory (decreasing telomere length with subsequent divisions); altered gene expression due either to mutations (Martin, 1997) or altered DNA (methylation status); the network or immune theory of aging (where there is progressive increase in proinflammatory status); and the free radical (oxidative stress) theory (Robaire, 2002). Aging is associated with recruitment of immune cells into the epididymis. Oxidative stress is a natural phenomenon, occurring as a result of the body's respiratory processes, causing the reduction of molecular oxygen into free radicals, such as the superoxide radical ($\bullet O_2$), hydrogen peroxide (H_2O_2), the hydroxyl radical ($\bullet OH$) and water. Oxidative damage can increase dramatically under certain conditions, such as poor diet, smoking, inflammation, exposure to radiation and aging. It would appear that oxidative stress is a key factor in mediating the dramatic response of the epididymis to age. Oxidative stress is associated with specific accumulation of lipofuscin, changes in the distribution of glutathione S-transferase, formation of intracellular vacuoles and altered expression of genes (reviewed by Robaire, 2002). Future research is needed to evaluate how both gene and protein expression in the epididymal epithium are affected by aging.

Blood–epididymis barrier

As in other tissues, cell–cell interactions in the epididymis are complex and involve interplay between several multimember families of proteins to enable individual cells to form and operate in a continuous syncytium. These interactions are further complicated by the influence of testicular factors that regulate the expression of epididymal genes and cellular targeting of proteins. The complexity of these interactions is necessary for epididymal sperm maturation by creating an appropriate environment and by co-ordinating epithelial cell functions and their secretions into the lumen. The regulation of these interactions and the formation and function of the blood–epididymis barrier involve endocrine/paracrine parameters (Cyr *et al.* 2003). Further research is needed to evaluate how these cellular interactions in the epididymis function with respect to one another and their significance to epididymal physiology, which involves cellular recognition, interaction of structural proteins and complex intracellular signaling pathways.

In the epididymis, the extracellular matrix (ECM) exists in a specialized form, the basement membrane (BM), which is composed primarily of collagen IV and laminin isoforms. Interactions between epithelial cells and the BM are mediated primarily by the integrin family of cell-surface adhesion molecules. These proteins are anchors by which cells attach to the EMC, binding to molecules such as laminins. Tight junctions between epididymal epithelial cells regulate this luminal environment and distinguish it from blood. The regulation of epididymal tight junctions and the function and regulation of cadherins, cell adhesion molecules involved in junction formation, are essential. Gap junctions, also part of the epididymal junctional complex, establish communication between epididymal cells and therefore allow the co-ordination of luminal changes, which are necessary for sperm maturation and storage (Cyr *et al.* 2003).

Functions

The epididymis plays a key role in the maturation and protection of sperm. During their transit through this epididymis, sperm are exposed to the harmful presence of free radicals and electrophilic compounds both endogenous, generated by lipid peroxidation, and exogenous. Oxidative stress is correlated with male infertility, and the epididymis possesses a region-specific antioxidant capacity, which may protect spermatozoa from oxidative attack (Potts *et al.* 1999; Sharma *et al.* 1999).

Several enzymatic detoxification pathways may protect cells from harmful substances; for example, the mercapturic acid pathways transforms many xenobiotics in soluble derivates of mercapturic acid, which are easily eliminated. This is catalyzed by a family of enzymes, the glutathione S-transferases (GSTs), which have different affinities for a wide variety of compounds (Picket and Lu, 1989). γ-Glutamyl transpeptidase (GGT) is present in almost all tissues, including the testis and epididymis. Catalytic activity, protein level and different RNAs of GGT are expressed in a region-dependent manner and regulated by androgen and testicular factors (Palladino and Hinton, 1994; Lan *et al.* 1998). As in other species, fertilizing capacity of human spermatozoa increases as they pass through the epididymides (Mathieu *et al.* 1992). Also, this organ has been considered as an important target for male post-testicular contraception (De Paolo *et al.* 2000).

Functional role of estrogen in the epididymis

Testosterone is the primary sex steroid in humans and its metabolite, 5-dihydrotestosterone (DHT), is the primary hormone that regulates epididymal functions. Estrogen in the rete testis fluid is now thought to be derived from the conversion of testosterone to estradiol by P450 aromatase found in germ cells of the testis and sperm traversing the epididymis. The luminal estrogen targets estrogen receptors (ERs) present in the epididymal epithelium, particularly the efferent ductule region, where ERα is abundant. However, ERα and ERβ are both found in the various regions of the epididymal duct and vas deferens (Hess *et al.* 2002). Future research is needed to evaluate: sources of estrogen in the male; the possible presence of ERα and ERβ in the reproductive tract; estrogens and development; estrogen regulation of fluid reabsorption in the efferent ductules; and possible functions in the epididymis and vas deferens.

Epididymal structure following androgen withdrawal

Orchidectomy causes epididymal weight to decrease to 25% of control over a 2-week period, and a further 5% in the subsequent 2 weeks. The degree of weight loss of the epididymis is not as marked as that for the ventral prostate, which involutes more rapidly any diminishes to less than 10% of control by 4 weeks after orchidectomy. The ratio of nucleus/cytoplasm in the mouse epididymis decreases after birth, as the epididymis differentiates, and increases dramatically after orchidectomy, as the epididymis dedifferentiates. Unlike the

case with other androgen-dependent male reproductive tissues, testosterone replacement, even at supraphysiological levels, only partially restores epididymal weight, to approximately 50% of control, this is due to the large proportion (nearly half) of epididymal weight that is attributable to spermatozoa and the luminal fluid bathing them (Ezner and Robaire, 2002).

Administration of increasing doses of testosterone to adult non-orchidectomized rats caused a suppression (due to loss of spermatozoa) and then a maintenance of epididymal weight, whereas such treatment resulted in increased prostate weights.

Functional histology of the vas deferens

The vas deferens is the least understood and studied organ of the male reproductive system. Half the sperm in the human ejaculate are potentially derived from the distal vas and ampulla. Thus the vas deferens plays a role in the viability and protection of sperm from reactive oxygen species (ROS), proteases and complement during their storage. The vas deferens and ampulla play an active role in sperm nourishment and maturation. In non-human primates, only after sperm have reached the cauda and vas deferens do they attain their full vigor and ability to swim rapidly. Any obstruction of the vas causes significant changes in the synthesis of certain proteins by the caput epididymal epithelium. Vasectomy in men causes a reduction in the levels of a protein normally synthesized at high levels by the corpus epididymidis as a result of the presence of inhibiting factors caused by such obstructions. Sperm taken from an obstructed epididymis or vas deferens has a poor fertilizability/conception rate.

EPIDIDYMAL SPERM

Sperm transit through the epididymis

Remodeling of the sperm plasma membrane during passage through the epididymis produces vigorous motility and the ability to fertilize the egg (Jones, 1998). This remodeling includes the uptake of secreted epididymal glycoproteins (Liu *et al.* 2000), the glycosylation of some membrane proteins, the removal or utilization of specific phospholipids from the inner leaflet of the bilayer, the processing of existing or acquired glycoproteins by endoproteolysis and the re-positioning of both proteins (Hunnicutt *et al.* 1997) and lipids (James *et al.* 1999) to different membrane domains. Phosphorylation of sperm membrane proteins by endogenous protein kinases may be part of the remodeling (Devi *et al.* 1997). This is associated with morphological changes in the sperm head.

Like several other proteins of the sperm plasmalemma, mannose-6 phosphate receptors (MPRs) may undegro redistribution during sperm transit through the epididymis (Belmonte *et al.* 2000). These receptors, which reside in the trans-Golgi network and in the plasma membrane, are responsible for the intracellular targeting of proteins to the lysosomes (Pfeffer, 1988). MPRs are present in the male reproductive tract: in the trans-Golgi network of epididymal principal cells and pachytene spermatocytes and round spermatids. Sertoli cells secrete glycoproteins containing mannose-6-phosphate residues, which are then endocytosed by spermatogenic cells (O'Brien *et al.* 1991).

The repositioning of some surface proteins may follow redistribution of lipids in the plasmalemma, and thus represents a critical phase in the maturation of the gametes. Amongst the various affected proteins of the sperm plasmalemma, MPRs undegro redistribution as the gametes traverse the epididymis (Belmonte *et al.* 2002).

Active oxygen in epididymal sperm

Epididymal sperm is capable of spontaneous ROS generation that appears to involve both the leakage of electrons from the mitochondrial electron transport chain and, potentially, membrane-bound reduced nicotinamide-adenine dinucleotide (NADPH) oxidase. The ability to generate reactive oxygen metabolites poses a threat to the integrity of epididymal spermatozoa in terms of their susceptibility to DNA damage and disrupted membrane function (Aitken, 2002). The epididymis is well endowed with antioxidant defense mechanisms. Small molecular mass antioxidants such as vitamin E, taurine and zinc are present in epididymal plasma.

The caput epididymidis elaborates a peroxidase, GPX5, that is associated with sperm to protect these cells from oxidative stress. Indoleamine dioxygenase is another important antioxidant enzyme located in the epididymis to remove O_2 without generating H_2O_2. The secretory form of superoxide dismutase (SOD) is generated in the cauda epididymidis and may protect these cells during their storage in the epididymis (Aitken, 2002). Sperm capacitation is an extension of maturation, initiated in the epididymis. Therefore, sperm in the cauda is not able to fertilize the egg *in vitro*. Before the sperm becomes able to fertilize it has to complete its maturation in a receptive female reproductive tract or in simple defined media containing a protein source, calcium and bicarbonate. In biological terms, capacitation enables the spermatozoa to respond to physiological signals given out by the cumulus–oocyte complex by undergoing the acrosome reaction, an exocytotic event that releases enzymes involved in penetration of the egg investments. ROS represent a mechanism for effecting both the maturation and the devastation of mammalian sperm. Maintaining a physiological balance between these opposing forces so that sperm mature without excessive oxidative stress is one of the main functions of the epididymis.

Changes in the epididymal sperm membrane

The sperm are surrounded by a limiting plasma membrane containing lipids, proteins, glycolipids and glycoproteins arranged in a classic bilayer structure. Sperm are also highly polarized cells and their plasma membrane is compartmentalized into different regions (acrosome, equatorial segment, postacrosome, midpiece and principal piece) that reflect compositional and functional heterogeneity. Unlike somatic cells, the sperm are transported through widely different milieus, ranging from the unique microenvironment within the seminiferous tubules to those in the epididymis, seminal plasma, uterus, oviduct, cumulus oophorus and eventually the perivitilline space, The plasma membrane has to be sufficiently stable physiologically to withstand these varying conditions, while at the same time being sensitive enough to detect specific signals from different fluids and to react accordingly. Since sperm acquire their fertilizability during passage through the epididymis, extensive investigations have been conducted on the physicochemical characteristics of the plasma membrane during sperm transport in the infertile state (Jones, 2002). Future research is needed to elucidate the biogenesis of the molecules involved in fertilization itself to understand the etiology of infertility in humans and the plasma membrane remodeling events during passage of sperm through the epididymis. Unfortunately, classic transmission electron microscopy of the sperm plasma membrane during epididymal maturation has not been informative, possibly because the resolution is too low to reveal molecular structure and/or because the intrusive fixatives required destroy any subtle changes in this delicate membrane. Other techniques are more revealing: freeze–fracture analyses alone or in combination with filipin (a probe for sterol complexes). The density and arrangement of instramembranous particles not only vary between different plasma membrane compartments, but also change substantially during epididymal maturation. In some species the sperm from the distal corpus and cauda epididymidis show hexagonal or crystalline arrays of particles appearing on the plasma membrane around the margins of the acrosome and in a distinct band lying immediately below the equatorial segment, but are apparently absent from ejaculated sperm (Jones, 2002). Little is known about the physicochemical significance of the ordered arrangements and dispersal patterns of these particles. Filipin–sterol (primarily cholesterol) complexes in the plasma membrane vary in density and arrangement during maturation. Their highest concentration is found in the plasma membrane overlying the acrosome, showing a slight increase during maturation.

Ultrastructural differentiation of epididymal sperm

There are striking differences in the electrophoretic mobility of caput and cauda epididymal sperm, suggesting that a maturation-dependent increase in anionic residues on the sperm surface results from this interaction. This is confirmed ultrastructurally by cytochemical criteria demonstrating altered binding of charged colloidal iron particles and lectins to specific surface domains of the sperm, as they traverse the epididymis. The extensive biochemical remodeling of the protein, glycoprotein and lipid composition of the sperm plasma membrane is an important component of post-testicular sperm maturation. These maturation-dependent changes are not restricted to the sperm plasma membrane; structural change occur in several intracellular organelles. There are remarkable changes in the dimension and internal appearance of the acrosome, and changes in the dimensions of the

nucleus. These are associated with modifications in sperm organelles: the nucleus and perinuclear theca of the head and the connecting piece, the outer dense fibers, the fibrous sheath and the outer mitochondrial membranes of the tail (Olson et al. 2002).

Freeze–fracture reveals maturation-dependent domain-specific changes in the distribution of intramembranous particles in the sperm plasma membrane. The altered patterns of the intramembranous particles may reflect changes in lipid bilayer fluidity, altered interactions of neighboring particles or interactions of the cytoplasmic or extracellular domains of transmembrane proteins with cytoskeletal elements or glycocalyx constituents, respectively. The post-acrosomal plasma membrane domain also undergoes several intriguing maturation-dependent changes as sperm traverse the epididymis. Future research is needed to clarify whether this represents an anchoring of membrane proteins to the post-acrosomal sheath and a consequent reduction in their mobility. Also, little is known about the functional significance of the changes in the intramembranous particles with respect to the role of this membrane domain in sperm–egg fusion. Freeze–fracture revealed maturation-dependent particle reorganization in the flagellar membrane. In cauda epididymal sperm, the midpiece plasma membrane exhibits numerous circumferential particle strands, which overlie the gyres of the underlying mitochondria. The strands of testicular and caput epididymal sperm are shorter, suggesting that their assembly may correlate with the acquisition of forward motility. Membrane–cytoskeletal interactions may play a major role in maintaining the unique identity and function of specific sperm plasma membrane domains and in the potential regulation of underlying domain-specific cytoplasmic organelles (Olson et al. 2002). More research is required on the molecular nature of these assemblies, their roles in regulating sperm function and their contribution to the post-testicular maturation of sperm.

Molecular regulation of epididymal sperm motility

The mammalian sperm has a 9 + 2 axoneme, typical of most cilia and flagella, but is surrounded by accessory dense fibers. Extending from the A microtubule of each of the nine doublets are two rows of dynein arms (outer and inner) with ATPase activities, which allow attachment and detachment of the dynein arms to the B microtubule of the adjacent doublet, serving as the motors of flagellation. The outer and inner arms are distinct in their structure, chemical components and function. The acquisition of the potential for motility and development of the swimming pattern are the most obvious maturational changes of sperm in the epididymis.

The application of computer-assisted sperm analysis (CASA) enables relatively objective and quantitative descriptions of such changes in terms of velocities and other kinematic parameters. These kinematic parameters can serve as sensitive indicators of sperm maturation in the study of epididymal regulatory factors, and the profile of changes can also form the basis of reference for studying the development of other functional capacities of maturing sperm. Motility development involves first, the acquisition of the potential for flagellation; and second, the co-ordination and modulation of the flagellar waveform, resulting in the characteristic mature swimming pattern.

Maturational changes in the molecular endowment of the sperm axoneme, a permissive intracellular ionic environment and effective signal transduction mechanisms. In concert with the stiffening of the flagellum and alterations of the plasma membrane composition this modulates its transport properties in the milieu regulated by the epididymis. This enables immature sperm gradually to attain conditions for accumulation of an efficient force for translation into bend formation and co-ordinated flagellation (Yeung and Cooper, 2002). This results in the mature motion pattern of forward propulsion when released at the end of the epididymal sojourn.

BIOCHEMICAL/PHARMACOLOGICAL PARAMETERS

Protein secretion in the epididymis

Epididymal cells are able to synthesize and secrete proteins and glycoproteins, as judged by autoradiography. Characterization of epididymal proteins was achieved when uncontaminated samples were collected from rete testis fluid and caudal epididymal fluid and the proteins were resolved using sodium dodecyl sulfate (SDS) polyacrylamide gel electrophoresis. The complexity of protein secretions results from two particularities: continuous and progressive changes in their composition throughout the male excurrent duct; and the presence of components in unusual concentrations, some of them not found in other body fluids. This specificity is maintained not only by active secretion and reabsorption throughout the tract but also by the presence of significant restrictions in the exchanges between the luminal compartment and blood plasma. A blood barrier formed by tight junctions between the Sertoli cells in the testis and epithelial cells in the epididymis is functional until the sperm complete their maturation. The most important function of the blood barrier is protection from autoimmune attack. This can occur from new antigens that appear on the sperm during their differentiation; and from specific testicular and epididymal protein secretions associated with the terminal cellular differentiation of the gametes. The membrane of the principle cell divides into two distinct regions: the apical pole, which communicates directly with the luminal environment and is involved in both secretion and reabsorption; and the basal membrane, which is exposed to the systemic circulation.

The secretion of several proteins such as GGT, GPX, SOD or lactoferrin thus suggests the presence of a system of protection from superoxides adapted to sperm metabolism throughout epididymal transit. The continuous and/or successive presence of several proteins with binding and/or lipophilic properties probably contributes to the modification, stabilization, or protection of specific sperm membrane domains, particularly those involved in egg binding or sperm agglutination in the epididymis. Some of these proteins may also be involved in immunological protection during epididymal transit or in the female genital tract. Further research is needed to identify the enzymatic activity of the proteins found in the epididymal environment. It would appear that these enzymes are sequentially activated because several specific inhibitors such as protease inhibitor are secreted sequentially by the epithelium. The function of the protein may also be controlled by modification of their molecular conformation. For many proteins (e.g. clustering, PGDS, CTP/HE1), low molecular variants appear during epididymal transit. These isoforms are probably the results of protease or glycosidase activity secreted in downstream parts of the epididymis (Dacheux and Dacheux, 2001). The molecular characterization of epididymal proteins (proteins sequencing by mass spectrometry and genome information) will be applied to identify several hundred proteins and to evaluate the role of the protein interactions in sperm maturation.

Nuclear chromatin

Extensive investigation has been conducted on the relationship between sperm nuclei and birth defects/male infertility with reference to nucleic acid, and the entire DNA–basic protein complex. Several unique techniques have been applied, since sperm are highly resistant to common decondensing agents, owing to an extensive cross-linking of the protamines by disulfide bonds. Bandyopadhyay (2002) studied DNA–basic protein components of individual sperm to correlate the characteristics of both DNA and protamines of the caput and cauda epididymal regions. To avoid the use of trypsin, a proteolytic enzyme, experiments were conducted to identify a fresh set of decondensing agents. β-Mercaptoethanol (0.25 mol/l) along with 4 mol/l urea were the most effective reagent mixture for bringing about complete decondensation of the sperm head. Incubation of sperm nuclei for 2 h in the presence of these chemical agents released DNA– basic protein from the sperm. After decondensation, the reduced cysteine residues in the protamine were blocked by incubation with 50 mmol/l iodoacetamide. Protamines were isolated from the viscous suspension by repeated extractions with 0.5 N HCl at 4°C. Acid extracts were dialyzed and purified through carboxymethylcellulose (CM52) column chromatography. The protamines were eluted with a linear gradient of NaCl ranging from 0.5 to 1 mol/l in 50 mmol/l sodium acetate buffer (pH 6.0). The CM52 column chromatography pattern showed one peak. When subjected to polyacrylamide gel electrophoresis, the samples obtained of the protamine after CM52 column chromatography migrated as a single band, thereby proving the homogeneity of the protein isolated.

Enzyme system

The epididymis is particularly rich in acid hydrolases (Figure 4.4) concordantly with a developed and active lysosomal apparatus. In mice, the highest levels of α-D-mannosidase and β-hexosaminidase are expressed in the epididymis (Hermo et al. 1997). Expression of some proteins in the epididymis depends on both circulating androgens and testicular factors (Hinton et al. 1988). These factors include a variety of molecules found in the seminiferous tubular fluid, such as luminal androgens, androgen binding protein or sex-hormone binding globulins (Turner et al. 1995), estrogen (Hess et al. 1997), growth factor (Lan et al. 1998) and other organic molecules. Non-steroidal testicular factors stimulate protein synthesis and secretion by caput epididymal cells. Testicular factors participate in the maintenance of epididymal 5α-reductase enzyme activity and to affect the expression of several epididymal proteins and glycoproteins. Some of the glycosidases synthesized by the epididymal epithelium are secreted into the lumen in an androgen-dependent fashion (Jones et al. 1980; Abou-Haila et al. 1996).

Some of the epididymal enzymes become bound to sperm on transit through the duct. The gametes may transport the enzymes to an extraepididymal environment where conditions could favor hydrolytic activity. Although some of these enzymes originate from the testis, most of them are synthesized and secreted by the epididymal epithelium lining the duct (Mayorga and Bertini, 1985; Skudlarek/Orgebin-Crist, 1986). The dynamic of the epididymal secretion, as for the distribution of the different acid glycosidases, may be related to the role of each enzyme in the epididymis (Belomonte et al. 2001). Lysosomal enzymes are differently compartmentalized in the cauda epididymis. Most of the β-galactosidase and aryl sulfatase (approximately 70%) are found in soluble form within the fluid, whereas about 60% of N-acetyl-β-D-glucosaminidase and α-mannosidase become transiently bound to sperm, and β-glucuronidase is mostly concentrated in the epithelium (Belmonte et al. 2001).

Enzymatic detoxification pathway

Several enzymatic detoxification pathways protect cells from harmful substances. For example, the mercapturic acid pathway transforms many xenobiotics in soluble derivates of mercapturic acid, which are easily eliminated. This pathway starts with the conjugation of the xenobiotic with the tripeptide glutathione (GSH). This step is catalyzed by a variety of enzymes, the glutathione S-transferases (GSTs), which have different affinities for a wide variety of compounds. The second step comprises the γ-glutamyl transpeptidase

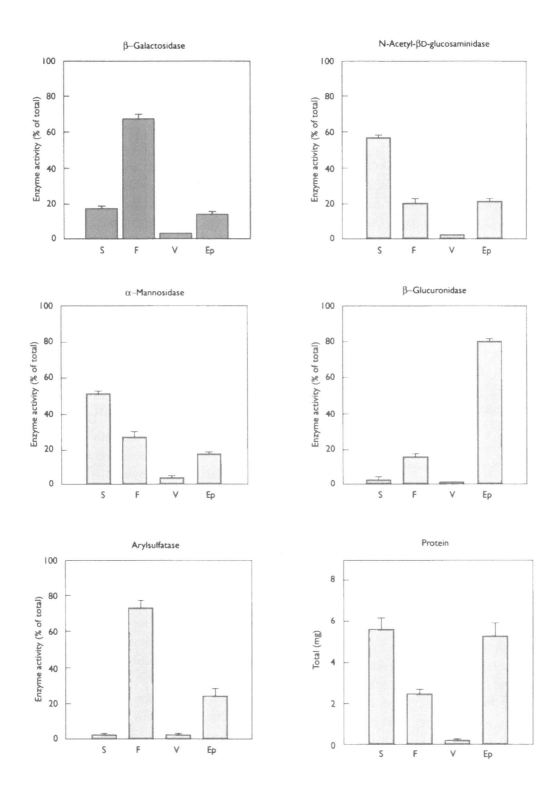

Figure 4.4 Distribution of acid hydrolases between compartments in the rat cauda epididymis. Values are expressed as means ± SD of six experiments. S, sperm; F, fluid; V, vesicles; Ep, epididymal tissue. (Reproduced with permission from Belmonte *et al.* 2002, *Arch Androl*, 48:193–201. www.tandf.co.uk/journals)

(GGT)-catalyzed removal of the γ-glutamyl portion, which protects GSH from peptidase action. The following steps include the elimination of the glycyl residue of the resulting conjugated compound by a specific dipeptidase, and a further acetylation of the cysteine for the final transformation to the mercapturic acid derivate (Montiel *et al.* 2003). Several immunocytochemical methods have been used to evaluate the expression of different isoforms of GST in the epididymis. Region-specific isoforms of GST have been found in the rat epididymis, and the expression of these isoforms showed significant changes during development and aging. On the other hand, GGT is also present in almost all tissues, including the testis and epididymis. Catalytic activity, protein level and different RNAs of GGT were found to be expressed in a region-dependent manner and regulated by androgen and testicular factors (Monteil *et al.* 2003)

Montiel *et al.* (2003) measured the activity of GGT and GST in epithelial cell cultures from human caput, corpus and cauda epididymides (Figure 4.5). GGT activity was highest in cultures from the cauda epididymis, both in conditioned media and in cell fractions, while GST activity did not show regional differences in conditioned media, but exhibited higher activity in cell homogenates from cauda cultures than those from corpus/caput epididymis. GGT and GST are present along the human epididymis, and a fraction of isoforms of these enzymes might be secreted to the luminal fluid to play a detoxificating role in sperm maturation (Montiel *et al.* 2003).

Pharmacology

Sulfated glycoprotein-2 (SGP-2), a major secretory protein of Sertoli cells, is synthesized in the same non-ciliated cell that takes up SGP-2 by endocytosis from the ductule lumen. Estrogens play a major role in the regulation of efferent ductule function. Estrogen receptors are expressed in this region of the male tract to an extent that exceeds even that of the female reproductive tract (Setchell, 2001).

Pharmacopathology

Dinitrobenzene, a chemical widely used in the manufacture of dyes, plastics and explosives, causes a limited number of obstructions in the efferent ductules,

which lead to fibrotic obliteration, calcification and granulomatous formations. Chloro-6-deoxyglucose also produces lesions in the efferent ductules and proximal portions of the epididymis. Quinazolinone, an antiarthritic and potent antitumor drug, induces sterility in animals by inducing occlusions of the efferent ductules and initial segment of the epididymidis. The disruption of blood flow to the epididymis is responsible for the effects on male reproduction. Cadmium alters the activity of several enzymes including that of carbonic anhydrase, which has its highest concentration in the epithelial cells lining the efferent ductules. Lead reduces sperm concentration in the epididymis without testicular effects, which suggests that there may have been an effect on fluid reabsorption in the efferent ductules. Young's syndrome, which involves a failure of efferent ductule function and infertility, is associated with mercury toxicity. High doses of fluoride cause the loss of cilia and the peeling of the epithelial lining in the epididymis (Setchell, 2001).

IMMUNOLOGICAL PARAMETERS

The epididymis contains cells of the immune system. There is an intimate relationship between both the epithelial and the interstitial compartments, which respond to functional changes in the epididymis. Future research is needed to evaluate: the nature of the chemical produced by the epididymal epithelium to attract immune cells to the tissue; the role of the immune cells in removing debris or damaged cells from the epithelium; and the consequences of the changes in the number of immune cells during aging or after drug treatment on sperm function (Figure 4.6).

Experimental autoimmune orchitis (EAO) is a model for studying cell-mediated autoimmunity and infertility. EAO can be induced in an animal by immunization with testicular extract and is often followed by autoimmune inflammation in both testis and the epididymis but not the vas deferens. After immunization of Lewis/NCr rats, there is an accumulation of CD4+ T cells, CD8+ T cells and macrophages in the epididymis and the rete testis. Interestingly, this EAO can be transferred to another animal using sperm antigen-specific CD4+ T cells clones. Activated T lymphocytes secrete interleukin (IL)-2, interferon-γ gamma (IFN-γ) and tumor necrosis factor (TNF), which are typical of the Th1 subtype.

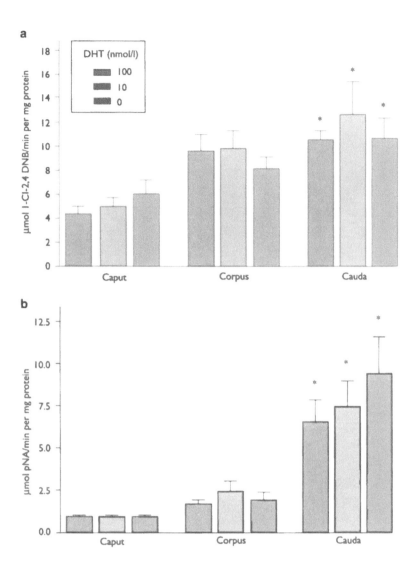

Figure 4.5 Glutathione S-transferase activity in cell homogenates from cultures obtained from caput, corpus and cauda epididymides. Cells were cultured in the absence or presence of 10 or 100 nmol/l of dihydrotestosterone (DHT) (DNB, dinitrobenzene). Cell homogenates were obtained on day 12 of culture. (b) γ-Glutamyl transpeptidase activity in conditioned media from cultures obtained from caput, corpus and cauda epididymides. Cells were cultured in the absence or presence of 10 or 100 nmol/l of DHT. pNA, p-nitro aniline. Media were collected every 48 h on days 4–8 of culture. Data are expressed as median ± SEM from nine patients. *$p < 0.05$ comparing cauda with corpus and caput; $p > 0.05$ between different hormone conditions. (Reproduced with permission from Montiel *et al.* 2003, *Arch Androl*, 49:95–105. www.tandf. co.uk/journals)

Transfer of the EAO is compromised by preliminary injection with an antibody to TNF, suggesting that this cytokine might play an important role in autoimmune infertility.

Mutant alymphoplasia (aly) mice have neither lymph nodes nor Peyer's patches. In this model, there is an accumulation of eosinophils and macrophages in tissues such as the liver and kidney. Within the male reproductive tract, the testis, efferent ducts, prostate and seminal vesicles do not show any accumulation of immune cells. However, in both the epididymis and vas deferens, extensive accumulation of lymphocytes (eosinophils and macrophages) occurs. These cells are found exclusively in the stroma and do not seem to enter the

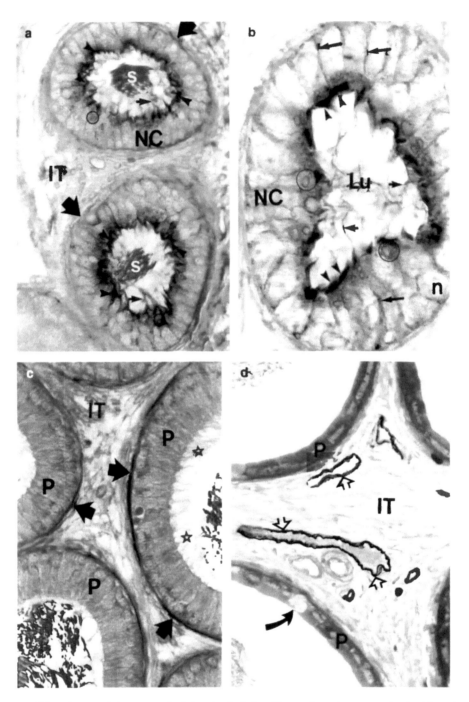

Figure 4.6 Low-power light micrograph in a normal adult animal of the efferent ducts immunostained with anti-aquaporin-1 (anti-AQP-1) antibody. An intense reaction is present over the microvilli (arrowheads) of the non-ciliated cells (NC) and cilia of ciliated cells (small arrows) extending deep into the lumen. Also reactive are apical endocytic vesicles (circles) of the non-ciliated cells. Sperm (S) in the lumen are unreactive. A faint reaction is visible over myoid cells enveloping the periphery of the tubules (large arrows). IT, intertubular space; magnification × 420 (b) High-power light micrograph in a normal adult animal of the efferent ducts immunostained with anti-aquaporin-1 (anti-AQP-1) antibody. The microvilli of the non-ciliated cells (NC) show a homogeneous thick band of reaction product (arrowheads). Also reactive are the tall cilia of the ciliated cells (short arrows) stretching into the lumen, the basolateral plasma membranes (long arrows) between adjacent epithelial cells, and the membranes delimiting large apical endocytic vesicles (circles) of the non-ciliated cells. Lu, lumen; n, nuclei of non-ciliated cells; magnification × 1048. (c) Initial segment of the adult epididymis immunostained with anti-aquaporin-1 (anti-AQP-1) antibody. While a reaction is absent from the principal cells (P), including their microvilli (stars); an intense reaction is present over the myoid cells enveloping the ducts of this region (arrows). IT, intertubular space; magnification × 420. (d) Cauda epididymidis of a normal adult animal immunostained with anti-aquaporin-1 (anti-AQP-1) antibody. Principal cells (P) and clear cells (curved arrow) show no reaction product, while the endothelial cells of vascular channels of the intertubular space (IT) are intensely reactive (open arrows); magnification × 262. (Reproduced with permission from Badran and Hermo, 2002)

epithelium or cross into the luminal compartment. Consequences of such infiltration on epididymal function have not yet been investigated.

PATHOLOGICAL PARAMETERS

Epididymal obstruction

The etiologies of ductal obstruction (in addition to vasectomy) include congenital absence or hypoplasia of the ductal system, ductal stricture following infection, iatrogenic injury and functional obstruction. Approximately 1.4% of all infertile men have congenital absence or hypoplasia of part or all of the ductal system including the corpus and causa of the epididymis.

Extensive investigations have been conducted on the autoimmune response to vasectomy with emphasis on antisperm antibody formation. Not only does an autoimmune response to sperm occur after vasectomy, but similar reactions occur after obstruction of the male reproductive tract at other points. Male rats in which the corpus epididymidis or vas deferens were obstructed prior to puberty developed systemic antisperm autoantibody responses after sexual maturation that were comparable in magnitude to antibody levels in adult vasectomized rats. Moreover, antisperm antibodies recognized certain 'dominant' autoantigens after both epididymal ligation and vasectomy, although sera from rats with epididymal ligations recognized some proteins that were not bound by most post-vasectomy sera and *vice versa* (Flickinger and Howards, personal communication).

Differences in autoantigens recognized after epididymal and vasal obstructions may reflect maturational changes in sperm components that take place during the passage of spermatozoa through the epididymis. Alterations in sperm proteins that would change the epitopes presented to the immune system could include proteolysis, changes in disulfide bonds, extension or removal of carbohydrate portions of glycoproteins, insertion of intracellular proteins into the sperm plasma membrane, unmasking of surface components and addition of proteins of epididymal origin to the sperm (Flickinger and Howards, 2002). Spermatic granulomas provide sites for presentation of large amounts of sperm antigens to cells of the immune system. Inflammation in the epididymal interstitial connective tissue resembles that seen after immunization with sperm or testis homogenates, and may provide a way in which sperm antigens can contact the immune cells. Macrophages can traverse the epithelium of the epididymis or the efferent ductules to reach the lumen and subsequently phagocytose spermatozoa, possibly beginning at sites of granuloma formation. On the other hand, if the epididymis ruptures, spermatic granulomas form and provide contact for sperm with the immune system.

Inflammation of the excurrent duct system

The complex excurrent ductal system, which includes the efferent ductules, epididymis and vas deferens, is subject to various pathological conditions that have a significant impact in sperm physiology/transport, resulting in subfertility or infertility. Pathologies may also occur in the male accessory glands: the prostate, seminal vesicles, and the bulbourethral (Cowper's) and periurethral (Little's) glands. Prostatitis and seminal vesiculitis are the common inflammatory conditions. A broad spectrum of inflammatory conditions of the accessory glands is referred to as male accessory gland inflammation (Chan and Schlegel, 2002).

Signs of chronic inflammation at the sites of stenosis in the epididymal tubules or, less commonly, vas deferens, are noted intraoperatively. Some of the patients may not be aware of a previous episodes of inflammation of the excurrent ductal system or sex accessory glands. The sequelae of these inflammatory syndromes have a severe impact on these organs, particularly in relation to male reproduction. While effective medical/surgical treatments are available for infections/their sequelae, recognition of the disease with prompt diagnosis is critical for successful management of these conditions and prevention of complications (Chan and Schlegel, 2002).

Pathology of epididymal cancer

Of resected primary epididymal tumors, only 25% are malignant, whereas the majority are benign. Primary malignancies of the epididymis include sarcomas, germ cell tumors, lymphomas and rarely adenocarcinomas. The most common benign epididymal neoplasm is the adenomatoid tumor, which usually presents as a firm well-circumscribed nodule that does not metastasize.

Adenomatoid tumors are of mesothelial origin, and have epithelium-like characteristics with no mitotic activity. Cells are cuboidal or flat, with a vacuolated but not clear cytoplasm, possess eccentric nuclei and often have a 'signet ring' appearance. Tubule formation may be observed, but the cells are not infiltrative as are adenocarcinomas. Epididymal adenocarcinomas are tubular, tubulocystic or tubulopapillary. Malignant cells may invade the stroma, periepididymal soft tissue or the adjacent testis. Epididymal cystadenomas are composed of multiple cysts and tubules or papillary fronds. Epididymal papillary cystadenomas in von Hippel–Lindau (VHL) disease are considered benign and are not resected. It may be that development of specific tumors resulting from the loss of the pVHL tumor suppressor depends on the tissue or organ that is affected. Other primary malignancies of the epididymis include sarcoma germ cell tumors, lymphoma and plasmacytoma.

Therapy of epididymal cancer

Because of the rarity of epididymal adenocarcinoma, guidelines for therapy have not been established (Ganem *et al.* 1998). If there is suspicion of malignancy, the epididymis should be explored from an inguinal approach. Abnormal retroperitoneal nodes detected on a computerized tomography (CT) scan should probably be resected. There is no evidence, however, that radiation therapy of chemotherapy is beneficial in advanced disease or in the adjuvant setting. Metastatic epididymal adenocarcinomas, similarly to adenocarcinomas that originate in other primary sites, appear not to be curable. Palliative measures such as radiation therapy or surgical resection of painful metastases may be indicated on an individual basis.

EPIDIDYMIS: HUMAN FERTILITY AND INFERTILITY

Little is known about the role of the 'normal' human epididymis in the development of male fertility/infertility. Future studies at the molecular level are needed to evaluate epididymal gene expression in humans and some animal models. Unfortunately, non-human primates are not suitable, owing to ethical and economic reasons. As compared to other mammals, human sperm production is poor, and the quality of sperm is highly heterogeneous. The requirement for post-testicular sperm maturation in humans may turn out not to be similar to that in other mammals. Sperm production/storage in humans does not seem to be under the same environmental/adaptive selective pressure. Absence of the products in the human epididymis, however, could reflect a loss of constraint for these gene products, specifically in human reproduction. Epididymal microsurgery as well as intracytoplasmic sperm injection (ICSI) in infertility patients have brought into question whether the human epididymis has the same essential role for the development of male fertility as it does in the rather few animal species tested. Little is known about mechanisms by which specific epididymal products implement the acquisition of the ability of sperm to fertilize.

In azoospermic men, 30% have 'obstructive azoospermia' while the remaining have a primary testicular failure, 'non-obstructive azoospermia'. In the obstructive azoospermia group, about 25% have congenital bilateral absence of the vas deferens (CBAVD), while the incidence among all infertile males is about 2%. Other obstructive conditions include vasectomy, failed vasectomy reversal operations, post-inflammatory scarring of the epididymis, inoperable ejaculatory duct blockage or distal vasal obstructions and functional obstructions in patients after extensive retroperitaneal lymph node dissections (Patrizio and Amin, 2002).

Anatomically, CBAVD is characterized by regression of variable portions of the epididymis, vas deferens and, in about 80% of cases, absence of the seminal vesicles. Epididymal sperm of men with vasectomy or failed vasectomy or reversal have a higher *in vitro* fertilization rate (without ICSI), as opposed to epididymal sperm of men with CBAVD, perhaps reflecting abnormal sperm interactions due to the effect of mutations in epididymal sperm. This difference is abolished with the use of ICSI; today it is common to report ICSI fertilization of epididymal sperm at about 50–60% (Patrizio and Amin, unpublished data).

Assisted reproduction for azoospermia

Several therapeutic approaches have been applied for irreparable obstructive azoospermia. These include ovarian stimulation and fertilization by ICSI in conjunction with epididymal sperm retrieval (microsurgical epididymal sperm aspiration (MESA) or percutaneous epididymal sperm aspiration (PESA). ICSI in conjunction with the less invasive PESA provides a pregnancy rate of about 45% per cycle. There are several advantages for the combined application of PESA plus ICSI (Patrizio and Amin, 2002):

(1) Waiting time is unnecessary for the appearance of sperm in the ejaculate, and sperm fertilization is quickly assessed; this point is particularly important when age is a factor in the female partner.

(2) Aliquots of epididymal sperm can be frozen for ICSI cycles.

(3) Excess embryos can be frozen and used in the future.

(4) There is no need for extensive scrotal surgery.

(5) There is no need to reconsider contraception (the man remains vasectomized).

The piece of one cycle of PESA plus ICSI with ovarian stimulation is more expensive than a vaso-to-vaso and comparable to a vaso-epididymostomy.

FUTURE RESEARCH

Very little is known about the physiology and pathophysiology of the human epididymis, mainly because of lack of proper experimental systems. A few studies carried out in normal subjects have demonstrated that, as in animal species, the fertilizing capacity of human spermatozoa increases as they pass through the epididymides. Extensive research should be conduction on the effect of drugs and metabolites on the functional ultrastructure of the epididymis, since it is an important target for male post-testicular contraception.

CHAPTER 5

Capacitation and fertilization

CAPACITATION

Sperm capacitation is functional reprogramming, in order to exhibit fertilizing ability (Yanagamachi, 1994). The fertilizing function of spermatozoa is accomplished by delivering a male genome into an oocyte and activating it, thereby initiating its development into an embryo (Figure 5.1). The mechanisms by which fertilizing spermatozoa provoke oocyte activation could be the activation of specific steroid binding sites in the nuclear matrix in response to an appropriate hormonal stimulus via the estrogen receptor. The nuclear matrix of sperm from men with idiopathic infertility is much less responsive to the stimulus of estradiol than that of spermatozoa from normospermic men (Figure 5.2).

The sequence of events during sperm hyperactivation, capacitation, the acrosome reaction and fertilization is as follows:

(1) Sperm subsets (capacitated active, capacitation latent, non-capacitated and dysfunctional) penetrate cumulus cells;

(2) Initial binding of sperm with zona glycoprotein, ZP3;

(3) Acrosome reaction follows sperm/egg recognition;

(4) Acrosomal cap discarded as sperm penetrates the zona pellucida (ZP);

(5) Acrosin exposed on the inner acrosomal membrane – may mediate secondary binding to ZP2;

(6) Fusion between plasma membranes of sperm and oocyte (Figure 5.3).

The organization of the nuclear matrix in the sperm (Nadel *et al.* 1995; Kramer and Krawetz, 1996) plays a major role in many dynamic aspects of nuclear function, including control of DNA supercoiling, formation of chromatin loops, regulation and co-ordination of transcriptional and replicational activities of DNA (Gerdes *et al.* 1994) and processing and transport of RNA (Ciejek *et al.* 1982).

The association of estradiol and the nuclear matrix, apparently through a receptor-mediated mechanism (Simmen *et al.* 1984), involves nuclear ribonucleoprotein (Peters and Comings, 1980), upregulation of estrogen receptor gene expression (Ing *et al.* 1996) and, probably, recruitment of RNA polymerase II cofactors (Ing *et al.* 1992). These events indicate that the activation of estradiol receptor binding in the nuclear matrix may be involved in the regulation of post-transcriptional mechanisms during fertilization.

The sperm undergoes a series of biochemical and functional modifications (functional reprogramming) collectively referred to as capacitation. A biochemical change could be the activation of the estrogen receptor (ER) binding in the nuclear matrix. Therefore, the measurement of the ER in the nuclear matrix of capacitated sperm of normozoospermic men could be an indicator of the prerequisites of human sperm to exhibit fertilizing ability. Calzada and Martinez (2001) measured the values of ERs in capacitated and non-capacitated sperm: they were 91 ± 21 fmol/10^8 sperm and 26 ± 7 fmol/10^8 sperm, respectively. The association of the ER with the nuclear matrix is an important factor in the regulation of the transcription of the sperm genome of capacitated sperm during the pronuclei stage.

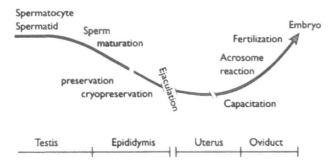

Figure 5.1 The progress of sperm through the male and female reproductive organs towards fertilization of the oocyte and formation of an embryo

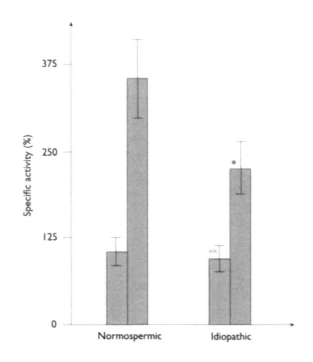

Figure 5.2 Specific activity in capacitated (■) and non-capacitated (■) sperm of normospermic men and those with idiopathic infertility. *$p < 0.0001$; **$p < 0.05$ as compared with values of normospermic men. (Reproduced with permission from Gonzalez-Unzaga *et al. Arch Androl*, 2003;49:77–88. www.tandf.co.uk/journals)

FERTILIZATION

Fertilization is a complex process associated with remarkable biophysical and molecular changes in the sperm before its fusion with the oocyte plasma membrane: capacitation, binding to the ZP, the acrosome reaction, penetration through the ZP and fusion with the plasma membrane of the oocyte. Little is known about the molecular mechanisms of capacitation, which was discovered in 1951 simultaneously by Austin in the UK and Chang in the USA. Capacitation is followed by the acrosome reaction, which involves the release of several proteolytic enyzmes.

Fertilizability

Fertilizability is associated with an increase in respiration and a subsequent change in motility (Hidiroglou and Knipfel, 1984), membrane cholesterol/phospholipid ratio, destabilization of the sperm membrane (Hammerstedt and Parks, 1987), increase in calcium level (Parrish *et al.* 1993), removal of zinc (Andrews and Bavister, 1989),

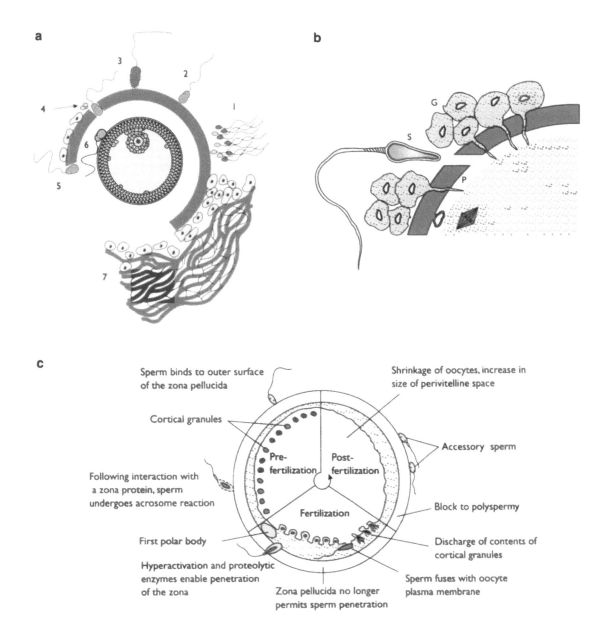

Figure 5.3 (a) Sequence of events during sperm hyperactivation, capacitation, acrosome reaction and fertilization. 1, Sperm subsets (capacitated active, capacitation latent, non-capacitated and dysfunctional) penetrate cumulus cells. 2, Initial binding of sperm with zona glycoprotein ZP2. 3, Acrosome reaction follows sperm/egg recognition. 4, Acrosomal cap is discarded as sperm penetrates the zona pellucida. 5, Acrosin exposed on inner acrosomal membrane; may mediate secondary binding to ZP3. 6, Fusion between plasma membranes of sperm; oocyte/sperm membranes fuse. 7, Cumulus matrix. (b) Sperm penetration of zona pellucida (ZP), and oocyte (O) and granulosa cells (G). Note the release of enzymes from perforations of the acrosomal cap. (c) Gamete interactions/fertilization

activation of the second messenger system (Duncan and Frazer, 1993) and activation of specific estradiol binding sites in the nuclear matrix of sperm cells of normospermic men (Calzada and Martinez, 2002). The measurement of the nuclear matrix–ER complex in human sperm plays an important role in predicting the fertilizing potential of a sperm sample (Calzada *et al.* 2001a,b).

Gonzalez-Unzaga *et al.* (2002) measured ER levels in the nuclear matrix of the sperm of normospermic fertile men and men with idiopathic infertility. In non-capacitated sperm cells, the ER in normospermic fertile men was present in 50% of the cases, whereas in infertile men it was present in 19% of the cases. In capacitated sperm, the ER in normospermic fertile men was present in 80% of cases, whereas in infertile men it was present in 31% of the cases. The concentration of ERs in capacitated and non-capacitated sperm cells of normospermic fertile men was 91 ± 21 and 26 ± 7 fmol/10^8 sperm cells, respectively, whereas in capacitated and non-capacitated sperm of men with idiopathic infertility, the ER values were 50 ± 17 and 22.5 ± 9 fmol/10^8 sperm cells, respectively. The diminution of the ER levels in the nuclear matrix is a biochemical indicator of male factor infertility.

Hypo-osmotic test

In the hypo-osmotic test (HOST) of sperm swelling, a score of < 50% correlates with extremely poor pregnancy rates in cycles not involved with *in vitro* fertilization (IVF) (Check *et al.* 1989). Abnormally low HOST scores do not correlate with poor fertilization rates following IVF (Avery *et al.* 1990; Chan *et al.* 1990; Enginsu *et al.* 1992). However, HOST scores of < 50% do correlate very well with extremely poor implantation rates following IVF–embryo transfer (ET) (Kiefer *et al.* 1990; Check *et al.* 1995; Katsoff *et al.* 2000). The poor implantation rates may be related to the transfer of a toxic factor to the ZP by the attached supernumerary sperm. Data supporting this hypothesis were provided by the demonstration of a very high pregnancy rate following intracytoplasmic sperm injection (ICSI) with semen specimens with low HOST scores, thus bypassing contact with the ZP (Check *et al.* 2001).

Redistribution of mannose-6-phosphate receptors on the sperm surface

Mannose-6-phosphate receptors (MPRs) are redistributed on the sperm surface following relocalization of other proteins during sperm maturation along the epididymal duct. The CI-MPRs, which were originally localized to the dorsal region of the sperm head, become redistributed over the entire acrosomal region as soon as the gametes enter the epididymis. The CD-MPRs extend their original distribution on the dorsal to the ventral region of the head when the sperm pass

from the corpus to the cauda epididymis. The number of cells immunoreactive to the CI-MPR progressively increases from the rete testis to the cauda, whereas the percentage of sperm immunostained for the CD-MPR increase to a maximum when the sperm enter the epididymis. The labeling on the dorsal region of the sperm head corresponds to that on the acrosomal region.

Possible roles of sperm mannose-6-phosphate receptors

These receptors may play one of three roles:

(1) The sperm may act as a vehicle to transport lysosomal enzymes to a site other then the epididymis (e.g. the female genital tract). The near neutral epididymal pH may favor the enzyme–sperm interaction but not the catalytic activity of the enzymes (Sosa *et al.* 1991). Subsequently, the female reproductive tract provides an optimal pH for acid hydrolase activity (Larsson and Platz-Christensen, 1991). It is possible that the enzyme may act there to modify glycoproteins on the oocyte, or the sperm itself, during the capacitation process prior to fertilization (Belmonte *et al.* 2002).

(2) The receptors recognize extraepididymal ligands (e.g. ZP glycoproteins). An essential step in the process of fertilization is the recognition and binding of the sperm to the egg's ZP. If glycoproteins of the ZP contain mannose-6-phosphate residues, a role for the MPRs in the primary sperm–egg binding could be postulated.

(3) Some receptors may play a role in the acrosome reaction. The CI-MPR recognizes insulin-like growth factor II (IGF-II), other growth factors and mannose-6-phosphate-bearing ligands; this interaction triggers a signal transduction cascade in other cell types (Belmonte *et al.* 2002).

Synthesis of YLP$_{12}$ peptide in sperm

The peptide, synthesized by solid-phase synthesis, is conjugated to tetanus toxoid, using 1-ethyl-3 (3-dimethylaminopropyl). Antiserum is raised in female rabbits and the antibodies are purified by using a protein A–Sepharose 4B column. The monovalent Fab are prepared using pepsin with further immunoaffinity

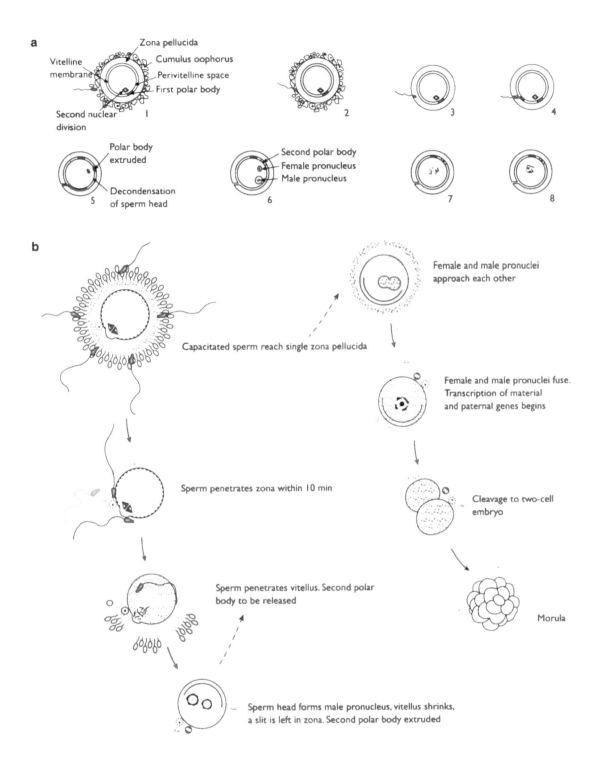

Figure 5.4 (a) Steps during fertilization: 1, Spermatozoon first encounters and penetrates the cumulus oophorus. The first polar body is present in the perivitelline space with the metaphase spindle of the secondary oocyte present in the cytoplasm. 2, A spermatozoon having undergone acrosomal activation. 3, The inner acrosomal membrane of a spermatozoon contacts the zona pellucida. 4, Enzymes exposed on the membrane surface allow penetration into the perivitelline space. 5, The equatorial region of the sperm head attaches and fuses with the vitelline membrane, stimulating completion of the second meiotic division. 6, The large male pronucleus and smaller female pronucleus form, following extrusion of the second polar body. 7, The pronuclei migrate to the oocyte center, where the nuclear envelopes disperse. 8, The prophase of the first mitosis division begins. (Reproduced with permission from McLare, 1980). (b) Nuclear changes during fertilization and formation of the two-cell embryo and morula

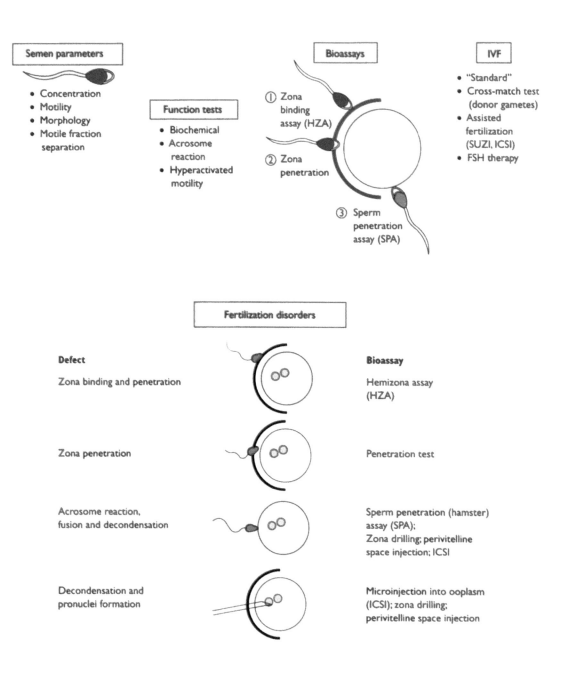

Figure 5.5 Diagnosis of failed *in vitro* fertilization (IVF) and sperm defects/fertilization failure. (a) Diagnostic scheme to establish a step-wise progressive diagnosis in cases of recurrent failed IVF. (b) Sequential analysis of specific sperm defects in cases of recurrent failed fertilization. ICSI, intracytoplasmic sperm injection. (Reproduced with permission of Elsevier from Oehninger *et al.* 1991)

purification with peptide–bovine serum albumin (BSA)–Sepharose 4B immunobeads. The acrosome reaction is determined by incubating fixed sperm with fluorescein isothiocyanate (FITC) conjugated to BSA. The slides are washed twice with phosphate-buffered saline (PBS), a drop of mounting medium (PBS containing 90% glycerol, 0.1% sodium azide and 10 mg/ml of 1,4-diazabicyclo (2,2,2) octane) is added to each well and the slide is examined using a fluorescence microscope. The dodecamer peptide sequence, designated as YLP_{12}, is present on the acrosomal region of the human sperm cell and is expressed only in human testis/sperm (Naz and Packianathan, 2000). Most of the sperm undergo the acrosome reaction when they are capacitated in the presence of 40–85 μg/ml of BSA or a control Fab. A significant reduction in the percentage of acrosome-reacted sperm is noted when the sperm are capacitated in the presence of YLP_{12}.

GAMETE INTERACTION

The bulk of the semen enters the uterus directly, or is forced through the cervical canal during momentary relaxation of the cervix assisted by the vaginal contraction resulting from copulatory stimuli. Most sperm are eliminated from the female reproductive tract. A few sperm are transported to the site of fertilization in the ampulla and/or ampulla–isthmic junction. The sperm/egg ratio in the ampulla during fertilization is 1 : 1 or even less. The female reproductive tract prevents morphologically abnormal sperm from reaching the site of fertilization. Not all fertilizing sperm are genetically normal. Normal embryonic development is maximal when eggs in the oviduct are fertilized soon after ovulation.

The gametes undergo a complex ultrastructural process of proliferation, chromosomal exchange and reduction at meiosis, differentiation, maturation and transport (Figure 5.4). Membrane fusion occurs between the sperm and oocyte. The oocyte–cumulus complex in the mature, ovulated oocyte is surrounded. Cumulus cells loosely attached to each other around the ZP and the radially expanded cumulus cells with the extracellular matrix of glycosaminoglycans. Their production is under the control of follicle stimulating hormone. This extracellular matrix is composed of granules that are trypsin-sensitive and filaments of mostly hyaluronic acid.

When sperm reach the egg in the ampullary region of the oviduct, substantial selective pressure has been exerted to present the optimal sperm to the egg. The cumulus matrix continues this selection process,

admitting only capacitated, acrosome-intact cells. Progress through the cumulus matrix is aided by the hyaluronidase activity of PH-20. Primary binding then occurs between ZP3 and proteins of the sperm plasma membrane. It is likely that several different proteins are involved in primary binding; some may act as 'glue' proteins, whereas others are predicted to have transmembrane signaling potential. Fertilization and pregnancy have been induced by using testicular, epididymal and immotile sperm (asthenozoospermia).

Gamete interactions occur in round-headed sperm at the functional level where fertility is impaired. Round-headed sperm were obtained from two infertile men whose semen analysis revealed this particular morphological condition in over 90% of their sperm.

Triple staining has shown that 100% of acrosomeless sperm have a complete absence of acrosome and various degrees of abnormality in chromatin condensation.

Immunochemical studies with monoclonal antibodies to acrosin exhibited an abnormal pattern of weak fluorescence in the post-nuclear region. Human ZP and zona-free hamster oocytes are used to study gamete interaction. Normal semen samples show an average of 46 sperm bound per zona. Round-headed sperm show no binding to the ZP. Certain acrosomal proteins are needed for this process; the acrosome is necessary for the correct organization of plasma membrane proteins.

There is complete absence of fusion with zona-free hamster oocytes, owing to the inability of reorganization of plasma membrane proteins in the post-acrosomal region as a result of the absence of the acrosome reaction in round-headed sperm.

IN VITRO FERTILIZATION, FERTILIZATION ANOMALIES AND SPERM FUNCTION TESTS

Figure 5.5 shows the method of IVF by microinjection and some parameters of fertilization failure. Sperm function tests include evaluation of zona binding and oocyte penetration.

CHAPTER 6

Reproductive failure in men

There are several causes of male infertility: gonadotropin deficiency, chromosome aberrations, genetic disorders, excurrent duct obstruction, environmental toxins, systemic and genital disease, neurological disorders and autoimmune disease. Stress, on any disturbance of homeostasis, has a profound effect on the reproductive physiology of men (Table 6.1 and Figure 6.1). Nutrition and environmental toxins exert an effect on male reproductive dysfunction. Several pharmacological agents cause sexual dysfunction (Table 6.2), whereas others are commonly associated with male hypogonadism (Table 6.3), which may be acquired before or after puberty. Ejaculatory disorders show various patterns: anejaculation, pseudoejaculation, premature ejaculation and retarded ejaculation (Table 6.4).

Male infertility can result from congenital, infective vascular, immunological or autoimmune reasons, as well as from unknown causes. Frungieri *et al.* (2002) conducted extensive investigations to identify cellular factors involved in local regulation of testicular function and their possible role in the pathophysiology of infertility. They examined mast cells in testicular biopsies of men with normal and abnormal spermatogenesis. Some of the biopsies were classified as 'mixed atrophy'. The seminiferous tubules represent various degrees of degeneration of the germinal epithelium, ranging from full spermatogenesis up to Sertoli cell only and seminiferous tubule fibrosis within the same biopsy.

Male infertility is manifested in several mechanisms: sperm production; viability and fertilizing capacity of the ejaculated sperm; and sexual desire. Causes of infertility include gonadotropin deficiency, chromosome aberrations, genetic disorders, excurrent duct obstruction,

Table 6.1 Etiological factors in male infertility

Congenital
Cryptorchidism
Immotile cilia syndrome

Vascular anomalies
Torsion
Varicocele

Infection
Orchitis

Immunological parameters

Antispermatogenic agents

Hormone imbalance
Hypogonadotropic hypogonadism
Hyperprolactinemia

Genetic
Chromosomal
Non-chromosomal

Coital disorders
Coital infrequency
Erectile dysfunction
    psychosexual
    endocrine/neuroendocrine
Ejaculatory failure
    psychosexual
    genitourinary surgery

environmental toxins, systemic and genital disease, neurological disorders, autoimmune mechanisms, stress, and disturbance of homeostasis and nutrition. Nutritional factors include caloric, protein and vitamin deficiencies, but minerals or toxic agents may also be important.

Sex differentiation is determined by genetic mechanisms. Genes on the short arm of the Y chromosome

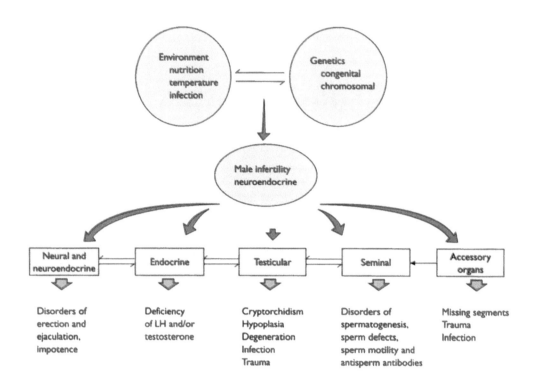

Figure 6.1 Some causes of reproductive failure. LH, luteinizing hormone

Table 6.2 Pharmacological agents known to cause sexual dysfunction

Impotence
Atenolol (Tenormin), Amitriptyline (Elavil), Chlorthalidone (Hygroton), Climetidine (Tagamet), Clofibrate (Atromid), Diazepam (Valium), Digoxin (Lanoxin), Disulfiram (Antabuse), Famotidine (Pepcid), Gemfibrozil (Lopid), Hydralazine (Apresoline), Indapamide (Lozol), Indomethacin (Indocin), Labetalol (Trandate), Leuprolide (Lupron), Lithium (Lithobid), Metoclopramide (Reglan), Metoprolol (Lopressor), Mexiletine (Mexitil), Naproxen (Naprosyn), Omeprazole (Prilosec), Phenytoin (Dilantin), Primidone (Mysoline), Propanolol (Inderal), Ranitidine (Zantac), Spironolactone (Aldactone), Thiazide (Diuretics), Verapamil (Calan)

Decreased/delayed libido/orgasm
Alprazolam (Xanax), Amiodarone (Cordarone), Amphetamine, Desipramine (Norpramin), Fluoxetine (Prozac), Lorazepam (Ativan), Methyldopa (Aldomet), Radiation therapy

Priapism
Psychotropic agents (Chlorpromazine), Antihypertensives (Hydralazine, Prazosin), Antidepressant (Trazodone), Vasoactive agents (Papaverine, PGE$_1$)

Courtesy of Professor Archibong

determine maleness. The testis determining factor is the male-specific histocompatibility (H-Y) antigen. Spermatogenesis is regulated by various genetic factors. Chromosomal anomalies are responsible for some 20% of male infertility. Disorders of the Y chromosome include cytogenic anomalies, such as translocations and numerical abnormalities, sex reversal, or ambiguous genitalia caused by mutations in the sex determining region of the Y chromosome. Several genes on the long arm play a role in spermatogenesis. Chromosomal aberrations play an important role in human reproductive failure. From a breeding point of view in animals, it is important to eliminate males that are affected by chromosomal aberrations, particularly those resulting in decreased fertility.

Extensive investigations have been conducted on the etiology, pathophysiology, genetics, biochemistry, biophysical molecular parameters and therapeutic approaches to male infertility (Lovell-Badger and Hacker, 1995; Rimini *et al.* 1995; Allen, 1996; Elliot *et al.* 1996; Lee *et al.* 1980; Weighardt *et al.* 1996; St John *et al.* 1997).

Table 6.3 Drugs commonly associated with male hypogonadism

Drug	
Primary hypogonadism	
Decreased Leydig cell production of testosterone	Corticosteroids
	Ethanol
	Ketoconazole
Decreased conversion of testosterone to dihydrotestosterone	Finasteride
Androgen receptor bolckade	Flutamide
	Spironolactone
	Cyproterone
	Cimetidine
Secondary hypogonadism	
Decreased pituitary secretion of gonadotropins	GNRH analogs (e.g. Lupron)
	Estrogens
	Medications that raise prolactin levels (psychotropic drugs, metoclopramide, narcotics)
	Corticosteroids
	Ethanol

Courtesy of Professor Archibong, Nashville, TN

Table 6.4 Ejaculatory disorders

Anejaculation (true impotentia ejaculationis)
Primary
    Lack of sexual education (no conditioning of the ejaculatory reflex)
Mechanical
    Retrograde ejaculation (retrospermia or 'le plaisir sec'), which occurs in diabetes, after prostatectomy, after pelvic fracture with rupture of the urethra, in some neurological disorders and during treatment with sympatholytic drugs
    Obstruction of excretory ducts
Organic
    In neurological disorders (such as spinal cord lesions), multiple sclerosis, eunuchoidism, primary and secondary hypogonadism, after pelvic operations, after pelvic fractures and in the event of local vascular disorders
Toxic
    alcoholism, morphinomania, cocainism and nicotine intoxication
Psychogenic
    Functional aspermia

Pseudoejaculation (incomplete ejaculation)
Primary, periodical
    Incomplete form of anejaculation caused by emotional stress such as at demand for an ejaculate for semen examination; stress situations may disturb the co-ordination of the ejaculatory reflex ('sham ejaculation')

Retarded ejaculation (ejaculatio retardata)
    Psychogenic, but mostly iatrogenic (phenothiazin, ismelin, monoamine oxidase inhibitors)

Premature ejaculation (ejaculatio praecox)
Permanent involuntary premature ejection of ejaculate, which occurs either:
    ante portas
    at intromission (immediately after contact of the penis with the labiae)
    immediately after intromission
    after short friction of the penis against vaginal walls

Almost 20% of idiopathic human sterility can be associated with immunological disorders (Hill, 1991). Either autoimmunity or isoimmunity can be found in infertile men of women having circulating antibodies directed against sperm cell antigens. Several studies have found a close relationship between immune system components and disorders affecting the function of male and female reproductive systems. Macrophages surrounding Sertoli cells (Calkins *et al.* 1988), T lymphocytes in the epididymis, macrophages in ejaculates (Wolff and Anderson, 1988), leukocytospermia and poor-quality sperm (Wolff *et al.* 1990), and increased levels of interferon-γ (IFNγ) in the cervical mucus of infertile women (Naz *et al.* 1995) are only some examples of these associations. Elevated concentrations of interleukin (IL)-2, IL-4 and IL-5 reduce the ova-penetrating ability of human sperm (Hill *et al.* 1989).

The expression of CD25 and CD122 correlates negatively with fresh sperm concentration but in sperm centrifuged on a Percoll gradient there was no correlation. Labeling with anti-CD25 and anti-CD122 antibody is evident on the head and the middle piece in fresh sperm, while in sperm centrifuged on a Percoll gradient a weak labeling is observed only on the principal piece. Fierro *et al.* (2002) have identified and localized cytokine receptors on human sperm. Cytokine receptors may be involved in the regulation of pathophysiological events in sperm cell functions and male infertility.

ETIOLOGY

Spermatogenesis disorders

Histological studies of the testes have revealed no significant differences between control and infertile men, either in the development of interstitial tissue or

Table 6.5 Intratesticular concentrations of steroids in control and infertile men (mean ± SEM) (Reproduced with permission from Marie et al. 2001)

	Control men	Infertile men
Pregnenolone		
(664–1767 ng/g)	175 ± 4	247 ± 80
Progesterone		
(30–99 ng/g)	81 ± 4	507 ± 132*
Dehydroepiandrosterone		
(11–424 ng/g)	132 ± 13	536 ± 459
Androstenedione		
(1–85 ng/g)	42 ± 3	180 ± 76*
Testosterone		
(451–1000 ng/g)	421 ± 11	1772 ± 384*
Estradiol	12 ± 2	175 ± 112**
Estradiol/testosterone ratio	0.028	0.098**

Normal range value is given between parentheses
**$p > 0.01$; *$p < 0.05$ when compared to the control group

in the spermatogenic score. Conversely, the testicular concentrations of pregnenolone, dehydroepiandrosterone, progesterone, androstenedione, testosterone and estradiol are higher in infertile men than in control men (Table 6.5) (Marie *et al.* 2002).

Sperm maturation arrest

Maturation arrest is the pathological condition wherein the development of the germ cell is arrested and therefore mature sperm are not formed (Wong *et al.* 1973; Levin, 1979; Coburn and Wheeler, 1991). However, the stage where this arrest of development will occur has not yet been specified. Some believe that it could occur at any level of spermatogenesis (Posinocec, 1976), whereas others believe that spermatogenesis can be halted only at specific stages. This debate has recently acquired clinical importance, since round cells with a haploid set of chromosomes from azoospermic men are now used to fertilize oocytes, with the methods of round spermatid injection (ROSI) or round spermatid nucleus injection (ROSNI) (Tesarik *et al.* 1973; Sofikitis *et al.* 1994; Papanicolaou *et al.* 2001).

Increased digoxin levels can lead to membrane Na⁺-K⁺ ATPase inhibition, a reduction in intracellular magnesium and an increase in intracellular calcium in the vascular smooth muscle cell. This can lead to vasospasm and a decrease in blood supply to the seminiferous tubules and Leydig cells (Altura and Altura, 1981). The increased nicotine levels documented in infertile

human males could also contribute to vaospasm and ischemia of the tubules (Kurup and Kurup, 2002).

Genes affecting male infertility

Germ-cell-specific proteins are expressed during meiosis, such as lactate dehydrogenase C4, phosphoglycerate kinase 2, cytochrome C and the heat shock protein HSP70-2. Gene targeting studies in the mouse have shown that several genes are expressed during specific stages of spermatogenesis and sperm function such as primordial germ cell development/migration (*C-kit*, SCF, TIAR, Lhx9), spermatogonial proliferation/survival (p27, Dazl), and various stages of meiosis (ATM, ATR, TLS, SCP3, Msh5, Hsp70-2). Some genes are important for successful formation of haploid spermatids and sperm and for the fertilization process *per se*. In their absence, there is partial to complete arrest in meiosis, leading to male infertility with no impact on the female phenotype (Feng, 2002). Decreased expression of the *c-kit* receptor and its ligand, SCF, in infertile men may alter the balance between cell proliferation/differentiation and cell death, resulting in increased apoptosis in spermatogenesis. Subsequently an inbalance in this equilibrium will result in male infertility.

Azoospermia

Azoospermia is caused by either failure of spermatogenesis or obstruction of the seminal tract. Most cases of azoospermia involve a disorder of spermatogenesis, with cases resulting from obstruction accounting for less than 15% of the total. Patients have various treatment options: intracytoplasmic sperm injection (ICSI), testicular sperm extraction (TESE) and surgical reanastomosis of the seminal tract (Belker *et al.* 1991; Niederberger and Ross, 1993; Schaysman *et al.* 1993; Mathews *et al.* 1995; Pavlovich and Schlegel, 1997; Matsuda *et al.* 1998; Matsuda, 2000).

Tsujimura *et al.* (2002) evaluated the efficacy of reanastomosis in 30 patients with obstructive azoospermia (19 post-vasectomy; seven with complicating inguinal herniorrhaphy; two with a characterized isolated congenital anomaly; one with young's syndrome). In cases of post-vasectomy, successful vasovasostomy was achieved in 15 of 18 cases (83%). The duration of obstruction in the three cases where anastomosis failed was 6, 9 and 20 years. In the group where obstruction followed inguinal herniorrhaphy, unilateral vasovasostomy was performed in six cases, and trans-epididymovasostomy was performed in one case. Success was achieved in three of six cases (50%). In all four remaining cases, microsurgical epididymovasostomy or trans-epididymovasostomy was performed, but success was achieved only in the patient with Young's syndrome.

Most patients with idiopathic azoospermia exhibit normal serum androgen levels (Simoni et al. 1997). This condition is due to a defective androgen response pathway. Some infertile men exhibit minimal androgen resistance (Aiman and Griffin, 1982). Azoospermic men may exhibit deletion of the AR gene in exon 4 (Akin et al. 1991), whereas in severe cases of oligozoospermia, there are missense mutations of exons 6 and 8 (Yong et al. 1994; Knoke et al. 1999). A point mutation of exons 6 and 8 has been detected in men with minimal androgen insensitivity (Tsukada et al. 1994). No mutations were detected for any azoospermic men in any of the AR gene exons 1–8 (Sasagawa et al. 2001). Chinese men manifest expansion of the CAG repeat length in the AR gene (Tut et al. 1997). The enhancements of CAG repeat lengths were detected also in Japanese men with idiopathic azoospermia and in patients from a mixed Australian multinational origin with idiopathic oligozoospermia or azoospermia (Sasagawa et al. 2002; Sasagawa and Nakada, 2003).

The main number of CAG repeats is much higher in men with reduced spermatogenesis than in fertile men, and this difference is highly significant in extremely severe cases of oligozoospermia (less than 1 million spermatozoa/ml semen) (Patrizio, et al. 2001). Sasagawa et al. (2002) reported that two infertile men had more than 28 CAG repeats, and none of the controls had a CAG repeat length greater than 28. Since defective spermatogenesis is due to heterogeneous mechanisms, analysis of large populations of men with unexplained male infertility may reveal a subgroup of men who have significantly longer CAG repeats.

Testosterone together with follicle stimulating hormone (FSH) plays a crucial role in the development and the maintenance of spermatogenesis. FSH modulates Sertoli cell function and germ cell development. Even though FSH receptors are present, the role of FSH is still obscure. With the availability of specific primers, reverse transcription–polymerase chain reaction studies have been developed and thus microdeletions of the Y chromosome have been discovered in infertile men. Marie et al. (2002) evaluated the hypophysogonadal axis measuring the intratesticular concentrations of several steroids in relation to the hormonal status; the data have been compared with those collected from men with cerebral death (stage IV coma), taken as a 'control' group. The histological studies revealed no significant differences between control and infertile men, either in the interstitial tissue or in the spermatogenic score. Conversely, the testicular pregnenolone, dehydropiandrosterone, progesterone, androstenedione and testosterone were higher in infertile men compared to control men.

Oligoteratozoospermia

Sperm flagellar pathology causes motility disorders that lead to male infertility. Sperm motility alterations are a common cause of male infertility. A high incidence of flagellar pathology was found to be the underlying cause of motility disorders that led to infertility. Motility alterations are associated with several numerical or positional anomalies of the microtubules and/or absence of inner or outer dynein arms of the axoneme (Bacetti et al. 1993; Staif et al. 1995). Peri-axonemal structures involve dense fiber (abnormal position or size) and a fibrous sheet of sperm flagellum (Chemes et al. 1987, 1998, 1990; Rawe et al. 2001).

Molecular parameters

Spermatogenic disorders

Little is known about the association of 5α-reductase type 2 gene mutations with the occurrence of cryptorchidism. Despite the presence of well-differentiated testicular tissue, patients with classic 5α-reductase deficiency have spermatogenic disorders. In vitro enzymatic studies showed deficiency in 5α-reductase activity in four among 24 oligospermic but otherwise healthy men. Future research is needed for systematic examination of this gene in males with idiopathic azoospermia. Suzuki et al. (2002a) performed mutation analysis of the 5α-reductase type 2 gene in patients with isolated cryptorchidism and idiopathic azoospermia.

Development of male genitalia

Dihydrotesterone (DHT), which is synthesized from testosterone by the membrane-bound enzyme 5α-reductase in androgen target and non-target tissues, is crucial for the development of male external genital organs during gestation. The androgen-dependent development of male genitalia can be divided into events requiring testosterone and those requiring DHT, both acting through the same AR protein (Suzuki *et al.* 2002).

Cell apoptosis

Cell death is mediated by increased intracellular calcium and ceramide-related opening of the mitochondria, causing a collapse of the hydrogen gradient across the inner membrane and uncoupling of the respiratory chain. This also leads to volume dysregulation of mitochondria, causing hyperosomolality of the matrix and expansion of the matrix space. The outer membrane of the mitochondria ruptures and releases AIF apoptosis-inducing factor (AIF) and cytochrome C. This results in procaspase 9 activation to caspase 9, which produces cell death (Ashkenazi and Dixit, 1998). Caspase 9 activates caspase-activated deoxyribonuclease, which cleaves the nuclear membrane laminins and several proteins involved in cytoskeletal regulation, such as gelsolin, which cleaves actin. Apoptosis is also implicated in spermatozoal death in human male infertility (Kurup and Kurup, 2002).

Testicular varicocele

Varicocele is implicated in infertility; its incidence in infertile men ranges from 20 to 40%. The incidence among screened prepubertal and pubertal boys (10–17 years) ranges between 9 and 25%. Grade I varicoceles are the most common and grade III the least common. Varicocele is not detected in boys younger than 9 years of age. There is a steady increase in the incidence of varicocele over the age range 9–14 years. This could be attributed to the gradual appearance and establishment of puberty, although the exact pathology is unknown. There was no correlation between varicocele and height, but there was a significant correlation with body weight.

Varicocele, the abnormal tortuosity/dilatation of the testicular vein within the spermatic cord, occurs in 16% of the normal adult population (Belloli *et al.* 1993;

Wyllie, 1985). Correction of the varicocele improves the semen characteristics in 50% of these men (Vermeulen *et al.* 1986). The Palomo technique, where both the testicular artery and vein are ligated, results in a good success rate in correcting varicocele (Palomo, 1949). With the advent of modern endoscopic surgery, the technique of laparoscopic varicocelectomy has progressively improved (Donovan/Winfield, 1992; Matsuda *et al.* 1992). Itoh *et al.* (2002) performed laparoscopic Palomo varicocelectony in 38 men with left-sided varicocele, with a mean operation time of 37 mins. There were no intra-abdominal visceral or vascular complications during the operations. Neither testicular atrophy nor recurrence was observed postoperatively. However, hydrocele formation was found in two (5.3%) patients. Laparoscopic Palomo varicocelectony is a safe and effective procedure for patients with varicocele.

Varicocele associated with testicular hypertrophy and infertility is the most common cause of male infertility. Extensive somatometric investigation has been conducted on the possible impact on later adult infertility of adolescent varicocele (Oster, 1971; Lyon *et al.* 1982; Kass and Reitelman, 1995; Paduch and Niedzielski, 1997).

Stavropoulos *et al.* (2002) detected left varicocele in 98 boys, aged 9–16 years. There was no difference in left and right testicular volume. Although six boys with varicocele had a left testicular volume ≥ 2 ml less than the right, there were also seven boys of comparable age who had a left testicular volume ≥ 2 ml larger than the right. It would appear that the use of left testicular hypotrophy (≥ 2 ml compared with the right testicle) should be reconsidered as an indicator for varicocele-induced damage of the testicle in this age group.

The early ligation of varicocele in affected adolescents can probably result in 'catch-up' testicular growth within 12 months of surgery. However, because only 13% of adults with varicocele are infertile, ligation should be performed only in adolescents considered to be at risk for infertility. Ultrasonography is the most accurate method for assessing testicular volume (Costabile *et al.* 1992). However, testicular size discrepancy in boys should not be considered as an established sign of varicocele. Other methods should be adopted for the detection of testicular injury in these boys: histology and testing of luteinizing hormone releasing hormone (LHRH) (Aragona *et al.* 1994; Aragona and Glazel, 1998).

Sperm dysfunction is associated with the excessive generation of reactive oxygen species (ROS) in 100% of oligozoospermic men. The most important ROS produced by human sperm are hydrogen peroxide, superoxide anion and hydroxyl radicals. Owing to a high polyunsaturated fatty acid content, human sperm plasma membranes are highly sensitive to ROS-induced lipid peroxidation, decreasing membrane fluidity and sperm fertilizing capability. Human seminal plasma and sperm possess antioxidant systems to scavenge ROS and prevent ROS-related cellular damage. Extensive investigations have been conducted on superoxide dismutase, catalase and reduced glutathione in human sperm and seminal plasma.

Ozbek *et al.* (2001) examined the seminal plasma antioxidant activity of patients with GII-GIII varicocele and compared the results with healthy control and infertile varicocele patients, finding it significantly lower in the varicocele group compared to controls ($p < 0.05$). It would appear that reduced ROS-scavenging enzyme activity in the seminal plasma of patients with varicocele is associated with impaired sperm function; antioxidant enzyme supplementation may be helpful in restoring this pathology.

Cryptorchidism

Cryptorchidism is associated with androgen insensitivity syndrome (AIS) (Levy and Husmann, 1995). Testicular descent occurs in two phases:

(1) The first stage is controlled by Müllerian inhibiting substance (MIS); the testes migrate down towards the lower abdominal wall and reach the site of the future internal inguinal ring by the 7th month.

(2) In the second stage, the testes traverse the abdominal wall via the inguinal canal and complete their passage into the bottom of the scrotum during the 28th week (Hutson, 1986).

The intra-abdominal portion of testicular descent is not androgen-mediated but the presence of functional androgens and the androgen receptor (AR) is required for the testes to descend through the inguinal canal into the scrotum. Patients with complete or partial AIS exhibit mutation of the AR gene (Marcelli *et al.* 1991;

Klocker *et al.* 1992). Molecular genetics analysis of boys with isolated cryptorchidism using tissue DNA showed no abnormalities of the coding sequences of exons 2–8 of the AR gene (Wiener *et al.* 1998). Screening for mutation of AR gene exons 1–8 using leukocyte DNA revealed no alterations within all exons in 48 patients with isolated cryptorchidism (Suzuki *et al.* 2001). The size of the CAG repeat in exon 1 of the AR gene did not differ between patients with cryptorchidism and control males (Sasagawa *et al.* 2000a, 2002). Although point mutations in the DNA and ligand domains of the AR are considered as a potential cause of cryptorchidism, it would appear that the association of AR gene alteration with the development of isolated cryptorchidism is rare (Sasagawa *et al.* 2002).

Molecular parameters of cryptorchidism

Androgens are required for testicular descent and normal spermatogenesis. Because androgens display their biological activities by binding to the AR, attention has been focused on abnormalities in the AR as a possible cause of cryptorchidism and impaired spermatogenesis in males with idiopathic infertility. However, tissue or leukocyte DNA molecular genetic analysis of males with isolated cryptorchidism showed no abnormalities of the coding sequences of exons 1–8 of the AR gene. The size of the CAG repeat in exon 1 of the AR gene did not differ between patients with cryptorchidism and control men (Suzuki *et al.* 2002). Based on molecular cloning parameters, there are two genes that encode the type 1 (mapped to chromosome 5) and type 2 (mapped to chromosome 2) isozymes 5α-reductase mutations in the type 2 gene (SRD5A2), causing the inborn error of 5α-reductase deficiency, which results in failure of development of normal external genitalia and prostate. Isolated cryptorchidism is much more common than clinical 5α-reductase deficiency (Suzuki *et al.* 2002). 5α-Reductase type 2 gene abnormalities do not constitute a major factor in the development of cryptorchidism or idiopathic azoospermia.

Priapism

Priapism (prolonged erection unaccompanied by sexual desire of stimulation) is manifested in two categories – high flow (non-ischemic) and low flow (ischemic) – depending upon the emissary veins involved, the severity of the disease involved and the duration of venous occlusion (Table 6.6). High-flow priapism is characterized by adequate (or increased) arterial inflow with normal venous outflow, but helicine arteriolar bypass, or a defect in their regulation, prevents detumescence.

Low-flow priapism includes sickle cell anemia, leukemia, secondary penile cancer, prostatitis, urethritis, prolonged sexual intercourse/erection, pelvic thromboses, congenital neonatal priapism, spinal stenosis and spinal cord injury.

In veno-occlusive priapism, blood stays trapped in the cavernous bodies; the erection is rigid and eventually painful. Usually, both cavernous bodies are affected, but partial priapism, restricted to a segment of one or two cavernous bodies, has been reported. In arterial priapism, erection is semi-rigid, because the venous system remains open, but arterial hyperflow overcomes it. The spongiosus body and the glans remain flaccid in both veno-occlusive and arterial priapism. The morbidity of priapism is caused by a lack of oxygen in the cavernous blood and by anoxic tissue injuries.

Table 6.6 Causes of priapism

Intracavernous injection of vasoactive agents

Thromboembolic or hypercoagulable states
  sickle cell trait or disease
  hematological diseases: polycythemia, thalassemia,
    thrombocytopenia
  leukemia and lymphoma
  inflammatory diseases: vasculitis and systemic infections
  total parenteral nutrition (high fat)
  dialysis
  infiltrative metastasis to the penis
  penile invasion of genitourinary or gastrointestinal tumors
  lipid infiltration (Fabry's disease)

Neurogenic
  central nervous system and spinal cord disorders: medullary
    trauma, lumbar spinal stenosis
  sexual hyperactivity

Drugs and medications
  antidepressants: trazodone
  antipsychotic drugs: chlorpromazine (phenothiazine group)
  antihypertensives: hydralazine, guanethidine and
    prazosin
  phosphodiesterase inhibitor: oral papaverine
  drugs of abuse: alcohol and cocaine

Gonadotropin-releasing therapy for hypogonadism

Trauma

Hypospadias

Hypospadias is classified into glandular, penile and scrotal/perineal types according to the anatomical location of the urethral meatus. Glandular and penile types appear as an isolated anomaly and account for the majority of cases of hypospadias, whereas a scrotal/perineal type frequently occurs in association with other genital anomalies such as microphallus, bifid scrotum and cryptorchidism (Sasagawa *et al.* 2000b, 2001, 2002). Mutations of the AR gene have been identified in six males from four families with this anomaly (Allera *et al.* 1995; Batch *et al.* 1993; Sutherland *et al.* 1996). However, mutation screening of the AR gene within exons 1–8 using the heteroduplex detection method showed no abnormal chromatograms in 25 patients with hypospadias (Muroya *et al.* 2001). The CAG repeat length genotype has no discernible effect on the development of hypospadias in these patients. Both the median CAG repeat length and the frequency of long CAG repeats were increased in 78 males with undermusculinization including 73 males with moderate to sereve hypospadies (Lim *et al.* 2000). Thus, CAG

repeat lengths could be variable among different patient populations with hypospadias.

Ejaculatory disturbance

Ejaculatory disturbance – transitory, intermittent, or permanent–may arise from direct blocking of nerve impulses or obesity, poor condition, or exhaustion. Ejaculatory disturbance may be due to failure of contraction of smooth muscles in the reproductive tract as a result of refractoriness of these cells to norepinephrine, exhaustion of the norepinephrine depots, or failure to release norepinephrine from the sympathetic nerve endings.

Klinefelter's syndrome

Klinefelter's syndrome is characterized by decreased testosterone production and subsequent hypersecretion of gonadotropins. The syndrome is treated with testosterone replacement. Eunuchs are not thought to be at risk for the development of prostatic cancer (Jackson *et al.* 1989). In contrast, supraphysiological androgen therapy has been implicated in the development of prostatic cancer in 40-year-old body builders (Roberts and Essenhigh, 1986). There have been significant increases in serum testosterone levels and prostate volume after testosterone replacement therapy. However, the serum level of prostate-specific antigen (PSA) did not change after testosterone replacement therapy (Shibasaki *et al.* 2002). It would appear that serum PSA is not influenced by exogenous testosterone in patients with Klinefelter's syndrome.

Nutrition/environmental pollutants

Estrogens play a major role in male reproductive function (O'Donnell *et al.* 2001). This concept is based on studies of men affected with congenital estrogen deficiency (Morishima *et al.* 1995; Carani *et al.* 1997) and the decline in sperm quality in sons of women exposed to the synthetic estrogen diethylstilbestrol during pregnancy (Stillman, 1982). Over the years there has been a consistent decline in sperm density, more prominent in the USA and Europe, and less so in non-Western countries, with a significant geographical variability in sperm concentration (Carlsen *et al.* 1992; Swan *et al.* 2000). Environmental factors, including estrogens, are related to these decreases in sperm concentration. Estrogen receptor-knock-out mice (ERKO) are infertile, presumably as a result of abnormal fluid resorption in the epididymal efferent ducts.

Cadmium is a highly toxic industrial and environmental pollutant that is cumulative and has a long biological half life. Apart from industrial exposure, other sources of exposure include inhalation of ambient air, cigarette smoke and emissions from combustion of fuels and plastic wastes. Additionally, cadmium is present in almost all food types, such as shellfish, liver, kidney, meats and rice. Exposure to cadmium causes anemia, hepatic, renal, musculoskeletal, Itai Itai and cardiovascular disorders, including hypertension. Exposure of men to cadmium reduces semen quality and sperm density, and causes asthenospermia. However, these effects are confounded by exposure to cigarette smoke, which contains heavy metals (lead, zinc and magnesium) other than cadmium.

Micropenis

The development of micropenis is due to inadequate production of gonadal androgens for stimulation of the target organ or an inadequate response of the target organ to stimulation. Mutation analysis failed unequivocally to identify a causative mutation in the AR gene of 64 Japanese boys with isolated micropenis (Ishii *et al.* 2001). There was only one patient with androgen insensitivity syndrome found in 45 patients with isolated micropenis, although the diagnosis was based on endocrine studies and family history. It would appear that a mutation of the AR gene is rare in children with isolated micropenis (Lee *et al.* 1980).

Since the CAG repeat length was not expanded in patients with isolated micropenis, nor was the frequently of long CAG repeats increased, the genotype of CAG repeat length was no discernible effect on the development of isolated micropenis.

DIAGNOSIS

Several methods have been used for differential diagnosis of male infertility (Table 6.7).

Sperm chromatin condensation

Semen analysis constitutes the most important investigation of male infertility, with sperm morphology, motility and concentration representing the three most important factors in the assessment of male reproduction potential. Although this holds true for natural conception, these parameters have not been equally important in assisted reproduction technologies (ART). There is still a need to develop more sensitive diagnostic techniques capable of identifying subfertile states that are amenable to the few therapeutic options available (Aitken, 1983). The presence of subtle sperm abnormalities that are unrecognized by conventional semen analysis may explain reproduction failure in men. Such structural or biochemical defects are associated with chromatin packaging in the sperm nucleus (Zamboni, 1992). Poor chromatin packaging and possible DNA damage may contribute to failure of sperm decondensation and subsequently fertilization failure or habitual abortion following fertilization (Ibrahim *et al.* 1988).

The degree of chromatin condensation can be assessed with the aid of acidic aniline blue staining,

Table 6.7 Differential diagnosis of male infertility

Reproductive failure mechanisms	Methods of diagnosis
Developmental	
Testicular or germinal aplasia	clinical history, physical examination, vasography, retrograde venography, scrotal thermography
Hypospadias	
Varicocele	
Ductal obstruction	
Genetic and chromosomal	
Hermaphroditism	karyotyping (buccal smear, sex chromatin)
Pseudohermaphroditism	
Klinefelter's syndrome	
Testicular	
Cryptorchidism	testicular biopsy (histology, histochemistry, tissue culture of seminiferous tubules)
Retarded descent	
Floating testis	
Pendulous testis	
Testicular hypoplasia (primary or idiopathic)	scrotal thermography
Testicular atrophy (trauma, inflammation, radiation injury)	ultrasonography
Endocrine	
Testicular insufficiency (primary, secondary)	endocrine profile (androgen, FSH, LH, GnRH, 17-hydroxysteroids, 17-ketosteroids, hCG stimulation)
Pituitary disorder (pre- and post-pubertal LH deficiency)	
Hypothalamic GnRH	
Neuroendocrine and psychological	
Disorders of erection	radiology (cervical vertebrae, lumbar vertebrae)
Disorders of ejaculation	
Impotence	
Semen factors	
Disorders in sperm concentration	semen analysis (counting, sizing, motility, live/dead, % abnormal)
Disorders in sperm morphology	
Disorders in sperm motility	
Infection	
Orchitis	incubation of cultures (gonorrhea, syphilis, mycoplasma, trichomonas, candida)
Epididymitis	
Prostatitis	
Urogenital tuberculosis	
Immunological	
Sperm agglutination	agglutination, microagglutination, immunofluorescence

LH, luteinizing hormone; GnRH, gonadotropin releasing hormone; FSH, follicle stimulating hormone

which discriminates between lysine-rich histones and arginine-and cystein-rich protamines (Auger *et al.* 1990). This technique gives a specific positive reaction for lysine and reveals differences in basic nuclear protein composition of ejaculated human spermatozoa. Histone-rich nuclei of immature sperm are rich in lysine and will take up the blue stain. On the other hand, protamine-rich nuclei of mature sperm are rich in arginine cysteine and contain relatively low lysine (Calvin, 1976; Gusse *et al.* 1986) and are not stained by aniline blue.

Hammadeh *et al.* (2002) conducted a study to evaluate sperm chromatin condensation in the assessment of male fertility. Chromatin condensation constitutes a valuable parameter in the assessment of male fertility, completely independent of conventional sperm parameters. Consequently, the inclusion of chromatin condensation to routine laboratory investigations of semen prior to assisted reproduction is strongly recommended.

THERAPEUTIC APPROACHES

Many drugs such as kallikrein, vitamins and Japanese herbal medicines have been employed in widespread oral administration as an empirical therapy for male infertility; however, the efficacy of these substances has not been established. The idea of treating male infertility with mast cell blockers is based on the observation of increased numbers of mast cells in the testicular tissue of infertile men. Hibi *et al.* (2002) examined whether long-term administration of tranilast improved semen in sereve oligoasthenozoospermia. Tranilast (300 mg/day) was administered until pregnancy was achieved or for a period of up to 12 months. Total sperm count was elevated, as expected. Although tranilast, a mast cell blocker, demonstrated a certain clinical benefit in terms of improvement of semen parameters involving severe oligoasthenozoospermia, it did not appear to afford clinical benefit in long-term administration.

The treatment of male infertility has improved dramatically, despite continued findings of a low level or absence of sperm in the ejaculate. One of the concerns, however, is that the infertile couples, regardless of whether they can really afford treatment, out of desperation for child, are prepared to undergo even the most sophisticated ART approaches such as ICSI, ROSI and ROSNI using germ cells from testicular sperm aspiration

(TESA). However, these approaches to treating male-factor infertility need to be carried out with extreme caution, in view of the possible risk of vertically transmitting defective fertility gene(s) to male progeny (when the etiology of infertility is genetic) (Feng, 2002).

Male accessory sex organs, composed of epithelial/mesenchymal components, require androgens for proliferation and maintenance of their function. There are three types of epithelial cell: secretory glandular cells, non-secretory basal cells and neuroendocrine cells:

(1) Basal cells, stem cells for secretory epithelial cells, are androgen-independent because they do not express androgen receptors. (ARs);

(2) Neuroendocrine cells play a role in regulating the growth and function of secretory cells;

(3) Mesenchyme comprises smooth muscle cells, fibroblasts, lymphocytes and neuromuscular tissue embedded in an extracellular matrix.

Infertility and its treatment is a stressful experience. Although the advancement in ART offers new hope to many infertile couples, the current treatment process is quite complex and uncomfortable. The costs are high and the probability of success is not as high as expected. The entire treatment process requires routine monitoring and a high degree of participation and co-operation. The physical and time demands of infertility treatment rest almost completely upon women. Women describe greater global and specific stress related to infertility than men in terms of sexual concerns and the need for parenthood. However, new treatment options for men are available, such as ICSI and microsurgical epididymal sperm aspiration (MESA), which requires more diagnostic tests and medical appointments for the male partners. Treatment by ICSI carries additional burdens for men, which causes them to express greater treatment-related stress.

Antisperm antibodies, especially sperm-immobilizing antibodies found in the sera of immunologically infertile women, cause infertility by interfering with fertilization and by blocking penetrance through the cervical mucus. There is an immunoglobulin binding protein capable of binding antisperm antibodies that trap any penetrating sperm. One of the mechanisms by which sperm-immobilizing antibodies exert their anti-infertility effect is the inhibition of the acrosome reaction. A spontaneous acrosome reaction is almost completely inhibited by sperm-immobilizing antibodies. The inhibitory effect on the acrosome reaction is abolished by incubation of antisperm antibody-treated sperm in antibody-free medium. This was demonstrated in an *in vitro* human fertilization test, in which the blocking effect of the antibody on the sperm–zona pellucida interaction was reversed by incubation of the antibody-bound spermatozoa in antibody-free medium. Only capacitated sperm undergo the acrosome reaction.

Chromosomal abnormalities and polymorphisms

Abnormalities in either sex chromosomes or autosomes are frequent in infertile men; therefore, disorders in spermatogenesis could be related directly to changes in the number or structure of chromosomes. Aneuploidy has been found in the sex chromosomes of sterile men. There is an association between alterations in gamete production and genetic disorders: Klinefelter's syndrome or 45, X/46, XY gonadal disgenesis. This may be due to the presence of the AZF gene (azoospermia factor) in the long arm of the Y chromosome, since deletion of the distal portion of that chromosomal region has been found in azoospermic patients. Other structural abnormalities in sex chromosomes, e.g. microdeletions, isochromosomes, translocations and ring chromosomes, have been found. Autosomal alterations, mainly Robertsonian translocations, have also been shown in infertile males. Cytogenetic analysis of sterile men is needed not only for the diagnosis of sterility, but also as the selection criterion for ART, e.g. ICSI.

Testosterone supplementation

Testosterone supplementation is indicated in patients with low testosterone levels to improve libido and sexual potency as well as to maintain bone mass, lean body mass and musculature. Side-effects include exacerbation of sleep apnea and prostatic symptoms, polycythemia, decreased high-density lipoprotein and increased risk of cerebrovascular accident.

Two oral formulations of androgens, methyltestosterone and fluoxymesterone, undergo significant first-pass hepatic inactivation, which decreases their efficacy and increases the risk for hepatotoxicity and altered lipid metabolism. Testosterone undecanoate has been used outside the USA with more effective results, as it is absorbed through the intestinal lymphatics, bypassing the hepatic circulation. Dehydroepiandrosterone (DHEA) is an oral adrenal androgen marketed at health food stores as a nutritional supplement; however, clinical trials in the use of DHEA have not been conducted, and high oral doses of DHEA can actually suppress serum testosterone levels.

Two parenteral formulations of androgens testosterone enanthate and testosterone cypionate, are effective and inexpensive modes of androgen supplementation. However, dosing intervals of every 2–3 weeks is required to maintain adequate serum levels and clinical

response. For this reason transdermal testosterone systems (Testoderm® (Alza) and Androderm® (Smith Kline Beecham)) are attractive, as they bypass hepatic inactivation and approximate physiological diurnal testosterone levels.

Significant improvements in libido, sexual arousal and frequency, duration and rigidity of nocturnal penile tumescence with testosterone supplementation have been demonstrated. However, only 35–60% of men can except a measurable improvement in sexual performance, with restoration of normal serum testosterone levels.

CHAPTER 7

Genetics and andrology

Although the difference in DNA content between X-chromosome-bearing and Y-chromosome-bearing spermatozoa is only about 3–8%, this small difference can be resolved using fluorescent staining and flow cytometric analyses. Furthermore, flow cytometers have been modified so that they can sort viable mammalian spermatozoa into relatively pure X and Y sperm populations. When these sorted sperm are inseminated into women, the sex ratio of the progeny is similar to that predicted by the ratio of X sperm to Y sperm in the flow-sorted inseminate. Considerable effort is being focused on developing this approach as a practical means of pre-determining the sex of domestic livestock and man.

CHROMOSOMES

Sperm chromosome aneuploidy (Figure 7.1) is elevated in some men whose partners have a history of recurrent pregnancy loss (RPL) and may cause RPL in some patients (Lowry *et al.* 1999; Carrell *et al.* 2002). Sperm chromosome aneuploidy, specifically disomy and diploidy, may be related to RPL (Rubio *et al.* 1999, 2001). There are also possible links to semen quality, including increased nuclear vacuolization, abnormal chromatin condensation and increased levels of CD4 and CD8 T lymphocytes in the semen. Carroll *et al.* (2002) evaluated the degree of sperm DNA fragmentation using the TUNEL assay on sperm from couples with unexplained RPL compared to sperm from two control groups – donors of known fertility and unscreened men from the general population. The percentage of sperm staining positive for DNA

fragmentation was increased in the RPL group (38 ± 4.2) compared to the donor (11 ± 1.0) and general population (22 ± 2.0) control groups. In the RPL group, no correlation was observed between semen quality parameters and the TUNEL data. Some RPL patients have a significant increase of sperm DNA fragmentation, which causes pregnancy loss in some patients.

Chromosomal arrangements occur during mitosis/meiosis. Normally the ovum (X) is fertilized by sperm X or sperm Y. In abnormal cases of non-disjunction of oogenesis or spermatogenesis, fertilization may occur between an abnormal sperm and/or an abnormal egg, resulting in various chromosomal anomalies. Structural anomalies of the chromosomes include translocation, deletions, rings and inversions of chromosomes during either mitosis or meiosis. Such anomalies effect individual autosomes or sex chromosomes.

The animal cell comprises a nucleus, protein-manufacturing units and energy-production points. Spiraling double strands of atoms are the DNA – the master chemical of genes. The sequence or layout of these atoms contains all the instructions the cell needs to function. Recent advances in genetic engineering have enabled scientists to uncover, rearrange and make copies, or clones, of genes. For example, each human or animal cell contains some 100 000 genes. At least 22 000 of these genes have been isolated, and some of their specific functions have been identified.

Genetic male infertility may be caused by chromosomal aneuploidies such as Klinefelter's syndrome (XXY), specific translocations and Y chromosome

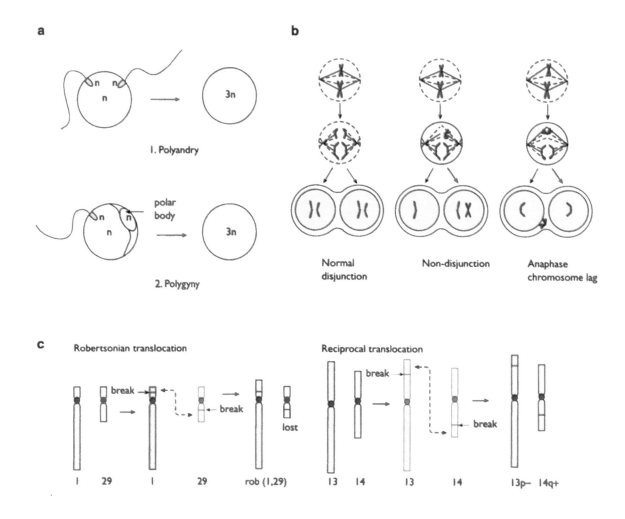

Figure 7.1 (a) Mechanisms resulting in triploidy by (1) polyandry and (2) polygyny. (b) Mechanisms of non-disjunction and anaphase chromosome lag leading to aneuploidy. (c) Reciprocal translocation and Robertsonian translocation. (Adapted with permission from Basrur, 1999)

microdeletions. Point mutations occur in the androgen receptor, and the cystic fibrosis transmembrane conductance regulator. Other pathogenetic defects associated with male infertility are microdeletions of the long arm of the Y chromosome (Yq), found in approximately 5% of men with severe primary testicular failure and a sperm density of less than 5 million/ml.

As new mutations associated with male infertility are discovered, traditional molecular techniques, such as restriction fragment length polymorphism and single nucleotide primer extension for the analysis of point mutations and small insertions and deletions, will be gradually superceded by non-gel-based solution detection systems that do not require time-consuming post-polymerase chain reaction (PCR) processing and

gel analysis. The most promising technology uses dual-color fluorescence detection with internal hybridization oligonucleotide probes on the Lightcycler that has the capacity to diagnose specific allelic mutations in real time.

GENES AND ANDROLOGY

There is a gene on the X chromosome linked to mental retardation. It may be possible to produce medication that could improve thinking skills and memory in mentally retarded children. This gene is much like the gene that regulates blood pressure. There is medication that can regulate blood pressure by blocking that gene's receptor. However, a medical solution to retardation is still a long way off. Nevertheless, there is a possibility of prevention. One mentally retarded patient had an abnormally arranged X chromosome and it appeared that a single gene was silenced by the rearrangement, causing disability. Several other genes have been linked to mental retardation, but this new discovery may account for more cases than all other known genetic mutations. Although this mutation is present in only a small percentage of the males with unexplained mental retardation; this finding is of special clinical and genetic significance. With a total of 30 000 to 35 000 genes in the human body, the discovery of even a single gene that may play a pivotal role in brain development could be extremely important.

Identification of genes that cause mental retardation and other human disabilities is a major focus of genetics research. More than 100 of the approximately 1200 genes on the X chromosome are involved in brain development and function.

Gene helps mice with muscular dystrophy

The crippling effects of muscular dystrophy were partially corrected in laboratory mice by the insertion of a new gene that restored to the muscles a protein lacking in victims of the fatal disease. Researchers fused a gene that encodes a muscle protein with a modified virus and injected the combination into the hind leg muscles of mice that had a disorder that mimics Duchenne muscular dystrophy. Within a month, the test mice had 40% improvement in muscle action compared to muscular dystrophy mice that received no injection. Researchers then measured the force produced before and after the muscle was stretched and the mice that were injected were much stronger than the uninfected control mice.

Duchenne muscular dystrophy is a muscle-wasting disease caused by the mutation of the gene that produces a muscle protein, dystrophin. The disorder, linked to the X chromosome, is inherited in about one of every 3 500 males born in the USA and some 12 000 patients live with the disease. The disease originated from a gene that fails to produce dystrophin, a protein that helps the muscles stretch and contract normally. Without this protein, the muscles tear faster than the body can repair them, a process called contraction injury. Over time, the muscles waste away. Patients generally are diagnosed by the age of 4, and they are usually

Table 7.1 Normal and abnormal sex chromosome constitutions arising at fertilization

Sperm		Ova		
		Normal	Non-disjunctive	
		X	XX	O
Normal	X	XX(normal female)	XXX	XO
	Y	XY(normal male)	XXY	YO
Non-disjunctive	XY	XXY		
	XX	XXX		
	YY	XYY		
	O	XO		

An O sperm or ovum is one that carries neither an X nor a Y chromosome. Non-disjunctive gametes arise through faulty sharing-out (non-disjunction) of the sex chromosomes. YO individuals are probably not viable; XXX individuals, in humans, are abnormal females. (Reproduced with permission from McLaren, 1980)

using a wheelchair by the age of 12. Most die in their twenties, although improved care has allowed some patients to live until their early thirties. Muscles in the heart and pulmonary system are affected, generally leading to death.

GENETIC DEFECTS

Genetic defects have been implicated in the pathogenesis of spermatogenic failure. (Tables 7.1, 7.2 and 7.3; Figures 7.2 and 7.3). The azoospermia factor (AZF) on the long arm of the Y chromosome (Yq), originally defined by cytogenetic findings in azoospermic men has been widely studied. Yq11 deletions encompassing three non-overlapping regions (AZFa, AZFb, and AZFc) disrupt spermatogenesis. Most studies of causes have used sequence-tagged site (STS) primers, and the incidence of Y microdeletions has varied widely, from 1 to 55%. Deletions vary in both extent and location, and no genotype–phenotype correlation has been easily recognized. The STS map in the euchromatic region of the Y chromosome has been revised several times, and most of the STS primers used thus far amplify anonymous sequences. Most STS markers do not belong to specific genes. Therefore, a microdeletion of an STS could represent a clinically irrelevant polymorphism rather than the cause of spermatogenic failure.

More than 30 genes and gene families have been identified thus far in the human Y chromosome. Some of these genes are located in AZF deletion intervals. Excluding genes located in the pseudoautosomal

Table 7.2 Basic types of chromosomal alteration. (Reproduced with permission from Rosnina et al. 2000)

Type of alteration	Definition	Example
Numerical	alteration in chromosome number	
Aneuploidy	inexact multiples of haploid number in eggs (2n ± 1; 2n ± 2)	39,XXY (Klinefelter-like syndrome)
		63,XO (Turner-like syndrome)
Euploidy (polyploidy)	exact multiples of the haploid number (e.g. 3n, 4n, 5n)	180,XY
Mosaic	two or more cell populations (different karyotypes) derived from a single zygote which differ in chromosome number and/or structure	60,XY/59,XYrob(1,29)
Chimera	two or more populations of cells derived from two or more zygotes	60,XX/60,XY
Structural	alteration in structure of the chromosome	
Deficiency	a segment of a chromosome that is lost	38,Xyt(7q−;11q+)
Duplication	a chromosome segment exists in excess of the normal	
Inversion	a segment is in a reverse sequence	
Translocation	a segment or a whole arm of one chromosome is transposed to another chromosome	59,XY rob (1,29)
		38,XY rcp (13q−;14q+)

Table 7.3 Follow-up observations on patients with sex chromosome aneuploidy. (Data from Ratcliffe and Paul, 1986; Rovert et al. 1995)

Disorder	Karyotype	Phenotype	Sexual development	Intelligence	Behavioral problem
Klinefelter syndrome	47,XXY	tall male (see text)	infertile; hypogonadism	learning difficulties (some patients)	may have poor psychosocial adjustment
XYY syndrome	47,XYY	Tall male	normal	normal	frequent
Trisomy X	47,XXX	female, usually tall	usually normal	learning difficulties (some patients)	occasional
Turner syndrome	45,X	short female, distinctive features (see text)	infertile; streak gonads	normal (but see text)	rare

region, two general types of gene exist: Y-specific multicopy genes and X-Y homologous single-copy genes. Two potential AZF candidates, RBM1 and DAZ, have been implicated in testis-specific RNA metabolism. Lin et al. (2002) used 15 Y chromosome maps in 19 patients presenting with spermatogenic failure (Figure 7.4).

GENETIC SCREENING

Azoospermia and severe oligospermia may be associated with genetic abnormalities. Genetic abnormalities may cause infertility by affecting sperm production or sperm transport. The three most common genetic factors known to be related to male infertility are cystic fibrosis gene mutations associated with congenital absence of the vas deferens; chromosomal abnormalities resulting in impaired testicular function; and Y-chromosome

microdeletions associated with isolated spermatogenic impairment. Chromosomal abnormalities have been found in karyotypes of 10–15% of men with azoospermia and 5% of men with oligospermia but less than 1% of normal men. Microdeletions of the Y chromosome have been found in 10–15% of men with azoospermia or severe oligospermia (Sharlip et al. 2002). Men with non-obstructive azoospermia and severe oligospermia should be informed that they might have chromosomal abnormalities or Y-chromosome microdeletions. Karyotyping and Y-chromosome analysis should be offered to men with non-obstructive azoospermia or severe oligospermia.

Microdeletions in the Y chromosome

Genes located on the euchromatic region of the long arm of the Y chromosome, such as those in AZF

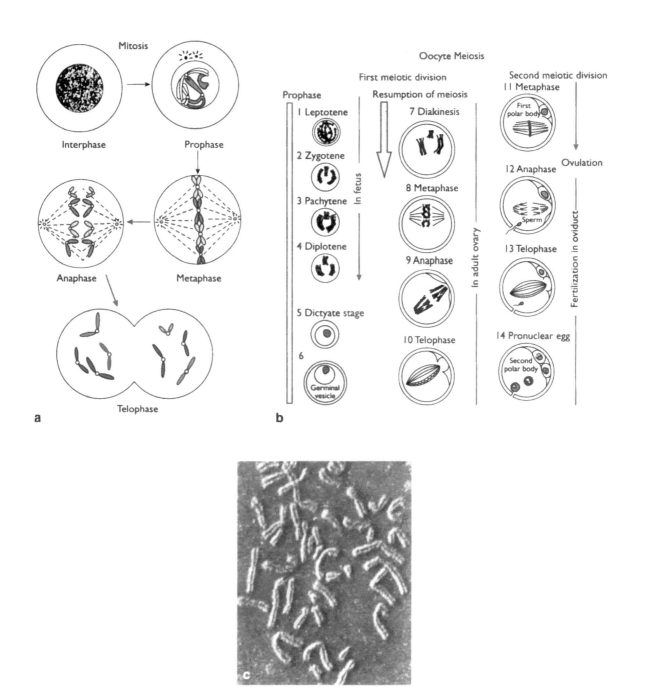

Figure 7.2 Chromosome arrangement during mitosis and meiosis. (a) Chromosome arrangement during mitosis. (Reproduced with permission from Feingold and Pashaya, 1983). (b) Oocyte meiosis. For simplicity, only three pairs of chromosomes are depicted. Prophase stages (1–4) of the first meiotic division occur in most mammals during fetal life. The meiotic process is arrested at the diplotene stage (first meiotic arrest), and the oocyte enters the dictyate stages (5–16). When meiosis is resumed, the first maturation division is completed (7–11). Ovulation occurs usually at the metaphase II stage (11), and the second meiotic division (12–14) takes place in the oviduct only following sperm penetration. (Reproduced with permission from Tsafriri et al. 1983). (c) Scanning electron micrograph of chromosomes

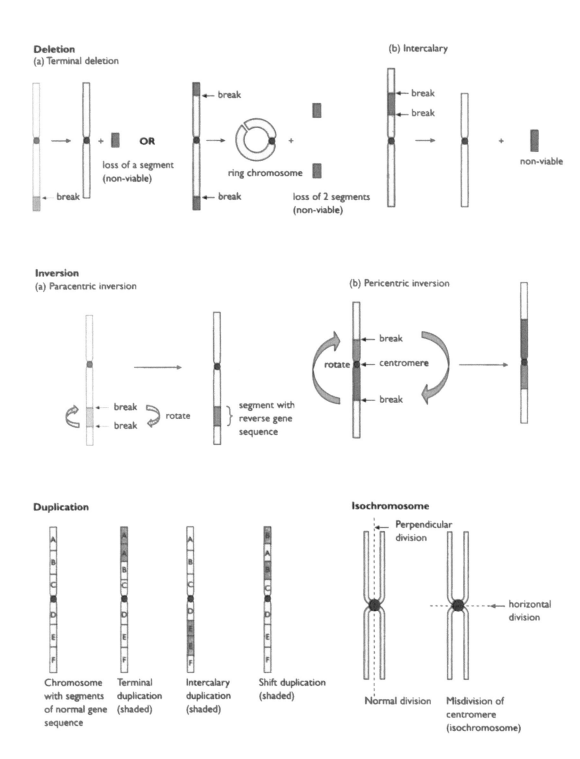

Figure 7.3 Illustrations of various structural aberrations: deletion, inversion, duplication, isochromosome. (Adapted with permission from Basrur, 1999)

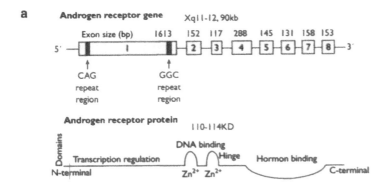

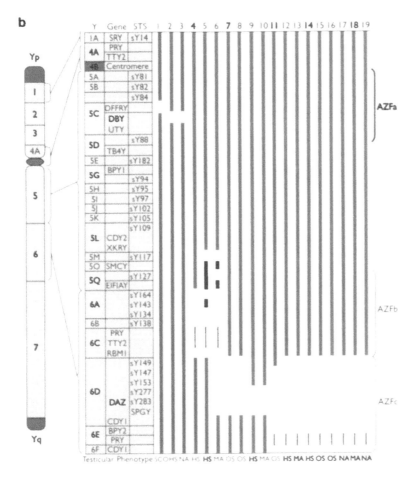

Figure 7.4 (a) The androgen receptor gene and protein. Exon 1 encodes the transactivation domain and contains a highly polymorphic CAG repeat encoding a polyglutamine tract. Exons 2 and 3 encode the DNA binding domain. The 5′ portion of exon 4 encodes the hinge domain, and the 3′ portion of exon 4 and exons 5 to 8 encode the ligand-binding domain. (Reproduced with permission from Sasagawa et al. 2002; Qungley et al. 1995). (b) Gene-specific primers to detect deletions of Y chromosome genes in men with spermatogenic failure. A multiplex polymerase chain reaction amplification system was developed to facilitate rapid screening. Another 24 markers for sequence-tagged sites (STS) were used to ensure the adequacy of gene-based screening. Of 180 patients evaluated, 19 (11%) had deletions of one or more genes, including DEFRY, DBY, RBM1, DAZ, CDY1, and BPY2. A second round of STS-based screenings did not show an increase in the deletions. Gene-based screening with multiplex polymerase chain reaction is a rational alternative for detecting deletions of Y chromosome genes in infertile men. (Reproduced with permission from Lin et al. 2002, *Arch Androl*, 48: 259–66. www. tandf.co.uk/journals)

regions, play an essential role in spermatogenesis. There are four regions in the AZF (AZFa, AZFb, AZFc and AZFd) on the Y chromosome, and gene deletions in these regions have been shown to be pathogenically involved in male infertility associated with azoospermia or severe oligozoospermia. AZFa was found in the proximal portion of deletion interval 5; AZFb was located at the proximal end of deletion interval 6, extending into the distal part of deletion interval 5; AZFc was found in the distal portion of deletion interval 6. The type of deletion (AZFa, b or c) has been proposed as a potential prognostic factor for sperm retrieval in men undergoing testicular sperm extraction (TESE). Infertile men with proximal deletions, which include AZFa and AZFb

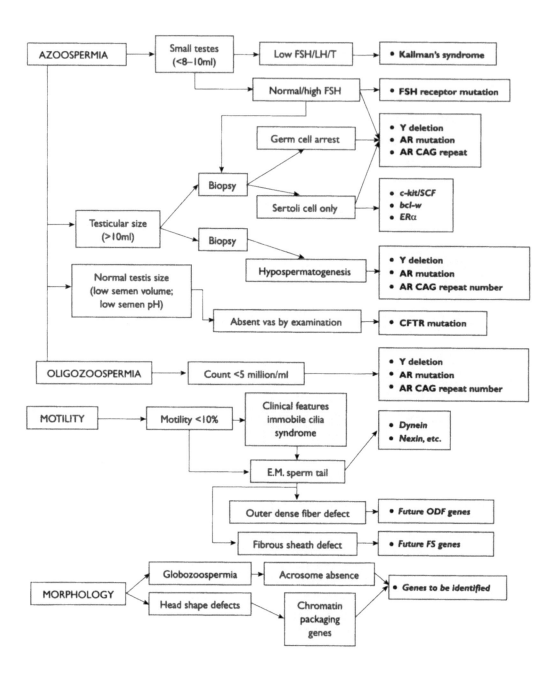

Figure 7.5 Schematic approach to identifying groups of patients with a potential genetic basis for infertility. Tests indicated in bold are currently available, whereas those in bold italics point to future directions. FSH, follicle stimulating hormone; LH, luteinizing hormone; CFTR, cystic fibrosis transmembrane conductance regulator; T, testosterone; SCF, stem cell factor; ODF, outer denser fibres; FS, fibrous sheath. (From Cram and de Kretser, personal communication)

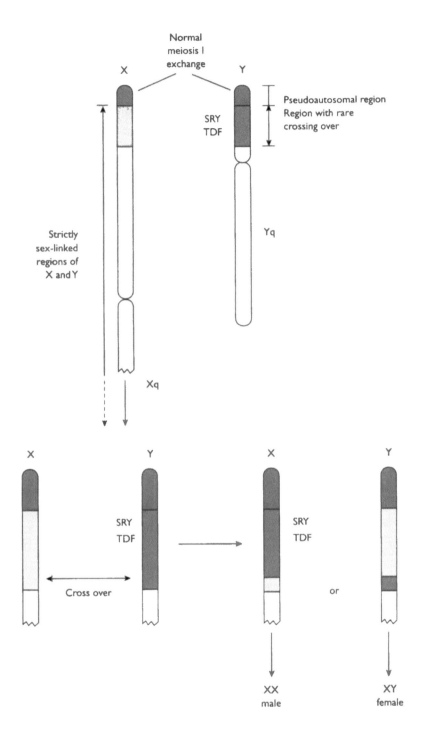

Figure 7.6 Etiological factors of XX male or XY female phenotypes by aberrant exchange between X- and Y-linked sequences. X and Y chromosomes normally recombine within the Xp/Yp pseudoautosomal segment in male meiosis. If recombination occurs below the pseudoautosomal boundary, between the X-specific and Y-specific portions of the chromosomes, sequences responsible for male sexual differentiation (including the SRY gene) may be translocated from the Y to the X. Fertilization by a sperm containing such an X chromosome leads to an XX male. In contrast, fertilization by a sperm containing a Y chromosome that has lost the SRY will lead to an XY female. (Reproduced with permission from Nussbaum *et al.* 2002)

regions, show severe defects in spermatogenesis, with high prevalence of Sertoli cell-only syndrome, whereas deletions of the distal AZFb and of the AZFc region can be compatible with residual spermatogenesis. Deletions including and extending beyond the AZFc region (AZFb+c and AZFa+b+c) are associated with a total absence of testicular spermatozoa. The presence of an AZFb deletion with spermatogenic arrest at the pachytene spermatocyte stage is a significantly adverse prognostic finding for TESE (Feng, 2002).

The DAZ gene

The *DAZ* gene family is reported to be the most frequently deleted AZF candidate gene and is located in the AZFc region. Originally thought to be a single-copy gene, DAZ is now known to be a multicopy gene family, which includes DAZ2, formerly known as spermatogenesis gene on Y (SPGY) and its autosomal copy on the short arm of chromosome 3 (DAZLI). The DAZ genes are expressed exclusively in testicular tissue and encode proteins that contain an RNA recognition motif, thereby suggesting that they have a regulatory role in RNA metabolism. Men with DAZ deletions are incapable of producing mature sperm; however, some men with oligospermia carry DAZ deletions. DAZL is expressed only in male and female germ cells in mice and men and is associated with spermatogenesis. Knockout-female mice with the DAZL gene show a failure of proper development of the female genital tract.

RBM genes

This gene family consists of 20 to 50 genes and pseudogenes that are distributed over both arms of the Y chromosome. Deletions of the AZFb region of the Y chromosome encompass at least one functional copy of the RBM1 gene. The multicopy nature of RBM1 has made it difficult to assign the gene with a specific function in spermatogenesis. An immunohistochemical study has shown that the RBMY1 protein is localized in the nucleus of human male germ cells, specifically at the AZFb region of the Y chromosome. The RBM1 gene cluster in the AZFb region may thus contain the only functional copies of the RBM1 gene, and their presence in male germ cells indicates their testis-specific expression (Feng, 2002).

PROGRAMMED CELL DEATH

In most mammals certain cells are destined to die during various stages of development. Programmed cell death occurs in well-defined steps under the influence of mutations of specific genes controlling cell death. These findings were first described in the mechanisms of cell specialization and organ development of the transparent worm *Caenorhabditis elegans*.

One American and two Britons won the Nobel Prize in medicine for discoveries about how genes regulate organ growth and about a process of programmed cell suicide. Britons Sydney Brenner and John Sulston, and American Robert Horvitz shared the 2002 prize, worth about $1 million. All three had worked together in the 1970s at Cambridge University in the UK. These remarkable findings shed light on the development of many illnesses, including AIDS and strokes. Information about programmed cell death has helped scientists understand how some viruses and bacteria invade human cells. In conditions such as AIDS, stroke and heart attack, cells are lost because of excessive cell death. In other diseases such as cancer, cell death is reduced, leading to the survival of cells that are normally destined to die. The laureates identified key genes regulating organ development and programmed cell death, a necessary process for pruning excess cells. Many cancer treatment strategies are now aimed at stimulating the cell-death process to kill cancerous cells.

DIAGNOSTICS OF GENETIC ABNORMALITIES IN MALE INFERTILITY

The study of Yq microdeletions will help in the development of better diagnostic methods and the expansion of the current knowledge of spermatogenesis. Many factors, including the many repetitive sequences on the Y chromosome, complicate the interpretation of the results from Yq microdeletion assays and the study of candidate genes that have critical functions in spermatogenesis.

Men with severe male infertility should be screened for Yq microdeletions as a part of their pretreatment investigations. The spermatogenic loci AZFa, AZFb and AZFc on the Yq11 chromosome control spermatogenesis in men and have an effect on fertility and genomic imbalance. When intracytoplasmic sperm injection (ICSI) is applied, AZFc-deleted spermatozoa are capable of fertilizing oocytes and eliciting full developmental potential. However, sons derived from use of the ICSI technique are most likely to inherit the Yq microdeletion, which may result in subsequent infertility (Feng, 2002). Diagnostic testing of deletions should be performed by multiplex PCR amplification of the STS locus in AZFa, AZFb and AZFc regions of the Y chromosome, which includes the following markers: sY84, sY86, sY127, sY134, sY252, and sY255.

The use of this primer set allows the detection of over 90% deletions in the three major AZF regions.

DIAGNOSTICS/THERAPEUTIC STRATEGY

Figure 7.5 shows an approach to identify groups of patients with a potential genetic basis for infertility.

There are various levels of treatment that are relevant to genetic disease with the corresponding strategies used at each level.

Figure 7.6 shows the etiological factors of XX male or XY female phenotypes by aberrant exchange between X- and Y-linked sequences.

CHAPTER 8

Immunoandrology

BACKGROUND

Rumke and Hellinga (1959) first reported the presence of sperm agglutinins in the sera of infertile men and that 3.3% had positive serum titers of 32 or greater of sperm agglutinins as determined by the macroscopic gelatin agglutination method. None of the fertile men had serum titers of that magnitude. Several other studies have reported incidences of 4–7% of infertile men positive for sperm agglutinins by the gelatin agglutination procedure. Differences in titers appear when serum samples are tested with more than one semen sample, but this is usually attributed to variation in semen quality.

Other studies utilizing microscopic observation have detected sperm agglutinins in the sera of infertile men but also with a fairly high incidence in fertile men. However, evidence from one laboratory has suggested that some sperm agglutination detected by this method may not be due to immunoglobulin, but to a β-macroglobulin in serum (Boettcher et al. 1970; Menge, 1976). The sperm immobilizing activity of some sera from infertile men is due to complement-dependent antibody.

Extensive investigations have been conducted on immunological techniques (Canadian Networking Tox Center, 1998), methods of cellular immunology (Fernadez-Botran and Vetvicka, 2000, 2001), immuno-gold–silver staining (IGSS) (Hayat, 1995; Hacker and Gu, 2002), basic methods in antibody production/characterization (Howard and Bethell, 2001); innate/acquired immunity, the mucosal immune system, T cell and B cell activation, kidney damage in autoimmune disease (Rao, 2002), the molecular structure of cytokines, histocompatability molecules and immunoglobulin, immune and receptor assays to measure analytes (Englebienne, 2000), vascular manifestation of systemic autoimmune diseases (Asherson et al. 2001), skin immune system (SIS) and clinical immunodermatology (Bos, 1997), cell wall-deficient forms of pathogens, nutrition/exercise immunology (Nieman and Pedersen, 2000), development and clinical testing of vaccines for human use (Paoletti and McInnes, 1998) and artificial DNA (Khudyakov and Fields, 2002).

BASIC IMMUNOLOGY AND CELLULAR COMPONENTS OF THE IMMUNE SYSTEM

Figure 8.1a shows the monomeric, dimeric and pentameric structure of immunoglobulin (Ig)G, soluble IgA with secretory component and pentameric IgM. Human secretory IgA travels through the epithelium aided by the secretory component. The two heavy chains are bound via the J chain, as in IgM. The variable regions of heavy and light chains are on the amino-terminal end of the peptide chains. The constant region of IgG is divided into three structurally discrete regions: C_H1, C_H2 and C_H3. These globular regions are stabilized by disulfide bonds and are called domains. The variable domain binds to the antigen; the constant regions are responsible for different effector mechanisms (Figure 8.1b). The in vivo population of T cells constantly recirculates to many different tissues. Local immune responses result in redistribution of T cells to the site of immune activation and thus heterogeneous distribution among body compartments (Figure 8.1c).

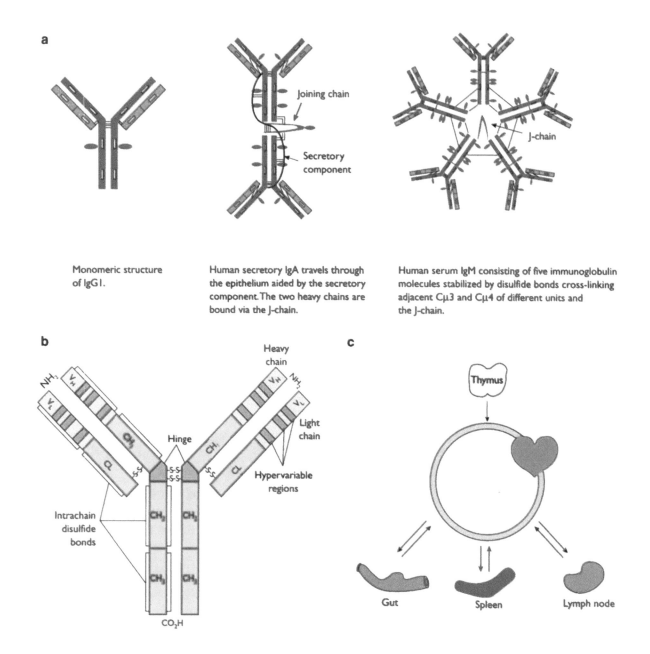

Figure 8.1 (a) Monomeric, dimeric and pentameric structure of immunoglobulin (Ig)G, soluble IgA with secretory component and pentameric IgM. (Reproduced with permission from Kunert and Katinger, 2002). (b) The basic structure of IgG. The variable regions (V) of heavy (H) and light (L) chains are on the amino-terminal (NH$_2$) end of the peptide chains. The constant region (C) of IgG is divided into three structurally discrete regions: CH$_1$, CH$_2$ and CH$_3$. These globular regions are stabilized by disulfide bonds and are called domains. The variable domain binds to the antigen; the constant regions are responsible for different effector mechanisms. CO$_2$H, carboxy-terminus. (Reproduced with permission from Nussbaum et al. 2002). (c) The in vivo population of T cells constantly recirculates to many different tissues. Local immune responses result in redistribution of T cells to the site of immune activation. (Reproduced with permission from Bucy and Golpfert, 2002)

The testis produces testis- and sperm-specific antigens, which are absorbed after trauma. The seminiferous tubules can be invaded by immune lymphocytes, whereas antibody enters the rete testes and efferent ducts; autoantibodies can cause agglutination and immobilization of sperm. The epididymis has two major functions: secretion of coating antigens; and phagocytosis of non-ejaculated sperm by macrophages.

The prostate secretes prostatic antigens, and the seminal vesicle secretes sperm-coating antigens. Any inflammation causes occlusion of the ejaculatory duct and absorption of prostatic and sperm antigens. Autoantibodies against seminal and prostatic secretions cause sperm agglutination.

Reproductive failure may result from primary and secondary immune responses as follows:

(1) Sperm elements are absorbed by macrophages and taken to the reticuloendothelial system which produces the large IgM antibody or primary response;

(2) This protects the body by attacking the immunogen;

(3) On repeated exposure to this antigen the macrophages stimulate lymphocytes to produce many circulatory antibodies of the IgG type which attack the antigen.

The plasma cells secrete immunoglobulin A into the circulation and into external secretions of epithelial membranes.

Anatomic sites for immune responses

Activation of immune responses can occur at several levels in the body, including the site of entry of microorganisms (skin, lungs, etc.). Antigens that enter the blood stream are concentrated in the spleen, where T and B cell responses can be initiated. Similarly, in the lymphatic circulatory system, the lymph nodes, which contain both T and B cells, capture the antigens. Activated effector and memory T cells leave the spleen and lymph nodes, circulate throughout the body, and home specifically to sites of antigen entry. B cells also can be present in peripheral organs, particularly mucosal tissues such as the intestine and reproductive tract. However, many activated cells remain in the spleen and lymph nodes, where the B cells produce antibodies, which circulate in the blood.

CELLULAR IMMUNE FUNCTION IN THE REPRODUCTIVE TRACT

The key cellular components of the immune system are: phagocytes (macrophages, dendritic cells, neutropils); and lymphocytes (T-helper lymphocytes, cytotoxic T lymphocytes, B lymphocytes, etc.). The B lymphocytes

Table 8.1 Some key cellular components of the immune system. (Reproduced with permission from Hansen, 2000)

Cell type	Key function
Phagocytes	
Macrophage	phagocytosis; antigen presentation
Dendritic cell	endocytosis and phagocytosis; antigen presentation
Neutrophil	phagocytosis
Lymphocytes	
B lymphocyte	secretion of antibody; antigen presentation
T-helper-1 lymphocyte	secretion of cytokines that stimulate macrophages and cytotoxic T cells
T-helper-2 lymphocyte	secretion of cytokines that stimulate B cells and antibody responses
Cytotoxic T lymphocyte	lysis of target cells
Gamma–delta (γδ) T lymphocyte*	lysis of target cells; secretion of cytokines and growth factors

*The T cell receptor is of the γδ type; other T lymphocytes have the αβ type

and T lymphocytes have a variety of immunological functions (Table 8.1).

The massive numbers of sperm introduced into the female reproduction tract have to be removed by a mechanism that does not lead to permanent immunity of the female against these cells. The immune response in the reproductive tract and associated lymph nodes adjusts to these requirements since lymphoid cells in the reproductive tract are regulated by ovarian steroid hormones, regulatory molecules in seminal plasma and locally produced factors from the reproductive tract and conceptus.

Generation of cell-mediated immune response

For activation of naïve T-helder and cytotoxic T lymphocytes, professional antigen-presenting cells (e.g. dendritic cells) are required. Dendritic cells process the antigens and present the immunogenic peptides in an MHC context with simultaneous delivery of co-stimulatory signals (e.g. B7/CD28 or CD40/CD40 ligand signals) to activate T lymphocytes. Two antigen-processing pathways are generally accepted. In the cytosolic pathway, endogenously synthesized antigens (cytoplasmic proteins) are digested in proteosomes and

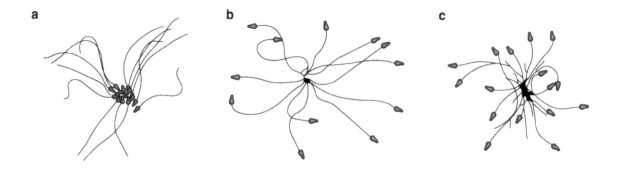

Figure 8.2 Typical sperm agglutination patterns caused by human serum agglutinins (a) Head-to-head; (b) tip of tail-to-tip of tail; (c) tail-to-tail. (Reproduced with permission of Elsevier from Abbas *et al.* 1997)·

transported into the endoplasmic reticulum by transporters associated with antigen processing, where they complex with MHC class I molecules for presentation to CD8+ cytotoxic T lymphocytes. In the endosomal pathway, extracellular antigens are phagocytozed, digested in lysosomes and then complexed with MHC class II molecules in vesicles for presentation to CD4+ T-helper lymphocytes.

CD44 glycoprotein

CD44 is a widely distributed polymorphic transmembrane glycoprotein with a molecular mass of 70–95 kDa. The predominant human hemopoietic form, CD44H, has a molecular mass of 80–90 kDa and is expressed by cells of both mesodermal and neuroectodermal origin. CD44 acts as a hyaluronan receptor, and this is consistent with the hypothesis that CD44 is a cell adhesion molecule. CD44 is also a signaling receptor for hyaluronic acid in T cells, and antibodies directed to the hyaluronan-binding region of CD44 inhibited the activation of T cells (Bains *et al.* 2002).

ACQUIRED IMMUNE SYSTEM

B and T lymphocytes are the two main types of cell of the acquired immune system. B cells are derived from the bone marrow. T cells also are formed from precursors in the bone marrow but undergo a period of differentiation in the thymus before seeding various lymphoid tissues. Both T and B cells express receptors

on their cell surfaces that are specific for a particular antigen. For B cells, the antigen receptor is an immunoglobulin, while for T cells, the receptor is a protein, the T cell receptor. Lymphocytes have the capacity for immunological memory. When a lymphocyte recognizes an antigen specific for its receptor, it undergoes activation whereby the cell proliferates. Some of these daughter cells differentiate into effector cells that perform various activities such as antibody production or lysis of target cells (Hansen, 2000).

THE IMMUNOLOGY OF SPERM

Sperm are antigenic if injected subcutaneously into the female. There are several physiological mechanisms to remove sperm from the reproductive tract following sexual intercourse in a way that will not lead to the development of humoral or cellular immunity to sperm. The deposition of sperm induces an influx of phagocytic cells (neutrophils, macrophages and dendritic-like cells) into the reproductive tract. Most of the sperm undergo phagocytosis by neutrophils. Seminal plasma contains various molecules that can inhibit lymphocyte activation. In contrast, lymphocytes in the lymph nodes draining the uterus become activated by seminal plasma, perhaps because immunosuppresants are inactivated as sperm antigens reach the lymph nodes (Hansen, 2000). Sperm undergo different types of agglutination (head to head, tail to tail, tip of tail to tip of tail) (Figure 8.2), which may be related to reproductive failure.

Sperm and seminal antigens

Sperm carry several antigens, including sperm-specific antigens, histocompatability antigens (i.e. those responsible for the rejection of tissue grafts), blood-group antigens and other somatic tissue antigens. Sperm antigens may be antigenic within the reproductive system of the male (autoantigens) or the female (isoantigens). Of the sperm antigens, those on the surface of the plasma membrane are probably responsible for reproductive failure (Hansen, 2000). The 'blood–testis barrier' functions as an autoimmune response, which isolates the testes from the rest of the body. If the barrier is breached, antisperm antibodies are produced that might attack sperm. Autoimmune antibodies against sperm are found in the seminal plasma and serum of infertile men. Antisperm antibodies can prevent fertilization by immobilizing sperm, impairing sperm penetration of cervical mucus and inactivating acrosomal enzymes.

Semen is a complex of antigenic components originating in the testis, epididymis, ejaculatory duct and accessory glands. These structures contribute different qualities and quantities of antigens. The antigenic components can be broadly classified as those in the seminal plasma or those that are sperm bound. Sperm, as they travel through the epididymis and ejaculatory duct, become coated with antigenic secretions from the ducts and accessory glands. These sperm-coating antigens adhere firmly to the sperm membrane. One such coating antigen, designated as sperm-coating antigen (SCA), originates in the seminal vesicle, is relatively heat stable and is a mucoprotein of high molecular weight. An iron-binding protein, lactoferrin, has also been found in seminal plasma and bound to ejaculated sperm. This material is secreted by the seminal vesicles but is not found in the testes or epididymis (Behrman and Menge, 1979). Some 7–19 antigenic components have been reported for human semen, as determined by precipitation methods in agar diffusion and immunoelectrophoresis. Absorption and cross-reaction studies have indicated that the majority of the seminal antigens are of serum origin and non-specific for the male reproductive tissues.

In semen, serum components have been identified: albumin, and α-, β- and γ-globulins, although in lower concentrations. Of the γ-globulins, IgG, IgA, and some degraded immunoglobulin molecules have been noted.

In addition, protease enzymes (aminopeptidases, acid phosphatase and hyaluronidase) are antigenically active in seminal plasma.

ABO blood group antigens have been readily detected in the seminal plasma of secretors. These antigens are rapidly adsorbed onto the sperm cells, which has resulted in confusion as to whether or not spermatozoa express ABO antigens in the membranes because of genic control or from adsorption of antigens from seminal plasma.

Antisperm autoantibodies

The formation of antisperm autoantibodies is related to temporary or permanent obstruction of the ejaculatory duct, testicular trauma or inflammation, and inflammation or infection of the epididymis and accessory sex glands. The incidence of men with antisperm antibodies is high after spontaneous or surgical obstructive azoospermia, vasectomy, epididymitis and prostatovesiculitis. Sperm extravasation, which does not normally occur, is a common event in cases of obstruction to sperm passage, thus providing an opportunity for a natural immune response. The body is normally protected from exposure to sperm antigens by the blood–testis barrier and normal cellular defense mechanisms in the epididymis. Sperm antigens are regarded as non-self because of their late appearance at puberty, which is after the immune system has become tolerant for self antigens. However, several cases of autoantibodies against sperm are not related to previous abnormalities or inflammatory conditions (Fjallbrant, 1968; Menge, 1976).

Several factors are responsible for the initiation of autoimmunity against spermatozoa. Men with unilateral or bilateral occlusions of the ductus deferens show an increased incidence of antisperm antibody. Similar results were observed in men who had had or were experiencing inflammation of the epididymis and accessory glands. These factors may result in insufficient drainage of seminal components, leading to increased absorption of antigens, initiating an immune response.

IMMUNOLOGY OF SEMINAL PLASMA

The seminal plasma from infertile men contains specific antisperm antibodies of the IgA and IgG classes.

Serum antibodies against sperm may belong to one or all of the three major immunoglobulin classes – IgA, IgG and IgM (Rumke, 1974). The IgG level of seminal plasma is 1% of that found in serum. Antisperm antibodies are found in seminal plasma only if present in serum and they are usually 2–4 dilutions lower. For spontaneous agglutination to occur in the ejaculate, the serum titer must be at least 64 (Friberg, 1974; Husted, 1975). Antibodies in the seminal plasma are detected by agglutination, immobilization, indirect immunofluorescence and antiglobulin methods. With serum, different immunoglobulin classes react to different portions of the sperm in indirect immunofluorescence and cause different types of sperm agglutination. IgM antibodies react to the acrosomal area and tip of the tail, causing head-to-head and tip of tail-to-tip-of-tail agglutination patterns, whereas IgG react with the equatorial segment and main tail piece, causing head-to-tail and tail-to-tail types of agglutination (Menge, 1976). In seminal plasma most sperm agglutination is caused by IgA antibodies, even though the serum agglutinins from the same individuals are of the IgG class.

Sexual intercourse is associated with microbial contamination, because the penis and sometimes the seminal plasma contain micro-organisms. Other mechanical or environmental insults may also lead to introduction of microbes into the reproductive tract. Despite these microbial invasions, micro-organisms can be rapidly removed from the reproductive tract and the tract usually remains free from infection. A sterile environment in the reproductive tract is maintained by the presence of an effective antimicrobial defense system that includes physical barriers, phagocytes that engulf and kill micro-organisms, B lymphocytes that produce antibodies against invading microbes and T lymphocytes that can kill virus and bacteria-infected host cells (Hansen, 2000).

Sometimes immunological defense mechanisms in the reproductive tract are not sufficient to prevent microbial colonization, and the resultant infections can temporarily or permanently cause infertility or sterility.

CLINICAL APPLICATIONS

For routine immunological evaluation of infertile men, antisperm antibodies should be sought using two methods on the sera and seminal plasma, as well as the gelatin agglutination and immobilization methods. The capillary cervical mucus penetration test and the indirect immunofluorescence method should be used for special projects, to obtain repeatable and reliable results. The availability of the microtechniques for agglutination and immobilization will permit convenient testing on a larger scale than with the tube methods. The evaluation of postcoital penetration of the cervical mucus and canal by sperm is a simple and practical method to evaluate sperm from infertile men and cervical mucus from infertile women. Control cervical mucus is obtained from healthy fertile or potentially fertile, normally cycling women at midcycle after a period of abstinence of at least 4–6 days, and it must be free of contamination by blood cells, bacteria and other cellular debris. Methods that reduce or eliminate exposure of sperm in the ejaculate to antisperm antibodies, i.e. by immediate washing and centrifugation of sperm cells and possible elution of antibodies by mild treatments with differing concentrations of salt and levels of pH, may be of value. The sperm would then be available for artificial insemination.

It is recommended that a laboratory establishing immunological testing for antisperm antibodies should consider performing two methods on the sera and possibly the seminal plasma of infertile men. In our own laboratory the gelatin agglutination and the immobilization methods are in routine use. We have also used the capillary cervical mucus penetration test and the indirect immunofluorescence methods for special projects, and obtained repeatable and reliable results. The availability of the microtechniques for agglutination and immobilization will permit convenient testing on a larger scale than with the tube methods.

Incidence of autoantibodies

Men may produce autoantibodies against seminal components capable of interfering with normal fertility. Infertile men contain sperm agglutinins in their ejaculates and sperm agglutinins in their serum samples. The spermatozoa from these men quickly lose motility in cervical secretions. Upon artificial insemination with donor semen, wives of these men have become pregnant. Antisperm antibodies have been detected in the sera of some men in infertile marriages, of which 4% had titers thought to be capable of interfering with fertility. Positive relationships were found between antibody titers with decreased motility and increased agglutination of sperm in the ejaculates; this reduced cervical mucus penetration by the sperm, lowering fertility. Treatment of sperm from fertile men with positive immune sera from infertile men inhibit their penetration of cervical mucus in capillary tubes.

Sperm antigens and antifertility vaccine

An 80-kDa human sperm antigen (80 kDa HSA) has been identified from human sperm extract as an antigen responsible for inducing immunoinfertility by using serum of an immunoinfertile woman as a probe in the Western blot technique. It has been purified to homogeneity from human sperm extract and its causal relationship with infertility has been demonstrated in actively immunized male and female rats (Bandivdekar et al. 1991, 1992, 2001). Immunofluorescent staining using rabbit anti-80 kDa HSA antibodies demonstrated its specific localization on the human and rat sperm head. Immunohistochemically, the antigen is localized only in the human testis and epididymis, but not in the other human somatic tissues such as brain, kidney, liver, heart, lung, spleen, intestine, appendix and nerve, suggesting that 80 kDa HSA is a sperm-specific antigen (Bandivadekar, 2002).

The protein was subjected to enzymatic digestion with endoproteinase Lys-C and endoproteinase Glu-C. The partial amino acid sequence of the major peptides thus obtained was determined. The digestion with endoproteinase Lys-C generated four major peptides, two of which showed partial sequence homology with lactoferrin. The 80 kDa HSA is a sperm-specific protein that is chemically distinct from any other protein involved in normal physiological processes. Earlier studies have demonstrated that it is antigenic, efficacious and conserved, and could be a promising candidate for the development of a contraceptive vaccine (Goldberg, 1990; Herr et al. 1990; O'Hern et al. 1995; Dickman and Herr, 1997; Primakoff et al. 1997; Tung et al. 1997; Naz, 2000).

Effect of vasectomy

After vasectomy, spermatogenic function of the testis apparently continues, causing the epididymis and often the proximal vas deferens to become turgid with packed sperm cells. The inhibition of sperm passage out of the ejaculatory duct increases the need for efficient elimination. Phagocytic activity, largely of macrophages and some epithelial cells in the epididymis, is responsible for sperm removal. Extravasation of sperm into interstitial tissues, often forming granulomas, has been reported occasionally in men with congenital absence of the vas deferens, vasoligation, vasectomy, testicular trauma and epididymitis. This causes inflammation, with infiltration of macrophages, lymphocytes and plasma cells. Sperm have occasionally been found in the blood vessels and lymph ducts of the spermatic cord. That these pathological conditions are conductive to induction of an immune response is demonstrated by the incidence of patients with a sectioned or obstructed vas deferens showing serum antibodies against sperm. After vasectomy, sperm agglutination occurred in 35% of cases, and in 25% of cases that had undergone successful correction of obstructive azoospermia. Some men may be more sensitive or responsive to sperm antigens, as well as to other antigens. Other factors, however, may also enter into the immune response. Therefore, there is a need for controlled research on sera of men before and after vasectomy.

EVALUATION OF SEMEN IMMUNOLOGY

The quality of semen samples used to evaluate anti-sperm antibodies is important. Samples should be obtained from healthy male donors whose ejaculates have been thoroughly examined and are consistently of high quality, as follows:

(1) Ejaculate volume 3–5 ml;

(2) Complete liquefaction within 20 min;

(3) Concentration of 80×10^6 sperm/ml;

(4) 70% initial motility and 50–60% after 2–3 h;

(5) Good forward sperm progression;

(6) No spontaneous agglutination;

(7) Sample free from debris and other cell types;

(8) Low incidence of abnormal sperm forms.

Whole and diluted ejaculates are protected from sudden changes in temperature and prolonged exposure to intence natural or artificial light. Ejaculates with a high concentration of sperm are diluted further than those with a low count, thus decreasing the concentration of seminal plasma, which may contain some competing cross-reacting antigens and anti-complement activity. Semen that is highly diluted (> 5 ×), centrifuged and washed or added to very diluted serum samples (> 100 ×) is diluted in a buffer containing 5–10% inactivated normal serum to maintain its viability. A thorough evaluation of the autoimmune response against spermatozoa in men should include the ejaculate as well as the serum. The ejaculate needs to be examined for its usual qualities, and careful attention needs to be paid to spontaneous agglutination and survival time of the sperm. For use in the following procedures, cell-free seminal plasma should be obtained by centrifuging the sample immediately after collection. Adequate controls, usually consisting of known negative serum and a positive serum, need to be run simultaneously with each test.

Antiglobulin method: mixed-cell antiglobulin reaction

This method (Coombs *et al.* 1973) may be useful in determining antibody and the immunoglobulin class of antibody bound to spermatozoa of infertile men. The principle is to use anti-immunoglobulin antibodies coated onto red cells to detect immunoglobulins attached to sperm cells.

(1) Human immunoglobulins, IgA, IgG and IgM, are attached to sheep red blood cells by chromic chloride (Gold and Fudenberg, 1967).

(2) Spermatozoa to be tested for the presence of antibody are washed twice and resuspended to a concentration of 7×10^6/ml of diluent. Hank's saline with 0.1% bovine serum albumin (BSA) or medium 199 with 0.25% BSA is the diluent.

(3) One drop each of the spermatozoa, the appropriate indicator red-cell suspension coated with an immunoglobulin and the class-specific antiglobulin reagent are gently mixed together and incubated together with examination at different times.

(4) The reaction is scored by placing a drop of the mixture on a siliconized microslide, covered with a siliconized coverslip and sealed with paraffin. It is

observed under phase-contrast microscopy. Mixed adherence of red cells and sperm cells indicates a binding of the corresponding immunoglobulin on the spermatozoa. Control sperm cells from fertile men must be included in the method.

Slide test (*in vitro* sperm penetration of cervical mucus)

This simple test is performed on donor semen and husband's semen on wife's cervical mucus as well as on a donor's cervical mucus as follows.

A drop of semen and a drop of cervical mucus are placed on a glass slide. A coverslip is placed on the slide and pressed slightly. Quantitative (number of sperm per high power microscopic field, × 400) assessment is carried out of sperm penetration in cervical mucus, in three consecutive high-power microscopic fields from the interface.

Two methods are used for cervical mucus penetration: capillary mucus penetration by Kremer (1965) as modified by Fjallbrant (1968) and the sperm cervical mucus contact test (SCMC) by Kremer and Jager (1976).

Capillary mucus penetration

(1) The cervial mucus is carefully obtained by forceps or gentle aspiration with a syringe and placed onto a clean glass slide in a humid chamber.

(2) The mucus is drawn up into capillary tubes (0.5 mm internal diameter, 40 mm long) and one end is sealed with modeling clay.

(3) The capillary tube is mounted on a special calibrated microslide with the open end placed into a chamber containing the semen sample.

(4) The slide is placed into a humid chamber and incubated at 37°C for 1 h.

(5) The slide is examined under low-power microscopy to determine the furthest penetration of the spermatozoa.

Penetration ratings: poor, ≤ 5 mm; fair, 6–19 mm; and good ≥ 20 mm. Spermatozoa from men with circulating and seminal plasma antisperm antibodies show poor penetration. Also, the *in vitro* treatment of spermatozoa with serum containing antibodies will inhibit normal penetration.

Sperm cervical mucus contact test

(1) Fresh semen from an infertile man is freed of large agglutinates by sedimentation for at least 30 min.

(2) Small amounts of semen and normal cervical mucus are mixed or placed adjacent to each other on a microslide and covered with a coverslip.

(3) The slides are incubated at 37°C for 15 min and observed under the microscope.

(4) It was reported that spermatozoa from men with sperm agglutinins (serum titers ≥ 64) upon contact with the cervical mucus quickly changed their forward motion into quick and jerky local movements.

The authors confirmed by other methods (indirect immunofluorescence and mixed cell agglutination) that sperm cells positive in the SCMC test had antibodies attached to them. They also found the same response using cervical mucus from a positive woman and semen from a control donor. If these results are confirmed, this would appear to be a relatively simple and rapid test for evaluating the presence of antibodies in semen or cervical mucus.

In the remainder of the chapter two techniques are described that are not readily suitable for routine clinical processing but may be of value for certain cases and for research purposes.

Two labeled antibody techniques are used: the indirect immunofluorescent method (Hjort and Hansen, 1971); and indirect immunofluorescence on swollen sperm heads (Kolk *et al.* 1974).

Indirect immunofluorescent method

(1) Spermatozoa in 0.2 ml of semen are suspended in 10–12 ml of physiological saline and centrifuged at 750 *g* for 10 min. The supernatant is discarded and the sperm washed twice more and finally resuspended to approximately 0.5 ml with saline. This gives a convenient concentration for smearing.

(2) Single drops of sperm suspension are smeared on microslides and air dried under a fan for 30 min.

(3) To aid in locating the desired area for staining throughout the procedure, a 1-cm diameter circle is etched in the center of the slide with a diamond-tipped pencil. The slides are fixed in absolute methanol for 30 min and then air dried or transferred immediately to phosphate-buffered saline (PBS) (pH 7.4) for 15 min.

(4) The area around the circle is blotted dry and the sperm area is then covered with the serum sample. The slide is placed in a humid chamber for incubation at room temperature for 30–60 min. The serum is rinsed away with PBS and the slide washed in two changes of PBS for 10 min each. With cervical mucus samples we have extended the incubation period an additional 6–18 h.

(5) The same process as in step 4 is repeated, except that the slides are incubated with fluorescein isothyocyanate (FITC)-conjugated antisera against human immunoglobulins for 30 min.

(6) After incubation, the slides are flushed and washed with three changes of PBS for 10 min. The slides are covered with coverslips using 10% glycerine in PBS.

(7) The immunofluorescent staining patterns are observed with a fluorescent microscope equipped with proper FITC interference filters.

Recently, these authors reported that agglutinating sera from some infertile males reacted in indirect immunofluorescence with heads of spermatozoa caused to swell by pretreatment with trypsin and dithiothreitol. The antibody appears to react with the nuclear protein, protamine.

Indirect immunofluorescence on swollen sperm heads

(1) Fresh semen is washed three times with PBS and the pellet is resuspended in 1–2 ml of a 50-mm Tris–HC1 (pH 9.0) buffer containing 0.4 mmol/l dithiothreitol.

(2) After a few minutes, a fresh trypsin solution in 1 mmol/lHC1 is added to a final concentration of 10 μ/ml.

(3) The reaction proceeds at room temperature with microscopic examination to determine the swelling response of the sperm heads. After the

desired amount of swelling is attained (1–30 min) the reaction is stopped with soybean trypsin inhibitor.

(4) The suspension is diluted with PBS to a concentration of 2×10^6 sperm/ml and smears are prepared on microslides. The slides are processed for indirect immunofluorescence.

Sperm agglutination technique

There are three methods: gelatin agglutination (Kibrick *et al.* 1952); microtray agglutination (Friberg, 1974); and tube-slide agglutination (Franklin and Dukes, 1964).

Gelatin agglutination

(1) Serum samples are inactivated at 56°C for 30 min to destroy complement activity. Unheated sera with strong immobilizing activity may kill the sperm before the agglutination occurs.

(2) A fresh semen sample meeting the above listed specifications is diluted in Baker's buffer to 40×10^6 sperm/ml.

(3) A 10% gelatin solution in Baker's buffer freshly prepared and warmed to 37 °C is mixed with an equal volume of warmed diluted semen to give a final volume necessary to complete the test. The mixture is kept at 37 °C until used.

(4) At this stage several possible methods can be used for mixing the serum and sperm–gelatin mixture:

  (a) Serum is serially diluted starting at 1 : 4 in serological tubes with Baker's buffer. Tubes are placed in a 37°C bath and an equal volume (0.2–0.3 ml) of sperm–gelatin mixture is added and mixed. Each sample is transferred to a Kibrick tube (3–5 mm internal diameter, 3–5 cm long).

  (b) The serum (0.3 ml) is serially diluted in the small tubes (5 × 50 mm) using 1-ml syringes with 1.5 inch × 20G needles and the sperm–gelatin mixture (0.3 ml) is firmly added to each tube to effect mixing.

(5) The tubes are read at 1 and 2 h after incubation at 37°C.

(6) Agglutination is observed as suspended white aggregates of spermatozoa or a settling of large aggregates resulting in a clearing of the medium.

Microtray agglutination

(1) Test serum samples (inactivated) are serially diluted with 0.01 mol/l PBS (pH 7.4) to give dilutions of 4-, 8-, 16- and 32-fold.

(2) 5 µl of each serum dilution is transferred to a 3 × 6 microchamber tray (Moller-Coates AS, Moss, Norway) under mineral oil by means of a Hamilton microsyringe. The microsyringe is carefully washed out with PBS between different serum samples.

(3) I µl of semen diluted (40×10^6 sperm/ml) in PBS is added to each 5-µl serum aliquot. It is allowed to stand at room temperature for 4 h before observation or at 37°C for 2 h.

(4) Degree and type of sperm agglutination is observed at 60–100 × and 600 ×, respectively, on an inverted microscope. The serum is considered positive for agglutinins if agglutinates are observed in at least two dilutions. If agglutination occurs at the 1 : 32 dilution, the serum should be diluted further and retested.

Tube-slide agglutination

(1) Serum samples are inactivated at 56°C for 30 min. Undiluted serum may be used, but more confidence is obtained if the serum sample is diluted 1 : 4 with Baker's buffer.

(2) A fresh semen sample is diluted to 50×10^6 sperm/ml with Baker's buffer. If a laboratory is performing other methods requiring 40×10^6 sperm/ml, this lower concentration is adequate for this method also.

(3) To 0.5 ml of diluted serum in a serological tube, 0.1 ml of diluted semen is added and incubated at 37°C.

(4) At intervals of 1 and 2 or 1 and 4 h, a drop of sperm suspension is carefully removed from near the bottom of the tube, placed on a microslide and covered with a coverslip.

(5) Upon examination, the degree and type of agglutination is scored. Two reported methods for determining positive sera are as follows:

   (a) The total number of freely swimming motile sperm, the number of agglutinated sperm and the type of agglutinates (head-to-head, head-to-tail, etc.) are recorded for 12 high-power fields; positive sera have ≥ 10% of motile sperm in agglutinates (Shulman *et al.* 1973).

   (b) The number of agglutinates per 100 motile freely swimming sperm is recorded. A positive serum has a score of 8/100 or higher (Boettcher *et al.* 1970).

(6) The test can be made quantitative by serial dilution of serum samples.

Sperm cytotoxicity methods

There are two common methods: the sperm immobilization test of Isojima *et al.* (1968); and the microtechnique for immobilization/cytotoxicity (Husted and Hjort, 1975).

Sperm immobilization test

(1) All serum samples are inactivated at 56°C for 30 min.

(2) An appropriate dilution is prepared of a known standard human serum or rabbit anti-human-sperm serum that, in presence of complement, immobilizes 90–95% of the sperm in 1 h and a control human serum that has no immobilizing activity.

(3) The complement source is pooled fresh guinea-pig serum stored in small aliquots either frozen (–20 to –60°C) or lyophilized. Human AB serum and rabbit serum have also been used. Commercial sources of complement often have added preservatives, which will be cytotoxic to sperm. Each new batch of complement needs to be tested without antibody for immobilization activity.

(4) Fresh human semen is diluted to 40×10^6 sperm/ml in Baker's buffer.

(5) The protocol for the test using small serological tubes is shown in Table 8.2. After the tubes are

arranged and dilution (*n*) made, 0.025 ml of diluted semen is added to each tube and incubated at 37°C for 1 h. When screening for immobilizing antibody, in many patients undiluted sera may be used initially with serial dilutions tested at a later date to obtain a more quantitative result.

(6) At the end of the incubation period the tubes are gently shaken. A drop is taken from each tube and placed on a microslide for microscopic examination at (100–400 ×). Several fields must be examined to obtain a reliable estimate of percentage of motile cells.

(7) Sperm immobilizing value (SIV) for each serum dilution is calculated as follows:

$$SIV = \frac{motility~(\%)~in~control~serum}{motility~(\%)~in~test~serum}$$

Positive sera have SIV ≥ 2.

Microtechnique for immobilization/cytotoxicity

(1) Dilutions of inactivated sera are made with 0.9% saline (undiluted, 1 : 3 and 1 : 9 for screening). Known sera with negative and positive activities are included in each test.

(2) A fresh ejaculate is allowed to stand for 15 min, and 0.5-ml portions are transferred to each of two centrifuge tubes and centrifuged at 170 *g* for 5 min. The pellet in one tube is resuspended in complement (human AB, Rh-negative serum) and the other pellet in inactivated complement. The suspensions are adjusted to 40×10^6 sperm/ml and kept at 37°C.

(3) The microtrays are filled with mineral oil and 1 µl of the serum dilutions are deposited in the 6×3 microchamber trays by means of a Hamilton syringe. Two rows of chambers are used for each serum sample.

(4) 2 µl of sperm suspension in complement is added to samples in one row and 2 µl of sperm in the inactivated complement is added to the other row.

(5) After incubation for 2 h at 37°C, 1 µl of an isotonic 0.8% trypan blue solution is added to each chamber.

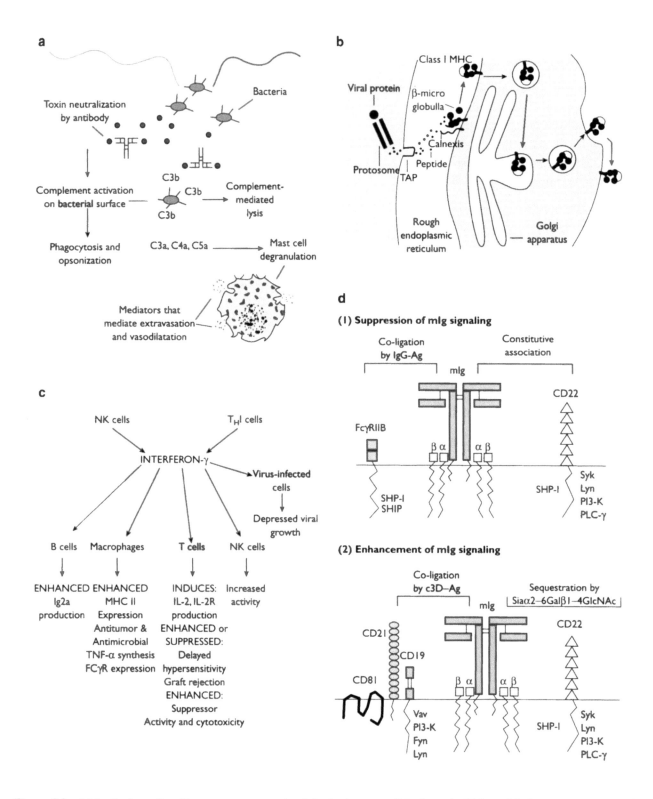

Figure 8.3 (a) Antibody-mediated immune response against infection by extracellular bacteria. (b) A model of antigen presentation for endogenous antigens. Note the association of class I MHC molecules with peptide. (c) Origins and targets of interferon-γ. (Reproduced with permission from Rao, 2002.) (d) Possible roles of B-lymphocyte co-receptors in membrane immunoglobulin (mIg) signaling. (1) Suppression of mIg signaling – FcγRIIB co-ligation with mIg by IgG–antigen (Ag) complexes exerts an inhibitory effect on mIg signaling through its association with the inositol polyphosphate 5-phosphatase SHIP and/or the tyrosine phosphatase SHP-1. (2) Enhancement of mIg signaling. Co-ligation of CD19– CD21–CD81 complex to mIg by C3D (CD21 ligand)–Ag recruits positive signal transduction effectors, which synergize with mIg to augment B-cell activation. (Reproduced with permission of Elsevier from O'Rourke et al. 1997)

Table 8.2 Protocol for the sperm immobilization test using small serological tubes. (Reproduced with permission from Isojima *et al.* 1968)

Samples	Volume (ml)	No. of tubes	Complement (ml)	Factors determined
Baker's buffer	0.25	l	0.05	immobilizing activity of complement
Control serum	0.25	l	0.05	base motility value
Standard serum	0.25	l	0.05	effectiveness of complement
Test sera	0.25	n	0.05*	immobilizing antibody independent of complement
Test sera	0.25	n	0.05	immobilizing antibody dependent on complement

*Complement serum heat inactivated

(6) The trays are mounted with a coverslip (28 × 53 mm) that is gently pressed into the mineral oil. It will slowly sink down, flattening the drops so that they fill the chambers.

(7) After an additional 1 h at 37 °C the microchambers are observed on an inverted microscope, preferably phase contrast. The percentages of immotile spermatozoa and stained spermatozoa are estimated on the basis of 0–25%, 25–50%, 50–75% and 75–100% and graded from 0 to 3⁺, respectively.

Molecular parameters of immunoandrology and related diseases

Molecular parameters of immunoandrology are illustrated in Figure 8.3.

FUTURE RESEARCH

Future research is needed into the purification and characterization of specific antigens of sperm. As this information becomes available, new methods will be developed for more critical evaluation of immunological infertility. Methods that reduce or eliminate exposure of spermatozoa in the ejaculate to antisperm antibodies (e.g. by immediately washing and centrifuging sperm cells and the possible elution of antibodies by treatments with differing concentrations of salt and levels of pH) may be of value and make sperm increasingly available for artificial insemination.

CHAPTER 9

Andropause: endocrinology, erectile dysfunction and prostate pathophysiology

ENDOCRINOLOGY OF ANDROPAUSE

Andropause is characterized by a decrease in sex hormones, growth hormone and insulin-like growth factor (IGF)-I and an increase in insulin levels, a consequence of the relative insulin resistance characterizing the aging process (Table 9.1). Sex hormones play a critical role in sex-associated congnitive abilities as well as interindividual differences within the sexes. Two decisive phases have been identified for the effects of sex hormones on brain structures and consequently upon behavior. Sex hormone levels in adult men activate neural structures and hence cognitive abilities. Andropause is associated with a decline in the serum level of testosterone, but not all men develop classic hypogonadal androgen levels. Many older men, however, could be relatively androgen deficient and might benefit from androgen supplementation.

The decline in testosterone levels during andropause leads to a rise in follicle stimulating hormone (FSH) and luteinizing hormone (LH) levels (Figure 9.1). The resultant high levels of FSH and LH act on the testes and the adrenals in an attempt to produce more testosterone. There is also a significant decline in growth hormone, melatonin, endorphins and dehydroepiandrosterone (DHEA; a precursor of testosterone). Certain metabolic disease such as diabetes may lead to symptoms akin to andropause. Diabetic men may

Table 9.1 Attempts to characterize an andropause syndrome that includes behavioral factors (data from Morley, 2000; 2001)

Werner (1946)
nervousness, decreased libido, decreased potency, irritability, fatigue, depression, memory problems, sleep disturbances, numbness and tingling, hot flushes
decreased libido, fatigue, depression, headaches
decreased general well-being, joint pain, muscular aches, excessive sweating, sleep problems, tiredness, irritability, nervousness, anxiety, physical exhaustion, decreased muscular strength, depressive mood, feeling past one's peak, feeling burnt out, decrease in beard growth, decreased ability to perform sexually, decreased libido, decreased morning erections
decreased libido, lack of energy, erection problems, falling asleep after dinner, memory impairment, sad or grumpy, decreased work performance, decreased endurance, loss of pubic hair, loss of axillary hair

Morley et al. (2000)
decreased libido, lack of energy, decreased strength/endurance, loss of height, decreased enjoyment of life, sad or grumpy, decreased work performance, decreased ability to play sports, decreased strength of erections, falling asleep after dinner

develop complications such as autonomic neuropathy (destruction of small blood vessels supplying the autonomic nerves). Therefore, diabetic patients should be treated appropriately, since proper management of

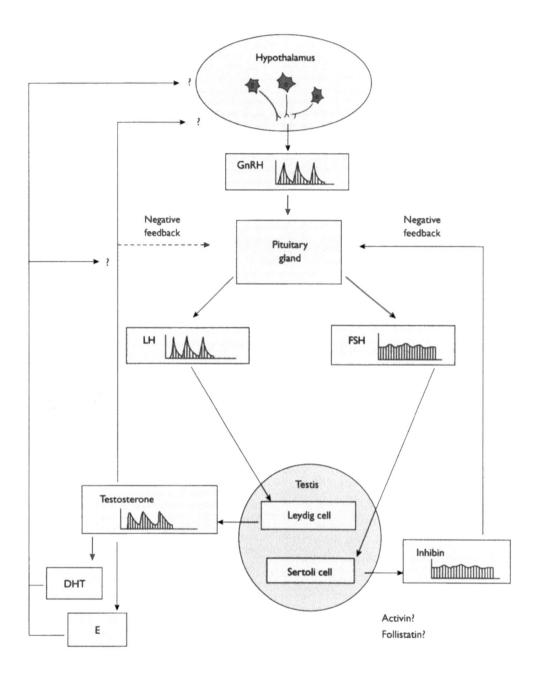

Figure 9.1 Hormonal interactions of the hypothalamic–pituitary–testicular axis. The pattern of secretion of gonadotropin releasing hormone (GnRH), luteinizing hormone (LH) and testosterone is pulsatile, whereas follicle stimulating hormone (FSH) and inhibin show non-pulsatile patterns of secretion. Solid lines indicate major sites of action and a broken line indicates a secondary site of action. Andropause is associated with asynchrony of this delicate hormonal balance. DHT, dihydrotestosterone; E, estrogen

diabetes may easily reverse some of the symptoms attributed to andropause.

The age-related decline in serum testosterone is associated with erectile dysfunction (ED). Bioavailable testosterone levels correlate significantly with nocturnal penile tumescence (NPT) (Vermeulen, 1991). Andropause is also associated with a rise in sex hormone binding globulin (SHBG), as well as a loss of the circadian (day versus night) rhythm of testosterone secretion. With more SHBG available, more testosterone is protein bound, and less is free bioactive testosterone. It is emphasized that the free bioactive testosterone is responsible for growth and sexual functions in men. The loss of the circadian rhythm results in a reduced ability of older men to cope with stress or challenging events.

This has implications for the delivery system of testosterone replacement. Testosterone administered by a skin patch or gel (transdermal form), is more favorable than injections, because absorption through the skin is more gradual and less erratic (Tan and Bransgrove, 1998).

Some 98% of testosterone, the main sex hormone in men, is bound to SHBG and albumin. Bioavailable testosterone comprises free and albumin-bound testosterone. With the onset of andropause, the albumin-bound fraction decreases while the SHBG-bound fraction increases, the free testosterone fraction remaining unchanged (Schiavi *et al.* 1993; Morley 1986; 2000; 2001) Serum testosterone levels should be evaluated in all men during andropause, but in men under the age of 50 only in those with decreased libido or physical signs suggestive of hypogonadism. Various types of testosterone supplementation have been used clinically to improve libido and to preserve bone mass, lean body mass and musculature. The two oral formulations of androgens methyltestosterone and fluoxymesterone, available in the USA, undergo significant first-pass hepatic inactivation, which decreases efficacy and increases the risk for hepatotoxicity and altered lipid metabolism. They are not recommended, for these reasons. Testosterone undecanoate, available outside the USA, has more effective results, as it is absorbed through the intestinal lymphatics, bypassing the hepatic circulation. Two available parenteral formulations of androgens, testosterone enanthate and testosterone cypionate, are effective and inexpensive (Tenover, 1992; Van den Berg and Hellstrom, 1997).

Growth hormone deficiency

Deficiency in growth hormones causes various symptoms:

(1) Reduction in lean body mass (voluntary musculature), associated with decreased overall strength and exercise performance as well as accumulation of subcutaneous fat;

(2) Lowered metabolic rate, causing further fat accumulation and possible elevated blood pressure;

(3) Increased unfavorable low-density lipoprotein (LDL) cholesterol associated with decline in favorable high-density lipoprotein (HDL) cholesterol;

(4) Loss of skin tone, associated with premature wrinkles and dry, itchy skin;

(5) Loss of bone mass, causing osteoporosis, reduced sex drive, poor general health, memory loss, hair loss and graying.

Andropause is associated with several pathophysiological changes: loss of bone and muscle mass, increased fat mass, impairment of physical, sexual and cognitive functions, loss of body hair and decreased hemoglobin levels. These changes are similar to those associated with androgen deficiency in young men.

Short-term testosterone administration is relatively safe in androgen-deficient men. The risks include erythrocytosis, induction or exacerbation of sleep apnea and breast tenderness or enlargement. Little is known about the clinical benefits or long-term risk of testosterone administration during andropause. For example, testosterone administration to older men with microscopic prostate cancer who are otherwise asymptomatic and doing well may lead to intensive monitoring of prostate-specific antigen (PSA) during the course of testosterone replacement therapy. An increase of PSA levels detected during the course of the more intensive screening dictated by the initiation of testosterone replacement therapy may necessitate a prostate biopsy, leading to the detection of subclinical prostate cancer that would have otherwise remained silent.

Molecular parameters

Androgens are synthesized from cholesterol and joined into four fused carbon rings. Because of their high cholesterol content, seafood such as oysters, shrimp

Table 9.2 Comparative effects of various testosterone supplements (parenteral depo-testosterone (DPT), Testoderm® scrotal patches (TSD) and Testoderm-TTS non-scrotal patches (TTS)) on serum testosterone, improved libido, improved energy, improved erection and discontinuation rate in patients with erectile dysfunction. (Reproduced with permission from Monga *et al.* 2002, *Arch Androl*, 48:433–42. www.tandf.co.uk/journals)

	DPT	TSD	TTS
Months of follow-up	92	38	28
Serum testosterone (ng/dl) after therapy	662	443	488
Improved libido (%)	73	38	86
Improved energy (%)	53	38	86
Improved erections (%)	40	31	57
Discontinuation rate (%)	13	73	0

and lobsters are regarded as aphrodisiacs. DHEA is the principal androgenic steroid produced by the adrenal cortex and is a precursor of both testosterone and estradiol. Adrenal androgens with little intrinsic biological activity are primarily active only after conversion in the peripheral tissues to testosterone. Most effects of androgens are mediated through an androgen receptor, a protein of 919 amino acid residues. Once androgen is bound, active transcription occurs, producing messenger RNA. Messenger RNA encodes several enzymatic, structural and receptor proteins.

Menopause versus andropause

Unlike andropause, menopause has certain specific characteristics that vary in intensity in various populations of women. After a transitional period, which lasts for 4–6 years, the symptoms of menopause are missed menstrual periods and periods that are shorter or longer, heavier or lighter than usual. Less common are hot flushes, weight gain and bloating, urinary irritation/urgency and infections, vaginal dryness, loss of sex drive, insomnia, fatigue, mood swings, inattention and forgetfulness, hair loss, joint pain and backaches. In men, the rise in FSH and LH levels is much less dramatic than in women. Therefore, the onset of andropause is much more gradual. Therapeutic prescriptions, based on individual hormone levels, include low-dose birth control pills for non-smoking women with no heart disease

risk factors. If well tolerated, they can safely be taken with some long-term protection against ovarian cancer, possibly osteoporosis and definitely pregnancy. The menopause serves a useful purpose. It provides the opportunity to enroll patients in a preventive healthcare program. Contrary to popular opinion, menopause is not a signal of impending decline, but rather a phenomenon that signals the start of something positive: a good-health program.

ERECTILE DYSFUNCTION

ED is the inability to achieve and sustain an adequate erection for sexual intercourse. The penis might be erect, but the erection may not last long enough, before it fades away.

Extensive investigations have been conducted on the etiology of ED, the effect of testosterone supplements, the endocrinology of menopause, the endocrine parameters for screening for prostate cancer and experimental animal models. Monga *et al.* (2002) evaluated the long-term efficacy of testosterone supplementation for ED, using parenteral depo-testosterone and Testoderm® scrotal patches as compared to Testoderm-TTS non-scrotal patches (Table 9.2). They reported a better response with depo-testosterone and Testoderm-TTS non-scrotal patches as compared to Testoderm scrotal patches. Testoderm-TTS non-scrotal patches were significantly better than depo-testosterone with regard to satisfaction with sexual intercourse (Figure 9.2).

Several malleable, mechanical, inflatable (self-contained) and inflatable (multi-component) devices are used for various cases of ED (Figure 9.3). These devices are inserted in the corpora cavernosa through an incision between the penis and the scrotum. The inside of each chamber in the penis is stretched open to allow placement of the device. The chambers are then closed and the skin stitched closed.

Viagra® (sildenafil)

The scale of Viagra® helped the Pfizer Pharmaceutical Company skyrocket the value of its stock. When sexual stimulation occurs, there is release of nitric oxide into the penis muscle. The inhibition of an enzyme (phosphodiesterase) by Viagra causes a marked rise of cyclic GMP and this results in increased muscle relaxation and a better erection. Viagra has no effect on the penis if there is no sexual stimulation, or when the concentrations of nitric oxide and cyclic GMP are low. Viagra does not improve libido like testosterone but may be an elegant complement to testosterone during andropause.

Viagra is available in two doses (50 mg and 100 mg) and must be taken 1 h before sexual activity. Viagra is safe, although some deaths have been reported with its use. These were men that had bad coronary disease and died of a heart attack. Sexual activity is a risk factor for heart attack in less than 1% of patients. Rare side-effects include headache, flushing, stomach problems, nasal stuffiness and abnormal vision. It may also cause a rare retinal disease.

Caverject® (alprostadil)

Caverject® is a prostaglandin to be injected into the side of the penis to achieve an erection. For some, this may be a daunting task and requires some skill and training. This prostaglandin can be inserted into the urethra, where it involves a less daunting task than penile injection, and many men prefer this. However, it is less effective than the injectable method. It has few side-effects, which include pain in the penis.

Yohimbine

Yohimbine, obtained from the bark of yohim trees, acts on adrenergic receptors in the brain and helps libido as well. Side-effects include palpitations, a fine tremor, raised blood pressure and anxiety.

Drugs not yet approved by the Food and Drug Administration

Several drugs are available in other countries but not yet approved by the Food and Drug Administration (FDA) in the USA, owing to lack of funding to promote them or to the stringent process required by the government.

Papaverine is effective in 80% of men, but it is not recommended for men with a vascular cause for their ED. Like Viagra it also increases cyclic GMP, but is less expensive.

Phentolamine (Vasomax®) is effective 40% of the time and can be potentially used alone or in combination with papaverine. Its side-effects include headache, facial flush and nasal stuffiness, causing blood pressure to drop. The FDA is evaluating Vasomax for its potential to accumulate brown fat in animal models.

Apormorphine (Uprima®) is a type of morphine that acts on the dopamine receptors in the brain. An under-the-tongue preparation will be available soon. The possible advantage of Uprima over Viagra is the faster onset of action because of quicker absorption under the tongue. Uprima is also safe in patients with coronary artery disease and hypertension.

OSTEOPENIA AND OSTEOPOROSIS

Osteopenia, a non-specific term, refers to decreased quantity of bone regardless of the cause. Osteoporosis is a condition of diminishing bone mass with subsequent atraumatic fracturing of skeletal parts. The vertebrae, hip and wrist are the most common sites of fracture. Osteopenia is regarded as the precursor or early stage of osteoporosis. Osteoporotic fractures are associated with morbidity, mortality and public health expenditure. Age-related decrements in muscle, bone and the central nervous system (CNS) are a part of normal aging, and testosterone (and other androgens) are potential 'trophic factors' that might either slow or partially reverse some of these decrements (Tenover, 1992).

The number of osteoporotic patients will increase in the future, owing to increased life expectancy. Spinal osteoporosis is eight times less likely to afflict men than women. The rate of hip fractures is two to three times lower in men than in women.

There is an age-related increase in fractures in men. Only in the past few years has the problem of osteoporosis in men represented a serious public health concern. The proximal femur is the most important site of osteoporotic fracture. The incidence of hip fractures rises exponentially in men with age. However, the age at which the increase begins is slightly older (5–10 years) in men than women. In the USA, men older than 65 years have an incidence of hip fracture of 4–5/1000, compared with 8–10/1000 in similarly aged women. Bone mineral density measurements are useful in several ways: cementing the diagnosis of low bone mass and gauging the severity of the process. Some men have osteomalacia, which is present in < 4% to 47% of men with femoral fractures. The diagnostic yield and cost effectiveness of extensive evaluation of biochemical parameters in men with 'idiopathic' osteoporosis is questionable. The remarkable histological heterogeneity among men with osteoporosis is due to different

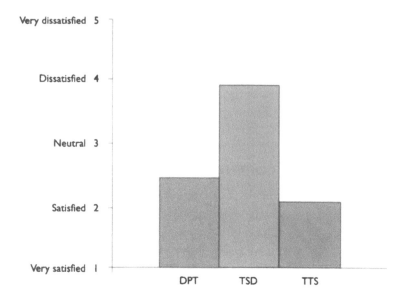

Figure 9.2 Comparative response of different testosterone supplements. DPT, depo-testosterone (Pharmacia and Upjohn, 400 mg intramuscularly 2–3 weeks); TSD, Testoderm® scrotal patches (Alza, 4–6 mg/24 h); TTS, Testoderm non-scrotal patches (Alza 5 mg/24 h). (Reproduced with permission from Monga *et al.* 2002, *Arch Androl*, 48:433–42. www.tandf.co.uk/journals)

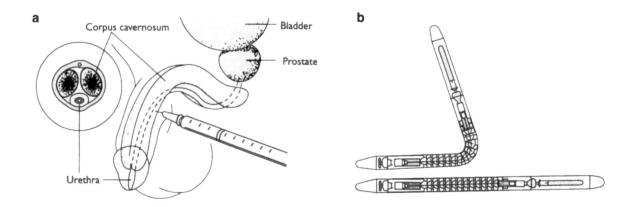

Figure 9.3 Penile anatomy and self-injection. Normal erection develops when blood flows into both corpora cavernosa within the penis. Penile self-injection is an effective technique to produce an erection by stimulating blood flow with medication injected directly into one of the corpora. After the medication is injected through a tiny needle, blood flow increases and an erection develops. (b) Mechanical penile implant. This movable device, also placed into the corpora, is easier to bend and stays in position better than the malleable penile implant. (Drawing courtesy Dacomed, Inc. Reproduced with permission from Marks, 1999)

stages of a single disease entity or separate subtypes of the disease. Several factors affect testosterone levels during andropause: genetic–environmental interactions, and psychosocial and socioeconomic factors. Plasma testosterone levels are below normal (defined as 250 ng/dl) in only 7% of men between the ages of 40 and 60. However, 20% of men between the ages of 60 and 80 have below-normal levels, and above 80 years, 35% have levels below normal (Vermeulen, 1991, 1993).

Testosterone and osteoporosis

Peak bone mass in men is achieved at age 25–29 years and declines gradually thereafter. The yearly loss of vertebral bone in healthy men is 1.3%. During late andropause more testosterone loss causes more fractures, particularly in hypogonadic men. Hence, after 80 years of age, fracture rates in men equal those of women. During late andropause, bone mineral density correlates better with serum estrogen than with testosterone. This is primarily due to amortization of testosterone. Weaker bones subsequently cause muscle atrophy; bone strength can be regained with testosterone replacement.

SUPPLEMENTATION DURING ANDROPAUSE

Administration of androgen

Flushing during andropause was first recognized in men who had experienced acute withdrawal of testosterone after bilateral orchidectomy. Testosterone falls with age in association with a parallel rise in gonadotropin concentrations. The rate of testosterone decline in men is much more gradual than is observed with estradiol in menopausal women. Men experience episodes of drenching sweats after orchidectomy that are similar to hot flushes of menopausal women, and exhibit circulatory changes similar to those in female flushing. Older men, with serum testosterone levels near or below the lower end of the normal range, may be a group in whom testosterone replacement therapy might benefit bone, muscle and psychosexual function (Tan, 1997; Tan and Bransgrove, 1997).

There are several testosterone preparations (Table 9.3). Testosterone propionate, a slow-release form of testosterone, is given by injection. Several alternative delivery systems are available: Testoderm, a patch applied to the scrotum; and Androderm, a patch applied anywhere on the skin. A gel form, Androgel is also easy to administer. The use of oral testosterone is limited because of the risk of damage to the liver. Testosterone pellets for subcutaneous implantation are not widely acceptable in elderly men. Short-acting testosterone propionate and aqueous testosterone injections are not practical for long-term use, because of the short duration of their effects.

Dosing intervals of every 2 to 3 weeks are required to maintain adequate serum levels and clinical response. Dosage and dosing intervals should be tailored to patient serum levels while on therapy. Androgen replacement using a non-scrotal permeation enhanced

Table 9.3 Testosterone preparations

	Preparation	Dosage
Oral		
Methyl testosterone	Android	10–50 mg/day
Fluoxymesterone	Halotestin	5–20 mg/day
Buccal		
Methyltestosterone	Oreton methyl	5–25 mg/day
Subcutaneous pellets		
Long-acting	Testopel	150–450 mg/3 months
Intramuscular		
Short-acting	Histerone	10–25 mg
	Tesamone	2–3 times a week
	Testandro	
Long-acting	testosterone enanthate	150–200 mg/2–4 weeks
	testosterone cypionate	
Topical		
Scrotal patch	Androderm	4–6 mg patch/22–24 h
Gel	Androgel	2.5–5 g/day

testosterone transdermal system increases the duration and rigidity of nocturnal erections, and increases libido and frequency of erections in men with hypogonadism. Testoderm TTS gives consistent improvement in symptoms including stronger libido, increased energy and consistently effective erections with the least adverse effects (Monga *et al.* 2002).

Possible risk factors of androgen administration

These include the following:

(1) Fluid retention caused by high blood pressure, edema or exacerbation of congestive heart failure;

(2) Effects of erythropoiesis (development of polycythemia);

(3) Exacerbation of sleep apnea;

(4) Changes in cardiovascular system through effects on lipoproteins and hemostasis;

(5) Effects on the prostate: promotion of benign prostatic hyperplasia (BPH) or pre-existent prostate cancer (Tenover, 1992).

Calcium supplement

When prescribing calcium, the andrologist should consider the individual patient's dietary habits and prescribe the dosage necessary to raise the daily calcium intake to the recommended level. The typical patient does not need concomitant magnesium supplementation. To minimize gastrointestinal side-effects and enhance absorption, patients should take calcium with meals and with a bedtime snack. The bedtime dosage may also counteract the parathyroid hormone-medicated calcium mobilization and excretion that occur during overnight fast.

Calcitonin may produce an analgesic effect and is useful during the immediate post-fracture period. Calcitonin is available in sterile solution for subcutaneous or intramuscular injection as well as glass bottles for nasal administration. For induction of maximal response, 100 IU/day administered subcutaneously or intramuscularly is the commonly used injection dosage. Lower dosages of 50 IU/day or 50 IU three times/week, or cyclic therapy in which the standard dosage is administered in 3-month intervals, may be used to prevent vertebral bone loss. A dosage of 300 IU/day of the nasal spray is recommended to produce the same response as 100 IU/day of the parenterally administered calcitonin.

Muscle mass

Androgens increase muscle mass by increasing the size of the muscle fibers. With testosterone replacement the myofibrils increase in number, leading to an enlargement of the muscle cell and mass. This is receptor mediated. The receptors in muscle are similar to those in the prostate. The conversion of testosterone to dihydrotestosterone is mediated by the enzyme 5α-reductase, found at very low levels in muscle.

ANDROPAUSE VERSUS MENOPAUSE: CLINICAL AND MOLECULAR PARAMETERS

There is no precise entity of andropause. Men 55–70 years of age may show a few or several symptoms: impotence, weakness, memory loss, osteoporosis, lack of intimacy and loss of muscle mass. Andropause and menopause are associated with fewer hormonal changes: an increase in the levels of FSH and LH and declines in testosterone and growth hormone levels. The estimated rate of decline in serum testosterone in aging men is 100 ng/dl per decade. A typical man of 45–70 years of age loses about 12–20 lb (5.5–9 kg) of muscle, 15% of bone mass and nearly 2 inches (5 cm) of height. Some environmental factors exert a negative impact on GnRH pulse regulation and gonadal function associated with declines in testosterone: smoking, alcohol and nutritional status.

There is a great deal of media publicity about andropause. However, little is known about the effect of lifestyle on the age of onset of andropause or the precise role of testosterone replacement. DHEA is easily available over the counter and many older men are taking this hormonal replacement. If unsupervised, testosterone replacement can lead to risks: prostrate carcinoma, atherogenesis and impotence. The age of onset of andropause is affected by confounding factors such as socioeconomic class and educational level, or by other pathophysiological mechanisms: hypertension, diabetes mellitus, cerebrovascular disease and/or memory loss. Physical stress may alter testosterone levels, as experienced by competitive athletes. In post-andropausal men, testosterone can sometimes reverse some of these responses. The effect on bone can also be influenced by testosterone.

PROSTATE PATHOPHYSIOLOGY

The prostate gland secretes a thin milky fluid which contains calcium citrate ions, phosphate ion, a clotting enzyme and a profibrinolysin. During emission, the capsule of the prostate gland contracts simultaneously with the contractions of the vas deferens so that the thin, milky fluid of the prostate gland adds further to the bulk of the semen. A slightly alkaline characteristic of the prostatic fluid may be important for successful fertilization of the ovum, because the fluid of the vas deferens is relatively acidic, owing to the presence of citric acid and metabolic end products of the sperm, consequently helping to inhibit sperm fertility. Also, the vaginal secretions of the female are acidic (pH of 3.5–4.0). Sperm do not become optimally motile until the pH of the surrounding fluids rises to about 6.0–6.5. Consequently, it is probable that the slightly alkaline prostatic fluid helps to neutralize the acidity of the other seminal fluids during ejaculation, thus enhancing the motility and fertility of the sperm.

Prostatectomy

Transurethral resection of the prostate (TURP) and radical prostatectomy may be associated with incontinence. The incidence of leakage after TURP is about 6% and after radical prostatectomy it ranges from 10 to 40%. Several pathophysiological processes may lead to post-prostatectomy incontinence and these may occur singly or in combination. General factors that may contribute include poor general cerebral function. Patients with Parkinson's diseases may have an increased risk of developing post-prostatectomy incontinence. Some specific causes of post-prostatectomy incontinence include persistent or recurrent bladder outflow obstruction. Continence after prostatectomy depends on a functioning distal urethral sphincter mechanism, since the bladder neck is generally rendered incompetent by the procedure. Secondarily, the bladder has to function as an effective low-pressure reservoir.

The close relationship between the prostatic apex and the distal sphincter mechanism is such that some degree of sphincter destruction is inevitable during prostatic resection. More significant damage to the sphincter may result if the resection is carried too far distally or as a result of diathermy or other trauma to the residual sphincter. Extensive urodynamic studies were conducted in patients who were incontinent after prostatectomy for BPH. Such patients exhibited unstable detrusor contractions.

Benign prostatic hypertrophy

The prostate can grow to many times its normal size. This growth, in part, is associated with the male hormone testosterone or its metabolites. Although not malignant, BHP can be very uncomfortable, as overgrowth of the prostate usually causes physical blockage of the urethra. This results in urinary tract problems because the urethra, which carries urine from the bladder, travels though the middle of the prostate. Also, bladder and kidney infections, as well as increased frequency of urination and discomfort, can result. BPH is diagnosed by closely examining a patient's urinary habits. Patients are often asked to keep a record or log of their urinary habits, recording any symptoms or problems and when they occur. This log provides more detailed information, and it can help a urologist evaluate a patient's symptoms. The American Urological Association has standardized this process by devising a checklist of symptoms to determine the likelihood of BPH.

Prostate cancer

The development and spread of prostate cancer is detected by the commonly used PSA test. PSA indicates if and when these PSMA appear. The presence of PSMA indicates that there are prostate cells circulating in the body. For cancer patients who have had their prostate removed, this is an indicator that cancer cells remain in the body. PSMA may be a more accurate predicator of cancer spread, because its expression is increased in hormone-refractory tumors following hormone-deprivation therapy, a common treatment for prostate-cancer patients, which seems to suppress PSA levels, possibly masking the cancer's spread. PSMA appears to be a more sensitive test, detecting cancer cells missed by PSA. Inhibin-related proteins (particularly activins) are present in the prostate, but their role in the progression to prostate cancer remains to be determined. The human prostate contains mRNAs for activin β_A and β_B subunits. The capacity to synthesize activins and follistatins has been supported by the localization of immunoreactivity for β_A and β_B subunit proteins, activin A and follistatin to the epithelial cells of men with advanced-stage carcinoma of the prostate.

Hormone-dependent cancers

For the palliative treatment of prostatic cancer, GnRH agonist therapy induces a transient rise in plasma testosterone levels during the first week of treatment, but a flare-up of disease. In a multicenter controlled study, the addition of an androgen receptor blocker, flutamide, prevented this adverse consequence of GnRH agonist treatment. The efficacy of GnRH agonists is comparable to that of surgical castration, with fewer side-effects. However, progression of tumor growth may occur despite castration.

BLADDER AND URETHRAL DYSFUNCTION

Andropause is associated with some degree of micturition disturbance. The basic types of bladder and urethral dysfunction include: disturbances of bladder control, voiding dysfunction and sphincter weakness. Incontinence is caused by aging both in the nervous system and in the lower urinary tract. Detrusor instability is the most common type of bladder dysfunction. Brain failure encompasses changes resulting from senescence as well as from disorders such as senile dementia and arteriosclerotic disease. There is an association between brain failure, incontinence and detrusor instability.

Neurological parameters

Lesions affecting the micturition pathway in the CNS above the sacral cord often results in unstable bladder activity. Where the frontal lobes of the cerebral cortex are affected by tumors, the normal sensation of bladder filling is usually lost and unstable bladder activity causes precipitant voiding. Bladder instability occurs in patients with multiple sclerosis, Parkinson's disease and Shy–Drager syndrome.

Urodynamics technology

Several laboratory techniques have been applied in urodynamics profilometry (Abrams, 1979; Abrams et al. 1979), cytometry (Farrar, 1994; Arver et al. 1996), endoscopy (Griffiths and Abrams, 1990), micturating cytography, synchronous flow cytography, uroflowmetry and electromyography. Unstable detrusor contractions are common in patients with a hypersensitive bladder. Although sphincter damage is an important factor in many cases of incontinence following prostatectomy for bladder outflow obstruction, abnormalities in bladder function are of special pathophysiological significance. Detrusor instability, poor bladder compliance and bladder hypersensitivity occur either in isolation or in combination with impaired sphincter function. Postoperative bladder dysfunction is of importance as a cause of incontinence following radical prostatectomy. However, sphincter weakness, and not bladder dysfunction, may be the principal factor leading to leakage. It would appear that the details of surgical technique are of importance in the preservation of continence after radical prostatectomy.

MODELS OF AGING IN MALE ANIMALS

The prostate gland is a seromucous gland except in the dog, where it is entirely serous. In the boar and ruminants, the prostate gland consists mostly of a disseminate portion (pars disseminata) in the form of a glandular layer in the submucosa of the pelvic urethra. In the stallion and carnivores the disseminate portion is represented only by scattered glands. The body of the prostate gland is well developed in the stallion and carnivore and is absent in the rat and billy goat (buck). It is an encapsulated, lobulated gland that partially or completely surrounds a part of the pelvic segment. In the rat, the prostate contains inhibin-related proteins. In aged mice, supplementation with DHEA sulfate (DHEAS) restores the normal responsiveness to growth factors and the capacity to elicit normal immune responses to foreign antigen, whereas in obese dogs and obese rats, DHEA reduces body weight by reducing food intake.

Animal studies demonstrate the importance of androgens for erectile function. The frequency and duration of penile erection are diminished after castration or androgen receptor blockade, and replacement of androgen in the form of testosterone restored this derangement.

Aged rats demonstrated the loss of the erectile response to external stimulation that could be restored with long-term implantation of testosterone. These animals exhibited a significant increase in the maximal intracavernosal pressure obtained following testosterone supplementation (Garban et al. 1995; Penson et al. 1996).

Androgens seem to regulate the activity of nitric oxide synthase (NOS) in penile tissue. There is a decline in NOS activity in the penis of castrated animals that can be reversed by androgen supplementation. Androgen supplements cause a dramatic increase in NOS mRNA. Testosterone induces calcium-dependent NOS (eNOS and nNOS) in several tissues in male animals. Castration decreased the levels of nNOS mRNA in the penis. Testosterone supplementation is accompanied by increases in the specific mRNAs for both eNOS and nNOS. However, stimulation of the erectile response in aged rats by androgens was not accompanied by a significant increase of penile NOS activity. Androgenic NOS expression occurs in the major pelvic ganglion in the rat (Chammness et al. 1995; Araujo et al. 1998).

Androgens may also modulate erectile response through nitric oxide-independent pathways. The molecular mechanism of the androgenic effect in the penis has also been investigated in the rat model. Testosterone stimulates cellular proliferation and DNA synthesis in the penis of castrated rats, while castration induces apoptosis of penile cavernosal tissues.

FUTURE RESEARCH

Emphasis on future research should focus on the following topics.

Functional anatomy

(1) Age-related changes in the hypothalamic–pituitary–adrenal axis, and sperm production;

(2) Changes in body composition during andropause;

(3) Body mass, bone mineral density and growth patterns of limb bones;

(4) Hormone receptors;

(5) Cell apoptosis;

(6) Mineral requirements, and calcium balance.

Pharmacokinetics of osteoporosis

(1) Biochemical measurements of bone mineral density;

(2) Genotype for fracture risk;

(3) Vitamin D: efficacy and metabolism;

(4) Fluoride: anabolic action and side-effects;

(5) Diseases that accelerate andropause;

(6) Replicative senescence.

Endocrinology, neuroendocrinology and autosomal anomalies

These include chromosomal anomalies and X chromosome anomalies.

Supplementation during andropause

(1) Need for testosterone supplementation. Comparative aspects of various supplements–those approved or still under evaluation by the FDA;

(2) Relationship between low serum levels of testosterone and ED;

(3) Efficacy of various medications for ED;

(4) Expansion of public health services to include problems of andropause;

(5) Legality of consuming drugs such as DHEA without a prescription;

(6) Risk/benefit profile for testosterone therapy in hypogonadal older men.

Experimental animal models

(1) Cellular models;

(2) Rat model;

(3) Non-rodent models;

(4) Non-human primates;

(5) Multicenter multidisciplinary future.

The negative stereotypical view of andropause is that the initial characterization is derived from men presenting with physical/psychological difficulties. The variability in andropausal reactions makes the cross-sectional study design unsuitable. More and larger longitudinal studies are needed to educate men and andrologists about the physiology and pathology of andropause.

CHAPTER 10

Stress: endocrine profile and reproductive dysfunction in men

Extensive investigations have been carried out on the biology and physiology of stress, the pathophysiology of aging, sexual dysfunction and adrenal insufficiency.

STRESS

Definition and concepts

The extensive investigations of the biology, pathophysiology and consequences of stress are reviewed in an elegant three-volume encyclopedia (Fink, 2000).

Psychological stress

Exposure to chronic and acute psychological stress may play a role in the development and/or triggering of cardiovascular pathology: coronary heart disease (impairment of cardiac function), myocardial infarction (heart attack) and myocardial ischemia (inadequate supply of blood to cardiac tissue). Cardiovascular pathologies are the interaction of physiological, environmental and behavioral factors, most of which are a function of the individual's life style, which can be modified. The activation of the autonomic nervous system induced by behavioral factors may increase the risk of cardiovascular pathologies.

Stress is a real or interpreted threat to the physiological or psychological integrity of an individual that results in physiological and/or behavioral responses (Selye, 1936, 1955). In biomedicine, stress often occurs in situations in which the adrenal glucocorticoids and catecholamines are elevated because of an experience (McEwen, 2000).

Stress involves a stressor and a stress response (Van er Kolk, 1996). A stressor may be a physical insult, such as trauma or injury, or physical exertion, particularly when the body is being forced to operate beyond its normal capacity (Mason, 1995). Other physical stressors include noise, overcrowding and excessive heat or cold. Stressors also include psychological experiences such as time-pressured tasks, interpersonal conflict, isolation and traumatic life events. These types of stressor may produce behavioral responses and evoke physiological consequences such as increased blood pressure (BP), elevated heart rate, impaired cognitive function and altered metabolism.

The physiological consequences of stress include self-damaging behaviors (such as smoking, drinking, overeating or consuming a rich diet) or risk-taking behaviors (such as driving an automobile recklessly). The physiological stress responses include the activation of the autonomic nervous system and the hypothalamic–pituitary–adrenal axis, leading to increased blood and tissue levels of catecholamines and glucocorticoids.

Experiences throughout the life course resulting in memories of particularly unpleasant or pleasant situations combined with genetic and developmental influences produce large differences among individuals in how they react to stress and what the long-term consequences may be.

Stress causes disturbance of homeostasis of the body by entropic forces (Bornstein and Chrousos, 1999; Bornstein and Ehrhart-Bornstein, 1999). The individual displays a complex set of behavioral and physical

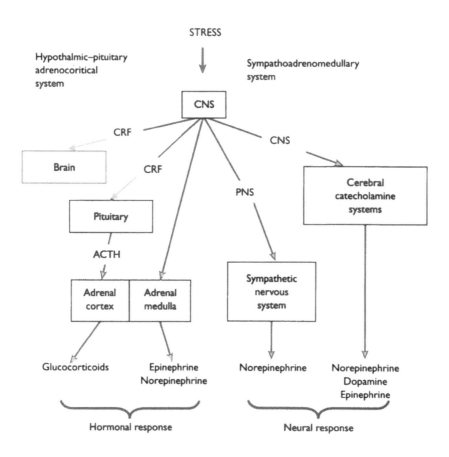

Figure 10.1 The hypothalamic–pituitary–adrenocortical and sympathoadrenomedullary systems. The central noradrenergic system is activated in parallel with the peripheral (PNS) sympathetic nervous system and is considered a central nervous system (CNS) counter-part. The cerebral catecholaminergic system (i.e. dopamine and epinephrine (adrenaline)) is also activated in stress. CRF, corticotropin releasing factor; ACTH, adrenocorticotropic hormone

reactions to stressors: adaptive responses to re-establish balanced physiological conditions (Chrousos, 1998). Stress may be a transient and time-limited state, well balanced by the adaptive responses of the organism, whereas excessive and prolonged stress may alter the physiological and behavioral defense mechanisms, rendering them inefficient or deleterious (Willenberg *et al.* 2000a).

Although stress and emotion are two different enti-ties, they both create physiological responses: increased perspiration, heart rate and arousal (Golberger and Breznitz, 1993). Stress is induced when the individual is in a difficult social situation (e.g. making a public speech), whereas emotion is induced by the feeling in words, pictures or films.

Stress-induced pathological conditions such as burnout and chronic fatigue are associated with memory impairments, which can be temporary or permanent.

Stress plays a major role in the progression of infec-tious diseases, by exerting a profound effect via the central nervous system (CNS) on the immune system, including the mechanisms necessary for resistance to microbial infections. Many response signals are medi-ated by soluble factors, such as cytokines produced by lymphoid cells of the immune system as well as factors important in control of the CNS, including steroids, neuropeptides and neurohormones produced by neu-ronal cells (Figure 10.1). The antimicrobial activities of monocytes/macrophage are depressed by the stabiliza-tion of lysomes by steroids, which prevents their fusion

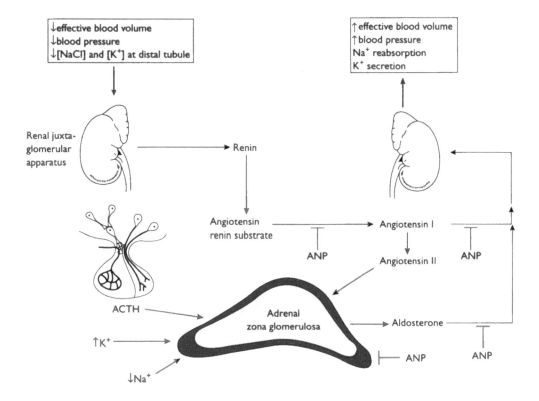

Figure 10.2 Regulation of the renin–angiotensin–aldosterone axis. ANP, atrial natriuretic peptide; ACTH, adrenocorticotropic hormone. (From Beishuizen, personal communication)

with phagosomes. Stress is also associated with increased risk of upper respiratory viral infection.

Acute mental stress is linked to myocardial ischemia and clinical coronary events such as heart attack or sudden death. Psychosocial risk factors for developing heart disease include accessibility to social and economic resources, the work environment and stressful life circumstances (Baker *et al.* 2000).

Anxiety and depression

Anxiety and depression are caused by complex alterations of the hypothalamic–pituitary–thyroid axis; of prolactin, growth hormone (GH) and melatonin irregularity; of sleep, activity, appetite and temperature disturbance; of the hypothalamic–pituitary–gonadal axis and dysregulation of the hypothalamic–pituitary–adrenal axis; and of multiple neurotransmitter disequilibrium. Stress and powerful emotions during everyday life play a role in the precipitation of mood disorders. Men are less susceptible than women to all forms of depression. Chronic subthreshold depression (dysthymia) and episodic major depressive disorder are at least twice as common in women as they are in men (Seeman, 2000). In childhood, depressive episodes are as frequent in boys as they are in girls.

Stress causes post-traumatic stress disorder (PTSD), or somatic realm, as in the various psychophysiological disorders. Both forms are more prevalent in women. When exposed to a major trauma, approximately twice as many women as men develop PTSD. Both sexes are subject to pulsatile changes in hormone levels and circadian fluctuations. It is not until old age, when the testes stop producing testosterone, that the hormonal environment of the male brain and the female brain approach the par that existed prior to puberty. Hormones determine how the male and female brains process experiences (Seeman, 2000).

Stress and blood pressure

There are remarkable individual differences in the response of BP; to stress. Some individuals may show essentially no change in BP; others may respond with an increase of 60 mmHg or more to exactly the same stressor. There are remarkable inter-relationships among BP, cardiac output and systemic vascular resistance (SVR). Since BP is the product of cardiac output and SVR, the concurrent measurement of BP and cardiac output permits the derivation of SVR, providing a more complete description of the hemodynamic response (Sherwood and Carels, 2000).

Acute stress causes a significant rise in BP for brief periods, within the range of 'hypertension' (Figure 10.2). The risk of hypertension development may be related to stress reactivity. Hypertensive individuals show greater BP reactivity than normotensives. There is some hereditary background for this phenomenon. Black men who are at increased risk for hypertension exhibit abnormally elevated vascular tone, indexed by SVR during exposure to several stressors. Men are more likely to develop hypertension than premenopausal women.

Stress can modify renal function, leading to sodium and fluid retention in some individuals, which may heighten and prolong stress-induced BP elevations. Altered function of the kidneys may be one of the target-organ effects of stress that could impact on long-term BP (Sherwood and Carels, 2000).

Stress and disease

Enlarged pituitary/adrenals cause pseudo-Cushing's syndrome manifestation, osteoporosis and opportunistic infections. Similar symptoms are noted in chronic active alcoholism, in anorexia nervosa, in individuals sexually abused in their youth and in obsessive–compulsive disorders. Stress also causes disturbance of the immunological hemostasis involving three major inflammatory cytokines: tumor necrosis factor-α, interleukin-1 and interleukin-6, produced at sites of inflammation to stimulate the hypothalamic–pituitary–adrenal axis.

The stress system utilizes several mechanisms that affect immune homeostasis. Besides the suppressive effect of glucocorticoids on the production of tumor necrosis factor-α, interleukin-1 and interleukin-6, glucocorticoids also inhibit the target tissue responses to cytokines through suppression of nuclear transcription factor-kB and AP-1 (Willenberg et al. 2000a, 2000b). In cases of hypersensitivity or hyposensitivity to stressors, disorders characterized by altered perception of signals to the stress system cause inefficient responses to natural challenges, with consequent development of secondary diseases. Several diseases such as Cushing's syndrome or Addison's disease cause disintegration of the stress system, which fails to mount an adaptive response.

Stress and nutrition

There are several interactions between stress and nutrition, and nutrition insecurity is one of the stressors in men who thrive to maintain optimal nutritional intake (McGrady, 1984). Malnutrition leads to immune dysfunction, including significant decline in CD4+ T lymphocytes, a syndrome similar to immunodeficiency in AIDS patients.

Malnutrition is also associated with several infections related to cytokine release, which leads to activation of the stress response. Thus, deficient nutritional intake is associated with both psychological and physical stressors. Approximately two-thirds of men become anorectic when stressed, whereas one-third overeat. Bulimia (binge eating, which may be associated with subsequent vomiting) is often precipitated by a traumatic event. Anorexia nervosa represents a classic pathological example of intrapsychic stress resulting in severe weight loss. Anorexia nervosa causes elevated levels of corticotropin releasing factor (CRF) in the cerebrospinal fluid.

The effects of nutrition as a stressor and stress alleviator, as a response to food ingestion increase or decrease, depends on the nature and duration of stress. Several psychiatric diseases, such as depression and anorexia nervosa, produce alterations in food intake secondary to activation of the classic stress response. Obesity is associated with several psychological stressors. Release of stress hormones, such as cortisol, can alter fat deposition, resulting in an increase in visceral obesity. Visceral obesity is associated with an increase in diabetes mellitus, hypertension, myocardial infarction, stroke and mortality (Morley, 2000). Aging is a physiological stressor that is associated with anorexia (Figure 10.3).

Dopamine induces chewing behaviors, whereas opioids are involved in ingestive behaviors. The endogenous system (dynorphin) and corticotropin releasing hormone (CRH) are neurotransmitters, playing a role in the alterations in ingestive behavior produced by stress. A number of diseases have a predominant component of altered food ingestion, such as anorexia nervosa and bulimia.

Behavior therapy

Behavior therapy is a system of psychotherapy that views mental disorders as products of maladaptive learning, which are best treated by techniques derived from classical and instrumental conditioning principles.

Progressive relaxation is applied clinically to various medical disorders in which indicators of stress, such as sustained autonomic arousal or chromic muscle tension, are present. This is effective in the treatment of anticipatory nausea associated with chemotherapy, tinnitus, insomnia, low back pain, hypertension and tension headache. Evaluation of the specific contribution of progressive relaxation in treating these conditions is often complicated by the inclusion of other potentially therapeutic components in the treatment protocols (Orne and Whitehouse, 2000). Relaxation may lower the blood pressure, but the magnitude of the effect depends on the extent to which stress played a role in the first place. Classical progressive relaxation may not be appropriate for certain disorders, owing to its potential for exacerbating symptoms. For example, in some men suffering from tension headache or myofascial pain disorders, the practice of alternately tensing and relaxing relevant muscle groups actually increased their pain. When such complications arise, progressive relaxation can be modified to omit the muscle contraction component of the exercises, as a means to sensitize patients to the presence of tension in their bodies (Orne and Whitehouse, 2000). All hypnotic phenomena that can be elicited through suggestions administered by a therapist can also be induced by the patient using self-hypnosis. This is because heterohypnosis is fundamentally self-hypnosis, and *vice versa*. That is, the experience of hypnosis requires an appropriately hypnotizable individual who is motivated to accomplish the goals targeted by select therapeutic suggestions, administered in a distinctively hypnotic context (Orne and Whitehouse, 2000).

Molecular parameters

Stress involves several molecular mechanisms: cytokines, macrophages and substance P. Cytokines are soluble proteins of low molecular weight released by immune cells during the course of an immune response. They serve to mediate and regulate the amplitude and duration of immune/inflammatory responses. Cytokines exert their action by binding to target cell surface receptors, which may be on the surface of the secreting cell (autocrine action), on the surface of a nearby cell (paracrine action), or in the circulation (endocrine action). Macrophages, irregularly shaped white blood cells, are the major differentiated cells of the mononuclear phagocyte system. Substance P, a member of the tachykinin family of neuropeptides, has several immunological functions. Circulating levels of substance P become elevated in stressful situations.

Heat shock proteins and stress

Heat shock proteins (hsp) include several families of proteins found across species and are classified depending on their molecular size (in kilodaltons) into hsp16–30, hsp60, hsp70 and hsp90. They regulate cell and tissue homeostasis and are protective when this is threatened by stressors (Willenberg et al. 2000a, 2000b). The major stress system is located in the hypothalamus and the brain stem, the phylogenetically oldest parts of the brain. These centers receive information from internal and external origins and compute appropriate responses, which are effected by two main pathways: the endocrine hypothalamic–pituitary–adrenal axis and the neural systemic sympathetic–adrenomedullary and parasympathetic systems (Willenberg et al. 2000a, 2000b). Their central regulators and peripheral end-products, CRH, glucocorticoids and catecholamines, are key hormones in the re-establishment and maintenance of cardiovascular, metabolic, immune and behavioral homeostasis.

Nitric oxide

Nitric oxide (NO) plays a pivotal role in the function (including stress, aging and response to infection) of every organ system of the body. The acetylcholine-producing interneurons in the hypothalamus release acetylcholine that stimulates a muscarinic-type receptor, which in turn stimulates CRH release from the CRH neurons. Neural NO synthase (nNOS) is located in neurons in the paraventricular nucleus (PVN) of the hypothalamus. Stimulated CRH release can be blocked by N^G-monomethyl-L-arginine (NMMA), a

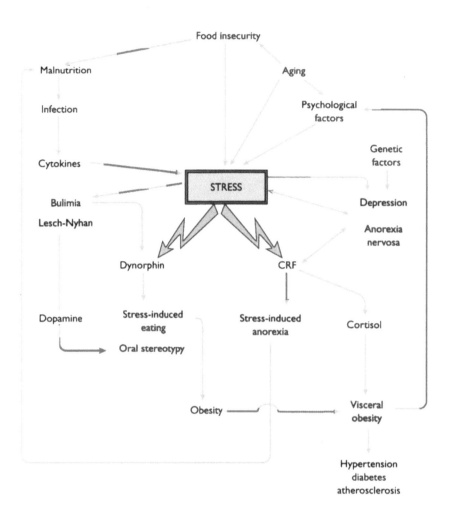

Figure 10.3 Nutrition and stress interrelate at multiple levels. Nutritional factors can produce stress and stress can lead to under- or overnutrition. Eventually a vicious cycle develops. CRF, corticotropin releasing factor. (Reproduced with permission from Morley, 2000)

competitive inhibitor of all forms of NOS. Consequently, CRH release from the neurons in the PVN is stimulated by cholinergic neurons that synapse on these NOergic neurons to activate NOS. NOS synthasizes NO that diffuses into the CRH neurons and activates CRH lease by activating cyclo-oxygenase I (COX-I), leading to the generation of prostaglandin E_2 (PGE_2) from arachidonate Vingerhoets and van Heck, 1990; McCann *et al.* 1994, 1998; Young, 1995; Stoney *et al.* 1987; Scanlan *et al.* 1998; McCann, 2000).

PEG_2 activates CRH via activation of adenylyl cyclase and generation of cyclic adenosine monophosphate (cAMP). cAMP activates protein kinase A, which induces exocytosis of CRH secretory granules into the hypophyseal portal vessels, activating ACTH release from the corticotrophs of the anterior pituitary gland. NO activates not only COX but also lipoxygenase (LOX), which plays a role in activation of CRH release (McCann *et al.* 1994, 1998; Wong *et al.* 1996; River, 1998; McEwen, 2000).

AGING

Extensive investigations have been conducted on biological aging, population aging, psychological aging and senescence (Gurland, 1983; Salzman and Leibowitz, 1991; Birren *et al.* 1992; Gatz *et al.* 1996; Lithgow, 1996; Fink, 2000). Biological aging refers to progressive

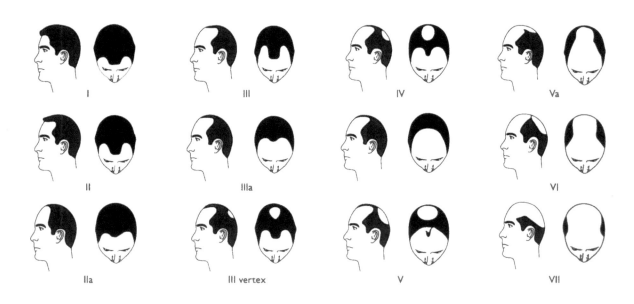

Figure 10.4 Hamilton–Norwood scale for androgenetic alopecia in males. (Reproduced with permission from Roberts, 2001)

deleterious changes occurring throughout adult life (Figures 10.4 and 10.5). Population aging is evaluated by the slope of the line relating the logarithm of mortality rate to age, expressed by the mortality rate doubling time about 8 years for humans and 3 months for laboratory mice. Population aging reflects the time-related changes in the age structure of populations. Owing to a combination of increased life expectancy and reduced birth rates, the relative and absolute numbers of old people has greatly increased. Psychological aging reflects the changes in behavior and mental processes that arise as individuals progress through life. Cellular senescence reflects the phenotype of those cells that are usually capable of mitosis but, after a number of cycles of cell division, have lost the ability to replicate but are not undergoing apoptosis (Horan and Little, 1998; Horan, 2000; Horan *et al.* 2000).

The rate of aging is governed by the rate of accumulation of macromolecular damage. Damage accumulates when repair or degradation of damaged molecules cannot keep pace with the rate of damage, which itself is determined by the production of damaging agents (e.g. reactive oxygen species (ROS)) and their subsequent detoxification (e.g. by antioxidant free enzymes). The decline in function and increasing mortality rate

associated with aging are due to ROS production and their subsequent reaction with cellular components, causing irreparable damage. It would appear that the aging rate is related to resistance to cellular stress. Oxidative damage is caused by free radicals generated mainly as a by-product of metabolism, by solar radiation, by a variety of stressors that elicit the heat shock response and by other toxic factors from the environment.

Survival depends on the ability of cells to sustain homoeostasis by being able to adapt to and/or resist stressors; and to repair or replace damaged molecules/ organelles. Some 4% of oxygen consumed by mitochondria is converted to the reactive peroxide and superoxide during oxidative phosphorylation. Aging individuals possess several defenses against oxidative stress including the small molecules uric acid, glutathione, ascorbic acid and vitamin E. Oxidative stress induces the synthesis of several antioxidant enzymes including superoxide dismutase (SOD), catalase and glutathione peroxidase.

Elderly population explosion

In 50 years, one out of three people will be older than 60. Those two billion seniors would outnumber the world's youth. Gain in longevity could bring worldwide

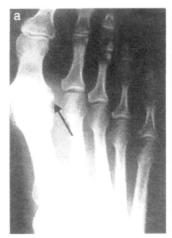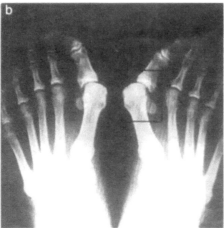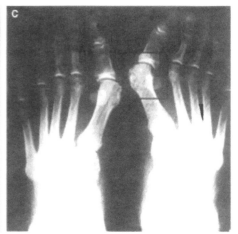

Figure 10.5   (a) Hallux rigidus joint space narrowing: arrow indicates dorsolateral osteophytes. (b and c) Severe hallux valgus deformity in a 68-year-old man: (b) weight-bearing. Note the aggravation of dislocation at the metatarsophalangeal joint; (c) non-weight-bearing. (From Dereymaeker and Mievis, personal communication)

economic crisis. With the population's proportion of taxpaying workers shrinking, national budgets could be overwhelmed in trying to provide retirement and health benefits for the elderly. Aging populations will significantly change patterns of savings, investment and consumption, labor markets, pensions, taxation, health care, family composition and living arrangements, housing and migration. In the developing world, the pace of aging is faster than in developed countries. The ramifications could be serious, as the elderly become an additional burden along with traditional scourges of disease and poverty. There are several aging-related issues that all governments should address: retirement and age flexibility; living with dependency; elderly benefits; technology and the aging process; and death matters such as euthanasia.

On the Internet

(1)   Second World Assembly on Aging: *www.madrid 2002-envejecimiento.org*

(2)   UN aging site: *www.un.org/partners/civil_society/ m-age.htm*

Pathophysiological and psychological aging

Aging is associated with several pathophysiological and psychological changes as well as various levels of depressive and anxiety symptomatology. Life expectancy has consistently been lower for men than for women. Consequently, the elderly population is composed of more women than men. Aging-related changes include losses in the sense of balance and movement, poorer hearing and vision, slower reactions and weaker muscles. Conditions such as heart disease, cancer, respiratory infection and kidney failure may arise. There are also losses in relationships, because of retirement, widowhood, or death of age-peers such as siblings or friends. Depression is the most common psychopathological disorder of aging. The American Psychiatric Association published the *Diagnostic/Statistical Manual of Mental Disorders* (DSM). The major depressive disorder involves significant depressed mood and loss of interest in activities in combination with three or four additional symptoms (loss of appetite, sleep disturbance, fatigue, feelings of worthlessness; these symptoms are not to be physiologically caused by a general medical condition and must extend for at least two weeks).

Anxiety disorders as described in the DSM include:

(1)   Panic disorders recurring in sudden episodes of intense apprehension, palpitations, shortness of breath and chest pain;

(2)   Phobias: fears and avoidance out of proportion to danger;

(3) Obsessive–compulsive disorder, consisting of repetitive thoughts, images or impulses experienced as intrusive, or of repetitive behaviors performed according to certain rules or in a stereotyped fashion;

(4) Generalized anxiety disorder: chronic and persistent.

Several pathological changes occur during depression: dysregulation of the monoamine system, increased monoamine oxidase activity, deficits in norepinephrine (noradrenaline) functioning, down-regulation of serotonin receptors and deep white–gray-matter disease. Age-related decreases in noradrenergic function provide one plausible biological mechanism that increases the predisposition towards late-onset anxiety (Penninx and Deeg, 2000).

Depression and anxiety are more common in older persons with unfavorable socioeconomic circumstances, such as low income or education. Minor depression has been associated with various different chronic diseases, such as lung disease, arthritis, cancer, stroke and myocardial infarction. Feelings of anxiety and depression are more frequent in older patients with osteoarthritis, rheumatoid arthritis and stroke as opposed to patients with heart disease, diabetes and lung disease. Physical disability may play an explanatory role in this disparity across diseases. Psychological stressors cause several physiological changes: altered autonomic balance, increased hypothalamic–pituitary–adrenal axis function, elevated resting heart rate and BP, decreased heart rate variability, increased ventricular arrhythmias and myocardial ischemia, hypersecretion of the adrenal steroid cortisol, adrenal hypertrophy and an increased cortisol response to adrenocorticotropic hormone (ACTH). Depressed persons engage less in physical activities such as walking and gardening and vigorous exercise activities such as sports.

Survival depends on the continuous provision of all body cells with fluid, oxygen, minerals, nutrients and the uninterrupted elimination of metabolic waste products to provide the cells and tissues with the essential conditions necessary for life. An intact vascular system is necessary to ensure these vital conditions; intact vascular and microvascular blood flow is a primary prerequisite. Circulatory failure has several symptoms: hypertension and tachycardia, measured eventually in the supine and sitting positions.

Endocrine and metabolic aging

Aging is associated with stimulation of sympatho-adrenal and hypothalamic–pituitary–adrenal systems together with secretion of glucagon and the pituitary hormones (GH), prolactin and vasopressin. In contrast, there is suppression of adrenal androgen production, and complex changes take place in the hypothalamic–pituitary–gonadal and hypothalamic–pituitaty–thyroid axes that lead to lower concentrations of some of their end hormones. The metabolites glycogen and fat are broken down so that the concentrations of glucose, lactate, non-esterified fatty acids (NEFA), glycerol and ketone bodies increase in the plasma. Persistence of stressful stimuli cause net protein breakdown in muscle, while in the liver the synthesis of plasma proteins known as the acute-phase reactants (APR) is induced (Horan and Little, 1998; Horan, 2000; Horan *et al.* 2000).

Growth hormone and aging

Human GH (hGH) is one of many endocrine hormones, like estrogen, progesterone testosterone, melatonin and dehydroepiandrosterone (DHEA), that decline with age. From the age of 20 to 70, GH levels in the body fall by more than 75%. Practically everyone over the age of 40 has a GH deficiency. Studies were undertaken in men between the ages of 61 and 80 who were overweight. These men did not alter their diet, exercise, or smoking habits. When they were given hGH, they gained an average of 8.8% in lean muscle mass while losing 14% of their body fat. They experienced localized increases in bone density and their skin became thicker and firmer. The subjects of this study reversed these parameters of aging by 10–20 years.

Supplements

There are several safe, effective, natural elements including glutamine, ginkgo biloba and grape seed that will stimulate the release of hGH. The problem has been that many of these elements are destroyed during digestion or trapped by the liver before the body can experience their benefits. The oral spray (sublingual) has an 8–9 times higher absorption rate than hGH pills. 'HGH Gold' is available at Cambridge Research Labs, Dept. HGH 256, 110 Vista Center Drive, Forest, VA 24551, USA, Tel: 800 456 2466.

Immunosenescence

There are two types of immunity: interactive innate (natural) immunity and acquired (adoptive or specific) immunity. Innate immunity involves polymorphonuclear leukocytes (neutrophils, eosinophils, basophils), natural killer (NK) cells and mononuclear phagocytes and uses the complement cascade as its main soluble protein effector mechanism. Immunosenescence (immunoaging) is a state of immunodeficiency that predisposes the individual to infections diseases and probably neoplasms. This condition may be associated with thymus gland involution, and is characterized by decreased proliferation of T lymphocytes and impaired T-helper activity, which lead to impaired cell-mediated and humoral responses to T cell-dependent antigens.

Cytokines regulate many cell types including cells of the immune system. In mice, aging has a pronounced effect on the pattern of cytokine secretion. In the young, interleukin (IL)-2 and IL-4 predominate, whereas in the old it is IL-10 and interferon-γ. Age-related changes in several body systems predispose to more general types of presentation known as the giants of geriatrics: immobility, falls, delirium and incontinence (Horan and Little, 1998; Horan, 2000; Horan *et al.* 2000).

Immunity ages throughout life: immune cell generation by the hematopoietic progenitor population diminishes while the ability of lymphoid/myeloid cells to perform their functions is blunted, owing to biochemical and molecular failures. The thymus gland atrophies after puberty and lumphokinesis (the flow of lymph through the lymphatic system and thus the transit of lymphocytes via the blood and lymph circulatory systems) declines.

Cellular and humoral immunity communicate via cytokines – growth factors produced by the diverse immune cell populations. These peptides are critical intercellular signaling molecules. They bring about multidirectional communication among immune cells, as well as cells from other systems of the organism; engage in host defense, healing and repair; and restore homeostasis (Chiappelli and Liu, 2000).

Heat shock proteins and aging

Aging is affected by heat shock proteins (hsp), stress proteins and antioxidants. On the other hand, aging

affects the extent to which stress proteins are synthesized in response to various stressors. The magnitude of the induced response declines with age and senescence. Such responses depend on the activation of the hypothalamic–pituitary–adrenal axis and the sympathetic nervous system. Heat shock proteins play a major role in the cellular actions of glucocorticoids, the archetypal stress hormones.

Heat shock proteins are produced by a family of highly conserved genes, found from bacteria to mammalian cells, that are rapidly transcribed and translated in cells and tissues exposed to various stressors. Heat shock protein genes are regulated by heat shock transcription factors (HSF), which are sensitive to several stressors. The hsp facilitate the disassembly and disposal of damaged proteins and the folding, transport and insertion of newly synthesized proteins into cellular organelles. The expression of hsp genes is sufficient to increase resistance to thermal stress (thermotolerance) in several situations (Horan and Little, 1998; Horan, 2000; Horan *et al.* 2000).

Aging and nutrition

Over the life span there is some 30% decrease in food intake due to a decrease in the central opioid feeding drive. There are peripheral alterations in adaptive relaxation of the fundus of the stomach due to decreased NOS activity. This leads to early antral filling and a greater degree of satiation for a given amount of ingested food. (Morley, 2000). Aging puts older men at greater risk for developing severe anorexia and weight loss when exposed to stressors.

Apoptosis

Apoptosis (programmed cell death) is a genetically controlled response for removing unwanted cells, which is triggered by various signals, including DNA damage, lack of survival factors and interaction of specific ligands with receptors that contain the 'death domain' (Besedovsky and del Rey, 1996; Chiappelli and Liu, 2000).

Hormone replacement therapy

Older men are treated with different types of testosterone replacement: injectables, transdermals, scrotal

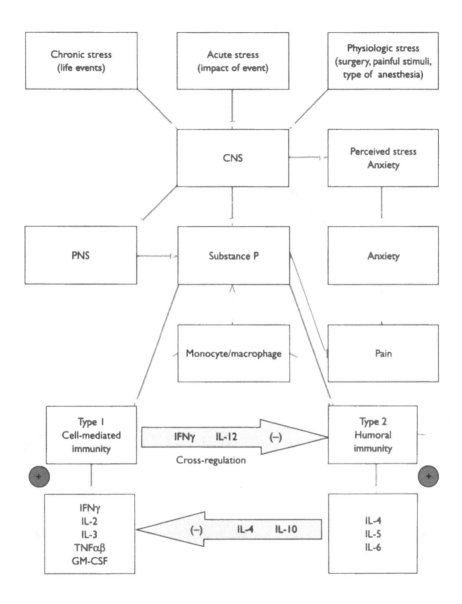

Figure 10.6 Interaction between endocrine system, immune system, stress and aging

patches (with or without enhancers), gels oral forms and testosterone undecanoate (not available in the USA). Other selected medications include tricyclic antidepressants, selective serotonin reuptake inhibitors, seratonin antagonist reuptake inhibitors, serotonin–norepinephrine reuptake inhibitors and dopamine reuptake inhibitors.

ENDOCRINE PROFILES

Figure 10.6 illustrates the interaction between the endocrine system, immune system, stress and aging.

Adrenal hormones

The adrenal axis is a complex of three cell types:

(1) Specialized cells in the hypothalamus that secrete the neuroendocrine peptide CRH;

(2) Cells in the anterior pituitary that secrete ACTH;

(3) The adrenal gland that secretes glucocorticoid and mineralocorticoid hormones in response to ACTH (Table 10.1).

Table 10.1   Pathological conditions associated with altered activity of the hypothalamic–pituitary–adrenal (HPA) axis. (Reproduced with permission from Chrousos, 1998)

Increased HPA activity	Decreased HPA activity	Disrupted HPA activity
Severe chronic disease	Atypical depression	Cushing's syndrome
Melancholic depression	Seasonal depression	Glucocorticoid deficiency
Anorexia nervosa	Chronic fatigue syndrome	Glucocorticoid resistance
Obsessive–compulsive disorder	Hypothyroidism	
Panic disorder	Adrenal suppression	
Chronic excessive exercise Malnutrition	Obesity (hyposerotinergic forms)	
Diabetes mellitus	Nicotine withdrawal	
Hyperthyroidism	Vulnerability to inflammatory disease (Lewis rat)	
Central obesity	Rheumatoid arthritis	
Childhood sexual abuse	Premenstrual tension syndrome	
Pregnancy	Postpartum mood and inflammatory disorders	
	Vulnerability to alcoholism	

The adrenal gland as the end-organ of the hypothalamic–pituitary–adrenal axis is subject to functional changes following stress. It responds quite rapidly to sustained stimulation with hypertrophy and hyperplasia, which can be monitored at the ultrastructural and molecular levels. In chronic stress, high levels of glucocorticoids and relatively low levels of ACTH are frequently observed. This dissociation between central activation of the hypothalamic–pituitary–adrenal axis and adrenal cortex function represents an adaptation to stress, whereby medullary input and hypertrophy and hyperplasia of the zona fasciculata of the adrenal cortex sustain elevated glucocorticoid secretion in the presence of low-normal ACTH concentrations (Willenberg *et al.* 2000a, 2000b).

Adrenocorticotropic hormone

ACTH and other peptides, including β-endorphin, a peptide known for its analgesic and euphoric effects in the brain, are produced in the pituitary from the chemical breakdown of a large precursor protein, proopiomelanocortin (Rhodes, 2000). The first 16 amino acids beginning with the N-terminal amino acid are all that is required for minimal biological activity. The regulation of ACTH secretion primarily involves the stimulatory effect of the hypothalamic hormones, CRH and AVP, and the inhibitory effect of glucocorticoids. Angiotensin II, catecholamines and immune factors have been shown to stimulate ACTH secretion. Novel stressors activate the

hypothalamic–pituitary–adrenal axis; with repeated encountering of the stressor, there is less and less response (Rhodes, 2000). The hypothalamic–pituitary–adrenal axis is regulated by two primary processes. One is 'closed-loop' negative feedback of cortisol to hormone receptors in the hippocampus, hypothalamus and pituitary gland. There are three types of 'closed-loop' negative feedback systems. In the 'long-loop' system, glucocorticoids exert a negative feedback on the anterior pituitary, hypothalamus and hippocampus. With the 'short-loop' system, ACTH itself feeds back on the hypothalamus, exerting negative feedback. With the 'ultrashort' system, the releasing hormone (CRH) acts directly on the hypothalamus to control its own secretion (Rhodes, 2000).

Adrenal insufficiency

Regardless of the etiology, adrenal insufficiency is characterized by hypocortisolism and/or the lesion that causes adrenal hypofunction, isolated or combined impairment of adrenal hormone secretion. The syndrome could be 'primary' due to 'adrenal', secondary due to 'pituitary' or 'tertiary' due to 'hypothalamus'. All forms of primary adrenal insufficiency are referred to as Addison's disease, where some 90% of the adrenal cortex is destroyed.

Autoimmune destruction of the adrenal glands is the most common cause of primary adrenal insufficiency. The destruction of the adrenal cortex can also be the consequence of chronic infectious diseases, such as tuberculosis, AIDS, toxoplasmosis and histoplasmosis.

Adrenal medulla

The adrenal medulla functions in concert with the sympathetic nervous system or it may function independently in meeting the homeostatic demands presented by stressful stimuli. The adrenal medulla secretes a complex of neuropeptides that exert effects within the adrenal medulla and throughout the body. The adrenal medulla is innervated by preganglionic sympathetic nerve terminals that release acetylcholine and various co-localized peptides, including substance P (Goldstein, 1995; Papanicolaou, 1997; Chrousos, 1998; Bornstein and Chrousos, 1999; Bornstein and Ehrhart-Bornstein, 1999).

Systemic sympathetic–adrenomedullary and parasympathetic systems

This axis originates from mostly norepinephrine cell groups of the locus ceruleus, medulla and pons. Efferent projections of these neurons terminate throughout the brain and spinal cord as well as in the peripheral ganglia of the autonomic nervous system. These systems perform various functions affecting cardiovascular tone, respiration and skeletal muscle movement. Certain stressors stimulate the hypothalamic–pituitary–adrenal axis producing adrenal corticosteroid secretions, followed by consequential increases in serum glucocorticoids and activation of the sympathetic nervous system, followed by the release of catecholamines.

Impairment of hypothalamic–pituitary–testicular function

In men, social stress may result in low testosterone secretion and oligoasthenozoospermia, which may remain undetected unless infertility issues arise. Severe male hypogonadism may include a decreased libido, diminished muscle mass and change in hair growth. While social stress-induced perturbations in gonadotropin releasing hormone (GnRH) pulsatility are a likely mechanism, direct effects of cortisol and serotonin on testicular function have to be considered (Shively, 2000).

Gonadotropin releasing hormone and gonadotropins

GnRH is a peptide with ten amino acid residues. It is synthesized in the hypothalamus and is transported by axonal flow to axon terminals within the median eminence, where it is released into capillaries. These capillaries collect into the long portal veins, which descend along the pituitary stalk to terminate in a second capillary plexus within the anterior pituitary gland. This direct vascular connection between the hypothalamus and the anterior pituitary gland allows for the rapid transport of undiluted hypothalamic GnRH to its target, the gonadotrope. Gonadotropins are released intermittently, in a pulsatile manner; each pulse of luteinizing hormone (LH) consists of an abrupt and brief release of the hormone from the gonadotrope into the peripheral circulation, followed by its exponential decrease, according to enzymatic degradation. A GnRH pulse generator is a structure responsible for the co-ordinated pulsatile secretion by the GnRH neurons (Ferin, 2000).

The development of the thymus is intertwined with the regulation of gonadal, adrenocortical, pituitary and other hormones. Hormones produced by the pituitary and adrenocortical glands have powerful modulating effects on immunity. Lymphoid organs are innervated with peptidergic and non-peptidergic neurons that secrete neurotransmitters locally and may carry information about the activated immune state of the organ to the brain by retrograde transport (Chiappelli and Liu, 2000).

The PVN is one of the main hypothalamic areas involved in the response to stress. CRH and vasopressin are produced in the parvocellular portion of the PVN. Stress increases the activity of CRH and vasopressin immunoreactive neurons in this nucleus. Little is known about the role of CRH of specific PVN origin in influencing LH secretion in stress.

Nitric oxide

Norepinephrine, glutamic acid and oxytocin stimulate LH releasing hormone (LHRH) release by activation of nNOS. The pathway is as follows: oxytocin and/or glutamic acid activate norepinephrine neurons in the medial basal hypothalamus that activate NOergic neurons by α_1-adrenergic receptors. The NO released diffuses into LHRH terminals and induces LHRH release by the activation of guanylyl cyclase and COX. In contrast to the NO stimulation of LHRH release, it has no effect on FSH release mediated by the FSH-releasing factor.

nNOS is present in folliculostellate cells, a cell type of the anterior pituitary not previously thought to produce hormones, but now known to produce several cytokines. nNOS has also been found in LH gonadotrophs (McCann *et al.* 1994, 1998; McCann, 2000). NO produced by this nNOS in the pituitary regulates pituitary hormone secretion. NO inhibits prolactin secretion: the principal prolactin-inhibiting hormone, dopamine, apparently acts on cell surface D2 receptors on folliculostellate cells to activate NOS followed by NO production.

The CNS pathology in AIDS patients bears a striking resemblance to aging changes and may also be largely caused by the action of iNOS. Antioxidants, such as melatonin, vitamin C and vitamin E, probably play an important acute and chronic role in reducing or eliminating the oxidant damage produced by NO (McCann *et al.* 1994, 1998; McCann, 2000).

Leptin

Leptin, the hormone encoded by the obesity (ob) gene, is a protein of 146 amino acid residues with a tertiary structure similar to that of cytokines. Leptin receptors (Ob-Rs) have been demonstrated in the hypothalamus, gonadotrope cells of the anterior pituitary and Leydig cells. The Ob-Rb isoform is highly expressed in the hypothalamus. Leptin accelerates GnRH pulsatility, but not pulse amplitude, in arcuate hypothalamic neurons in a dose-dependent manner. Leptin may facilitate GnRH secretion predominantly via indirect mechanisms acting through interneurons secreting neuropeptides, e.g. cocaine and amphetamine-regulated transcript peptide, galanin-like peptide and/or melanocortin-concentrating hormone (MCH) in the hypothalamic zona incerta. Leptin may directly release LH and, to a lesser extent, FSH by the pituitary via NOS activation in gonadotropes.

Leptin and the pathophysiology of male reproduction

Leptin exerts significant effects on interstitial cells and Lydig cells of the testis. Androgens suppress leptin production whereas estrogens and insulin induce leptin production.

Leptin at medium–high physiological doses (beginning from 10 ng/ml) appears to antagonize the augmenting effect of several growth factors (insulin-like growth factor (IGF)-I, transforming growth factor (TGF)-β) and hormones (insulin, glucocorticoids) on gonadotropin (FSH/LH)-stimulated steroidogenesis. These effects are related to its effect on peripheral metabolism by increasing uptake, hepatic glucoeogenesis, and carbohydrate and fatty acid oxidation. It would appear that leptin acts as the critical link between adipose tissue and the reproductive system, indicating whether adequate energy reserves are present for reproductive function (Moschos *et al.* 2002).

Paracrine mechanisms mediated by locally produced cytokines play certain roles in causing endocrine changes in inflammation or sepsis. Similarly, various neuropeptides including prolactin and GH are produced in immunocompetent cells.

Several cytokines, including IL-1 and tumor necrosis factor (TNF), can activate the hypothalamic–pituitary–adrenal axis when given by systemic routes. These cytokines seem to act through the hypothalamus via the release of CRH, which is the most important regulator of ACTH. IL-1, IL-2, IL-6 and TNF act directly on the adrenal cortex to enhance the biosynthesis of glucocorticoids, possibly contributing to the persisting hypercortisolism present in sepsis.

ANIMAL MODELS

The effects of behaviorally mediated stresses on reproductive dysfunction can be studied in non-human primates, which live in complex social groups and have higher cortical brain areas, similar to humans, making study of these species particularly useful in understanding how such stresses may impact on reproduction in men. In rodents and cats, eating is induced by gentle pinching of their tails. This is due to activation of dynorphin, an endogenous opioid. This is an excellent model of stress-induced eating which is predominantly dependent on the activation of dopaminergic and opioid neurotransmitters.

FUTURE RESEARCH

(1) The endocrine, immunological and metabolic consequences of physical stress or experimental infections on aging. For example, are glucocorticoids toxic to hippocampal neurons?

(2) The relationships between stress and aging. Do stressors affect the rate of aging, and does aging affect responses to stressors?

(3) Whether and how early recognition and treatment of depression and anxiety are able to prevent a downward spiral in the health status of older persons.

An increased understanding of the mechanisms by which psychological and social stresses suppress the activity of the reproductive axis may well be achieved by focusing future studies on the individual differences in response to stress.

1. Erectile dysfunction (ED)

Erectile dysfunction is the inability to obtain sufficient penile rigidity to allow vaginal penetration, regardless of the cause. ED is associated with advancing age and is related to medical conditions and psychological disorders associated with stress. Volitional erection usually begins with psychological arousal which involves all of the senses (sight, touch, smell, taste and hearing) as well as imagination. The sensory input arrives to special areas of the subconcious brain via afferent neural pathways (Gignac *et al.* 2000). This process is modulated by stress and hormonal imbalance. From the spinal cord the pathway leads to the paired cavernosal, nerves running alongside the prostate (neurovascular bundles), which are responsible for the induction of erection. The efferent neural activation leads to a change in the blood flow pattern to the penis whereby more blood is trapped in the paired erectile bodies (corpora cavernosum). Thus, there is greater inflow compared to outflow and the penis elongates, increases in diameter, and develops sufficient rigidity for vaginal penetration. This requires normally functioning arterial, cavernosal, and venous systems. (Gignac *et al.* 2000). There are three types of penile erection:

(1) Psychogenic erection: result of concious sensory input/fantasy;

(2) Reflexogenic erection: occurs by a reflex pathway in the spinal cord initiated by genital stimulation;

(3) Nocturnal erection: normal physiologic erections of the penis.

Psychogenic (nonorganic) ED is classified into five major categories:

Type 1: anxiety, fear of failure (e.g. performance anxiety)
Type 2: depression

Type 3: marital conflict, strained relationship
Type 4: ignorance and misinformation, religious scruples (e.g. about normal anatomy or sexual function)
Type 5: obsessive-compulsive personality (e.g. anhedonia) (Gignac *et al.* 2000).

The presence of ED, regardless of the cause, leads to psychological stress such as fear of underlying disease and loss of self-image. The intrinsic and extrinsic causes of psychological stress can lead to physiological changes altering the afferent/efferent pathways. Anxiety may be associated with higher circulating levels of catecholamines and these neurotransmitters can affect the erectile mechanism. Emotion exerts significant effects on how the senses are interpreted, potentially turning positive signals into inhibition of erection, thus stress can diminish libido profoundly. (Gignac *et al.* 2000).

2. Stress/reproductive dysfunction

Secretion of reproductive hormones is impaired by social and psychological stress. This impairment can be subtle, consisting of a mild suppression in reproductive hormone secretion, or can be dramatic, causing a complete suppression of reproduction. There are remarkable differences among men in the responsiveness of the reproductive axis to social stresses due to various factors: the type of stress, the magnitude and duration of stress, the perception of the stress by the individual, the social status, the concurrent level of aggressive behavior displayed by the individual, seasonal cues, and the prior level of activity within the reproductive axis.

The physiological mechanisms contributing to social stress induction of reproductive dysfunction include activation of the adrenal axis, increased secretion of endogenous opioids, increased prolactin release, and changes in sensitivity to gonadal steroid hormone feedback. Reproductive dysfunction is caused by various forms of physical stress: energy restriction, temperature stress, infection, pain, and injury. Little is known about the effects of behaviorally induced stresses, i.e. psychological and social stresses, on the activity of the reproductive dysfunction. The effect of a particular stress at a particular time on the reproductive axis of an individual animal can be modulated by various variables: social status, the magnitude and duration of stress, perception of the stress, aggressive behavior, seasonal cues, and the prior level of activity within the reproductive axis (Abbott *et al.* 1989; Sade *et al.* 1976).

Several acute psychological stresses cause the acute suppression of circulating testosterone and LH levels. In baboons darting and capture lead to an immediate suppression of testosterone in some animals, but to an initial increase in plasma testosterone levels followed by a much more subtle decline in other animals. In monkeys there is significant correlation between aggressiveness and testosterone titers, with the more aggressive males showing higher circulating levels of testosterone. Based on the ability of both acute and chronic social stress to suppress reproductive hormones secretion it would appear that social status (i.e. dominance rank) plays an important role in determining the lifetime reproductive success in primates, with subordinate animals experiencing a greater degree of social stress and having a lesser degree of reproductive success.

CHAPTER 11

Erectile dysfunction

Erectile dysfunction (ED) – persistent inability to achieve or maintain an erection sufficient for satisfactory sexual intercourse – is manifested in 10–60% of men, depending on age and demography of the population (Table 11.1).

Some 40% of diabetic men > 60 years of age have ED all the time (complete ED). Men with ischemic heart disease are 1.9 times more likely to have complete ED than those without ischemic heart disease. ED may lead to depressive symptoms, low self-esteem, other signs of psychological distress and decreased quality of life. ED can be due to organic or psychological mechanisms associated with psychological, neurological, endocrinological, vascular (venous or arterial), traumatic or iatrogenic factors (drugs or surgery).

ED is a common problem in general medical practice affecting especially the elderly and those with hypertension, ischemic heart disease, peripheral vascular disease and diabetes mellitus.

Penile erection, a psychological–neurological–endocrine–vascular phenomenon, involves three simultaneous steps: arterial dilatation with subsequent increase in flow; lacunar space dilatation with filling of the corpora cavernosa; and decreased venus outflow. Penile erection is associated with increased arterial flow, smooth muscle relaxation and increased venous outflow resistance. Psychological distress can have a grave detrimental effect on sexual function. Also, there is concern about the possible negative effects of psychiatric medications on erectile function and libido.

Table 11.1 Prevalence of erectile dysfunction (ED)

Country	Age (years)	% with ED
USA	40–80	10–12
France	18–70	39
Spain	25–70	73
Nigeria	21–84	34
Korea	> 50	59

ETIOLOGY

Penile erectile function is regulated by various neural, endocrine and enzymatic mechanisms including the penile dorsal nerve, intracavernous nerve, growth factors and nitric oxide synthase (NOS). There are several risk factors for penile ED: old age, cardiovascular disease, excessive smoking, arterial insufficiency, abnormal penile hemodynamics and diabetes (Monga and Rajasekaran, 2003). Abnormal penile hemodynamics are often associated with functional impairment of smooth muscle contraction or neurogenic relaxation of the muscle of the corpus cavernosum. Penile hemodynamics can be evaluated by monitoring functional impairment of smooth muscle contractility and relaxation to neurogenic stimulation in strips of cavernous muscle obtained from patients.

ED may be due to organic and/or psychogenic factors, including hypertension, hypercholesterolemia, atherosclerosis, myocardial infarction, pituitary/gonadal dysfunction, anemia, renal/hepatic failure, depression or anxiety. Measurement of testosterone does not help in assessing potency or libido, and low testosterone levels are not age related. Therapeutic correction of testosterone does not improve sexual function.

Two major psychopathological/emotional factors play a significant role in the etiology of ED: performance anxiety and relationship discord. Half of the men with impotence have an organic etiology, the majority being of vascular origin. The vascular problems result from arterial insufficiency and/or incompetence of the veno-occlusive mechanism (venous leak). Differentiating between the two has prognostic and therapeutic implications. Corporal fibrosis, which causes venogenic (venous leak) impotence, develops secondary to abnormalities in the regulation of collagen synthesis and degradation, probably related to chronic ischemia. Erectile/sexual functions are regulated by dopamine/oxytocin release by the neurons of the hypothalamus. However, hypogonadism does not seem to contribute to the impaired penile reflex, as replacement of testosterone did not recover the centrally mediated penile reflexes.

Potassium channels are key regulators of membrane potential, and therefore of transmembrane Ca^{2+} flux and, subsequently, the degree of contraction of many types of smooth muscle, including human corporeal smooth muscle. Corporeal smooth muscle tone, in turn, modulates penile blood flow and intracavernous pressure, and thus affects both penile rigidity and erectile capacity. At least four subtypes of potassium channel are present in human corporeal myocytes, with the large-conductance calcium-sensitive potassium channel (maxi-K or K_{Ca} channel) and the metabolically regulated potassium channel (K_{ATP}) being the most physiologically relevant (Wang et al. 2000). The low po_2 in patients with arteriogenic impotence and the subset of men with severe venous leak impotence support a concept of low cavernosal po_2 as a mechanism for both arteriogenic and venogenic impotence.

In humans and rodents, erectile and reproductive function is suppressed by hyperprolactinemia, but little is known about its effect on penile erection. Hyperprolactinemic men exhibit decreased libido and inability to either obtain or maintain a rigid erection. Although plasma testosterone levels are usually reduced in the hyperprolactinemic state, correction of the low testosteronemia with administration of intramuscular testosterone does not correct the erectile abnormality.

Factors that affect erections can be of five different etiologies or a mixture of any combination of these causes (Hancock, 2002). Psychogenic and organic are the major classifications of etiology for ED. Organic origin is further designated as neurological, hormonal, vascular, cavernosal and mixed. Historically, ED was thought to be only psychogenic in origin.

Psychogenic factors

Less than 50% of ED is attributed to a psychological diagnosis. Onset and duration of ED are key elements for determining whether the source of the dysfunction is psychogenic or organic. In general, men younger than 50 years are likely to have psychogenic dysfunction, while the dysfunction of those older than 50 will usually be of organic origin. In many cases there are elements of both. An example is the depression that follows coronary artery bypass grafting as a result of coronary artery disease. Anxiety, stress, depression, troubled relationships, job changes or loss, fear of performance, or troubled history of sexual relations can all contribute to ED. Unfortunately, the treatment for many of these conditions can also contribute to the problem. Special attention should be given to the medications used to manage these conditions. Referral to a psychotherapist or sex therapist is recommended to facilitate management.

Neurological factors

Neurological ED can occur as a co-morbid condition of many disease states. Neural control of erections is from the neuroeffector system. This can be adrenergic, cholinergic, or non-adrenergic and non-cholinergic. Patients with diseases at the level of the brain, such as Parkinson's diseases, Alzheimer's disease and cerebral vascular accidents, can all be affected by decreased sexual desire.

Interestingly, patients with a complete upper motor neuron lesion can in many cases get erections, while few of those with complete lower motor neuron lesions are capable of erections. Patients with diabetes, vitamin deficiencies, drug abuse or alcohol abuse syndromes frequently present with peripheral neuropathy and ED. Finally, damage to the pudendal or cavernosal nerves resulting from trauma to the genitals or surgery and/or irradiation to the pelvic floor as well as spinal cord injury can, and often does, affect penile erections.

Endocrine factors

ED of hormonal origin is often detected prior to diagnosis of the disease state. Abnormalities of the hypothalmic–pituitary–gonadal axis will often result in difficulties or inability to obtain or maintain erections. Diabetes mellitus and lack of control of blood sugar levels is the most common cause – of up to 39% of ED. Abnormalities of the thyroid, kidneys, or liver can also be the cause. These can all result in loss of nocturnal erections, low sexual interest or impotence. Considerations for management of the disease state may require referral for endocrinology assessment prior to initiation of treatment.

Arterial factors

Since erections are dependent on blood flow, vascular supply is essential for erections. The primary source of blood supply to the penis is from the pudenal artery and the periprostatic plexus. Tumescence is full with 100 mmHg. Atherosclerosis, hypertension, venous incompetence, uncontrolled diabetes and history of cardiac, gastrointestinal or urological surgery or irradiation can all contribute to the dysfunction. Patients with severe arterial disease show changes in the cellular structure of smooth muscle cells of the penis. The dysfunction can be in the form of lack of erection, slow tumescence, or early detumescence. Each of these are indicated in the onset of ED. The initial presentation of erectile issues should prompt investigation of the potentially associated disease state, as this may be the first sign of chronic vascular disease. A review of the medications used for these conditions is also recommended.

Venous and cavernosal factors

Injury to the cavernosa can affect the venous return of blood from the penis. The cavernous vein, which branches from the pudenal and periprostatic plexus veins, comprises the venous drainage of the cavernosum. Damage or incompetence of the venous drainage will create a scenario of erections that are not sufficient for penetration, or erections that cannot be maintained for completion of sexual activity. Some

injuries can result in Peyronie's disease, or a rupture of the tunica albuginea. This results in failure to obtain erections or pain during erections. Congential abnormalities may create difficulty with venous return as well as abnormal communication between the cavernosum and spongiosum or the glans penis. Finally, a history of priapism will indicate fibrotic tissue that will interfere with the venous blood flow.

Mixed etiology

Finally, a mixture of the aforementioned disease states or injuries, along with the treatment, can often be the cause of the dysfunction. Impotence occurs in 50% of patients receiving renal dialysis. Once transplantation is successful, there is a reversal of impotence in 75% of patients. Many medications for psychological diagnosis, hypertension and cholesterolemia will create ED. The most frequently associated medication for erection difficulty is the antihypertensives. Of these, the angiotensin-converting enzyme inhibitors or calcium channel blockers are the least implicated in ED. If medications can be identified and changed without jeopardizing the patient's well-being, the solution to the dysfunction may be found. Unfortunately, the majority of organically imposed dysfunction is irreversible and thus detection of the origin and selection of management to target this is paramount for successfully treating the patient with ED.

MECHANISMS

The erectile bodies of the penis are the paired corpora cavernosa on the dorsal aspect of the penis. The corpora cavernosa are covered by a thick fascial layer called the tunica albuginea. Parasympathetic stimulation from levels S2–S4 results in an erection. Nitric oxide (NO) from non-adrenergic, non-cholinergic neurons, cavernosal smooth muscle cells and cholinergic-stimulated endothelial cells (endothelial NOS, eNOS) is the primary neurotransmitter, acting through guanylate cyclase to increase cGMP levels, which alters intracellular calcium levels, resulting in smooth muscle relaxation of the corpora cavernosum and penile vasculature. Resultant increased arterial inflow and expansion of the cavernosal sinusoids compresses the emissary veins and subtunical venules against the fibroelastic tunica albuginea, causing penile tumescence. Somatic neural stimulation causes contraction of the bulbocavernosus and ischiocavernous skeletal muscles, which results in the rigidity of the erection. Sympathetic neural stimulation results in seminal emission, ejaculation and contraction of the lacunar space and return of the flaccid basal adrenergic-mediated cavernosal smooth muscle tone. Endothelin-1 is a potent vasoconstrictive mediator that helps to maintain a flaccid tone.

Penile cavernosal contractile tone is contributed in part by a calcium sensitizing mechanism involving a small monomeric G-protein called RhoA. This protein activates an enzyme called Rho-kinase; activated Rho-kinase is responsible for sensitization of myofilaments to Ca^{2+}. A specific inhibitor of Rho-kinase, (+)-(R)-*trans*–(1-amino-ethyl-*N*-(4-pyridyl)cyclohexacarboxamide dihydrochloride monohydrate (Y-27632) lowers the blood pressure of hypertensive rats but not of normotensive rats. This suggests that Y-27632 has vasorelaxing activity preferentially on vascular beds with high basal tone. Intracavernosal injection of Y-27632 in rats induces penile erection independently of the NO pathway. *In vitro* studies employing rabbit and human penile corpus cavernosum evaluated the effect of this Rho-kinase inhibitor on nonadrenergic-mediated contractions. This compound exhibits dose-dependent inhibition of these contractions, which indicates the involvement of the Rho-kinase mechanism in a nonadrenergic-mediated penile contractile pathway. The involvement of the Rho-kinase pathway in penile smooth muscle contractile mechanisms has been confirmed by *in vivo* studies in rats. Pretreatment with Y-27632 attenuated the endothelin-1-induced reduction in the neurogenic erectile response in rats. Thus, Rho-kinase antagonism represents a potential avenue of therapy for ED where abnormally high noradrenergic tone has been implicated. Furthermore, Rho-kinase antagonists would not require a functional nitrergic system and presumably would be efficacious in patients with full loss of nitrergic function. It would appear that studies targeting selective Rho-kinase antagonism might be a potential therapeutic avenue for the treatment of ED associated with aging as well as hypertension.

Priapism, prolonged erection unaccompanied by sexual desire or stimulation, is manifested in two categories: high flow (non-ischemic) and low flow (ischemic) depending upon the emissary veins involved, severity of the disease involved and duration of venous occlusion.

High-flow priapism is characterized by adequate (or increased) arterial inflow with normal venous outflow, but helicine arteriolar bypass, or a defect in regulation, prevents detumescence. Causes of low-flow priapism include sickle cell anemia, leukemia, secondary penile cancer, prostatitis, urethritis, prolonged sexual intercourse or erection, pelvic thromboses, congenital neonatal priapism, spinal stenosis, spinal cord injury, antipsychotics, clozapine, chlorpromazine, antihypertensives, hydralazine, guanethidine, antidepressants, marijuana, alcohol, cocaine, heparin and testosterone injection.

EVALUATION AND DIAGNOSIS

Several intracavernosus vasoactive injections have been used alone or in combination for the evaluation and diagnosis of ED: papaverine, phentolamine, prostaglandin-E$_1$ (PGE$_1$), vasointestinal peptide and moxysilite. High levels of state-anxiety, measured by psychological tests, are often present in newly diagnosed impotent patients and may lead to an incomplete pharmacologically induced erection with vasoactive agents. The veno-occlusive mechanism is highly susceptible to psychological factors and to the type and dosage of the vasoactive agent. Some authors therefore combine intracavernosus injections (ICI) with audiovisual sexual stimulation. Treatment of individuals with ED without adequately addressing the possible presence of psychopathology could account for treatment failures and has the potential for leaving serious emotional problems untreated.

Diagnosis

The major risk factors include tobacco abuse, atherosclerosis, alcohol or illicit drug abuse, diabetes mellitus, hypertension, pelvic irradiation or surgery and iatrogenic causes. A history of obstructive sleep apnea and pelvic surgery or trauma is also associated with increased incidence of ED. Another element that has a significant impact on the accuracy of the diagnosis is the general well-being of the patient.

Physical examination

In order for an erection to occur, there must be a co-ordination of anatomical, hormonal, neural and vascular components of the body. While the subjective portion of the visit gives enough information to narrow the differential diagnosis of the etiology, the objective segment is essential to be able to dismiss underlying or coincidental disease. The physical examination should include inspection of the bulbocavernosal reflex to assess neural response. The penis is examined for plaques, and the testicles for atrophy, infection, or mass. A digital rectal examination should be performed to assess size, shape and consistency of the prostate and rectal tone. Assessment of peripheral pulses, and vibratory sensation of the lower extremity could be instrumental in determining the neural and vascular status of the patient. The thyroid and the breasts of the patient are examined for potential indications of hormonal deficiencies.

Laboratory tests

At a minimum, a urinalysis, prostate-specific antigen (PSA) and complete blood cell count (CBC) should be obtained. Additional testing should include blood glucose, liver and renal function and cholesterol levels. Many clinicians recommend obtaining a stress test, since the correlation between artery disease and ED is so strong and the results could impact on management options. A low testosterone level will decrease libido or desire for sexual activity, but not the ability to have an erection. If the testosterone level is low, free testosterone should be tested, to confirm the level. Prior to initiation of exogenous testosterone, evaluation of the pituitary for tumor should be completed, with referral for endocrinology assessment. Testosterone rarely will improve ED if only mild deficiencies are detected. More importantly, there is significant risk for iatrogenic illness with the use of exogenous testosterone. A high luteinizing hormone (LH) level would indicate testicular failure and would respond to supplemental testosterone. If the LH level is low, the suspicion should be higher for a pituitary tumor.

A simple, inexpensive test is to provide the patient with test strips to determine nocturnal erections and the rigidity of the erection. This can be accomplished with commercially prepared strips or even with postage stamps placed on the penis at bedtime. Dorsal nerve conduction studies may be obtained if a neural origin is suspected and the patient wishes to pursue nerve grafting. Doppler color flow studies can help to assess the arterial flow to the cavernosa. This may provide benefit to those who are seeking surgical revascularization.

Basic research in hypertension-related ED is another challenging area for investigation. Hypertension is considered to be one of the most important vascular risk factors involved in the onset of ED; the precise mechanism of hypertension-related ED remains an enigma. Hypertension-induced vascular changes, endothelial dysfunction and hormonal abnormalities are regarded as the possible etiologic factors. Abnormal smooth muscle contractility may be a major cause of hypertension-related alterations, and a smooth muscle relaxant that modulates this process would be useful therapeutically. Clinical studies suggest, however, that antihypertensive drugs *per se* could affect the compliance of the erectile tissue. ED is a well-recognized adverse effect of several antihypertensive agents, possibly due to drug-induced penile arterial insufficiency. Few animal studies were conducted to evaluate the pathophysiology of hypertension-induced ED. Future research is needed to characterize the association between hypertension and male erectile function by monitoring the neurogenic erectile response and its correlation with systemic arterial pressure changes. This has been undertaken in a genetic spontaneously hypertensive rat (SHR) model. In SHR animals a significant impairment in the neurogenic erectile response is observed. A lower resting baseline intracavernosal pressure (ICP) and an elevated threshold to develop tumescence suggest a possible derangement in penile perfusion as well as in other hemodynamic mechanisms of the erectile tissue in the SHR species. The identification of agents that have a selective relaxant activity on the vascular beds with high basal tone and vascular remodeling capability would be ideal for the treatment of ED in this population.

THERAPY

Major therapeutic approaches for ED include vasoactive intracavernous pharmacotherapy, oral medication, a penile prosthesis and vacuum constrictor devices (Figure 11.1). The acceptance rate is higher for intracavernous pharmacotherapy than for penile prostheses, and vacuum constrictor devices have the highest dropout rate. In the Middle East, the acceptance and satisfaction with such devices are directly related to the degree of ED, number of wives and age difference between patients and spouses (range between 1 and 46 years). Vacuum constrictor devices and the disposable

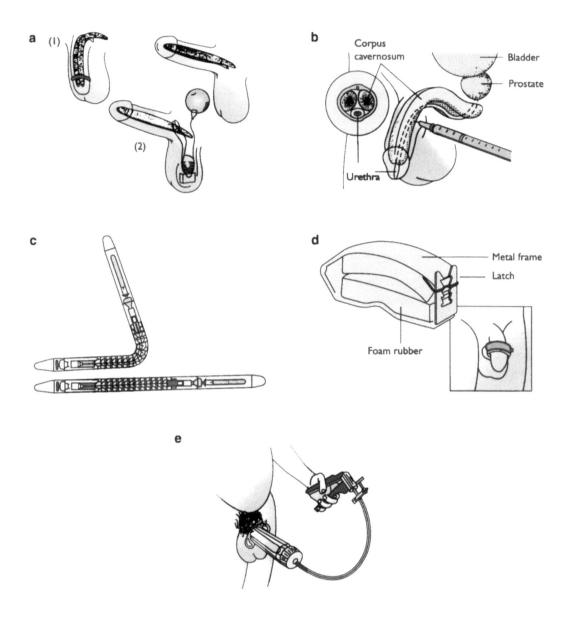

Figure 11.1 Major therapeutic approaches for erectile dysfunction. (a) Penile implants (1, malleable implant in normal and erect position; 2, inflatable implant). (b) Self-injection into one of the corpora to stimulate blood flow and produce an erection. (c) Mechanical penile implant. These are easier to bend and retain their shape better than malleable implants. (d) Penile clamp to prevent urine leaking from the urethra. (e) Vacuum device

cavernotome are used to induce corporeal dilatation during implantation of the penile prosthesis in patients with severe corporeal fibrosis. Electronic devices are applied to evaluate digitalized axial rigidometry, relative intracavernosal pressure and glans temperature.

The ICI of vasoactive drugs has been applied for improving erection and erection induction in certain types of ED. The mechanisms of action include a

psychogenic effect, improved cavernous hemodynamics, prostagladin-induced angiogenesis, improved cavernous oxygenation, cavernous smooth muscle hypertrophy and normal episodic fluctuations in erectile function. ICI is popular in spite of effective oral therapy or alternative methods of delivery of vasoactive agents. Chlorpromazine may be used as a substitute for phentolamine in a mixture with papaverine. Chlorpromazine is cheaper and just as

Table 11.2 Penile revascularization. Clinical criteria for patient selection

Patient history characterized by

(1) strong libido
(2) consistent reduction in erectile rigidity during sexual activity
(3) variable sustaining capability
(4) best maintenance of the rigidity during morning erections
(5) poor spontaneity of erections

Normal hormonal evaluation
Normal neurological evaluation
Increased arterial gradients during cavernosal artery occlusion pressure determination

effective as phentolamine. Use of artificial devices in delivering vasoactive agents has been successful. The devices avoided multiple corporeal punctures.

ED patients are classified into three groups according to the size of branches between the deep dorsal artery and cavernous tissue: adequate branching; inadequate branching; and complete lack of branching. The success rate with microscopic revascularization of the inferior epigastric artery to the deep dorsal artery was 100% in those with adequate branches to the cavernous tissue, 75% with inadequate branches and 40% with no branches. Penile revascularization is recommended for young males with arteriogenic impotence and no vascular risk factors (Table 11.2).

Oral medications

Viagra® (sildenafil) (Pfizer)

Viagra® selectively inhibits the enzyme phosphodiesterase (PDE) type 5, the enzyme responsible for breakdown of cyclic guanosine monophosphate (cGMP) in the corpus cavernosum. Persistence of cGMP leads to smooth muscle relaxation, resulting in an erection. The clinical effect of sildenafil on health-related quality of life was evaluated in 40 patients (61 ± 8 years old). Sexual satisfaction according to SF-36 scales was evaluated before and after treatment with sildenafil citrate at a dose of 25 or 50 mg. After treatment with Viagra, scores increased for all scales: physical functioning, general health and role-emotional functioning. Patients who evaluated effectiveness of the treatment as excellent showed significantly better physical functioning, role-physical functioning and general health scale scores compared with those who evaluated

their outcome as good or poor. In comparison with the scores at baseline, patients who considered outcome with Viagra to be excellent also showed significant improvements in physical functioning, general health and role-emotional functioning (Hafez, personal communication).

In the four months following Food and Drug Administration (FDA) approval of sildenafil, over 3.6 million out-patient prescriptions were written in the USA. The overall response rate (good or excellent effect) was 59%, while 15% reported no response. The response rate was better in men younger than 70 (78%) as compared to men older than 70 (43%). The response rate deteriorated with increasing degree of ED as classified by the erectile function domain score.

This success is not shown in patients with uncontrolled medical illness, those receiving specific medications, or those with low serum testosterone levels or alcohol or drug dependence. To be considered truly effective a therapy should not only provide an erection but also enhance overall sexual satisfaction. Studies therefore should determine the social and psychological effects of Viagra treatment in patients with ED.

New oral agents

Vardenafil (Bayer) is a more potent and selective PDE-5 inhibitor than sildenafil. Vardenafil has a more rapid onset of action (T_{max} 0.66 h) compared to sildenafil (1.16 h) or tadalafil (2.0 h). A more rapid clinical onset of an erection would more closely approximate the ideal 'on-demand' oral agent for ED. Men treated with vardenafil 5 mg and 20 mg reported (66% and 80%, respectively) that their erections had improved, compared to 30% on placebo. Seventy-five per cent of attempts at intercourse were successful in the treated group, compared to 40% in the placebo group. Side-effects included flushing (11%), headache (7% on 5 mg; 15% on 20 mg), dyspepsia (1% on 5 mg; 10% on 20 mg) and rhinitis (5% on 5 mg; 7% on 20 mg). In a study of 452 diabetic men, improved erections were reported by 72% of men on 20 mg compared to 13% of men on placebo.

Tadalafil (Cialis®, ICOS-Lilly) is also a more potent and selective PDE-5 inhibitor than sildenafil. Men taking 10 mg or 20 mg of tadalafil reported 56% and 64% improved erections, respectively, compared to 23% on placebo. Over 80% of sexual intercourse attempts were successful with 10 mg of tadalafil, compared to 40% of attempts on placebo. Side-effects include headache (23%), dyspepsia (11%), back pain (5%) and myalgia (4%). However, visual disturbances were not reported. Tadalafil has a long half-life (17.5 h), suggesting less dependency on accurate dosing prior to intercourse, and possibly 'more spontaneity'. Concerns exist that the long half-life of tadalafil may predispose to upregulation of PDE-5.

Apomorphine (Uprima®, TAP Pharmaceuticals) is a semisynthetic D1/D2 dopaminergic agonist that acts on the paraventricular nucleus of the hypothalamus and the lumbosacral spinal cord to stimulate a spontaneous erection. Phase III clinical trials in over 5000 patients have demonstrated that erections firm enough for intercourse were achieved in 54% and 47% of men on 4 mg and 3 mg apomorphine, respectively, compared to 32% on placebo. Side-effects include nausea (7% at the 3-mg dosage) and syncope (0.2%).

Alprostadil (MUSE®) through intracorporeal injection or the urethra is an effective alternative treatment for some men. Alprostadil is a form of a natural substance (PGE_1) and serves to open blood vessels to increase blood flow to the penis. It is effective in a wide range of medical disorders including diabetes, surgery and injury. It is not effective in those patients with severe circulatory or nerve damage. Clinically, MUSE is most effective in conjunction with an Actus Ring to restrict the venous flow. The most commonly used dose for patients at the Charleston V.A. Hospital has been 500 µg, with a range of 125–1000 µg. MUSE should be inserted into the urethra by pushing the button completely after urinating. Gently massaging or rolling the penis in the hand helps absorb the medication into the tissues. The effect is enhanced by standing for approximately 10 min and by sexual stimulation. Sexual positions can affect the erect penis. Standing or being on top help keep the penis erect. Generally, MUSE should not be used in those patients with bleeding disorders, e.g. sickle cell disease or trait, patients taking blood thinners, or those who are prone to blood clots. A MUSE trial is usually given in the clinic setting to evaluate the efficacy or potential complication of the medication. Primary complications could include hypotension, urethral bleeding, or priapism.

The other method is injection therapy with PGE_1; prostaglandin and papaverine D_2; and prostaglandin, papaverine and chlorapromazine D_3. It includes medical conditions such as diabetes, hypertension, injuries and post-surgical treatment for prostate cancer. The dose is individually adjusted for each patient and is effective 90% of the time. The primary side-effects of injection therapy are priapism (erections lasting longer than 4 h) and bleeding. These conditions may require emergency intervention. Injection therapy should not be used with any other sexual dysfunction treatment modality. It should also not be used in patients with bleeding disorders or those patients who are on coumadin or heparin.

FUTURE RESEARCH

Little is known about the effect of stress and related hormone changes on the neurobiological correlates of psychogenic impotence. Future research is needed to evaluate parameters of blood biochemistry, hormone profile and cavernosometry associated with ED. Patterns of ED were examined using frequency distributions and contingency tables generated with Microsoft Graph software. The relationships between various grades of ED and self reported co-morbidity were examined using logistic regression and EGRET software, with the final multivariate model being derived using backwards stepwise elimination. Color–power Doppler sonography is a valuable technique in the initial evaluation of penile circulation in ED. This procedure is employed to achieve a full penile erection and complete smooth muscle relaxation by an ICI of several vasoactive drugs for full evaluation of the morphodynamic features of the cavernous arteries and to obtain information about the cavernous veno-occlusive mechanism.

Future research is needed to evaluate the role of growth factors in ED. One such growth factor is vascular endothelial growth factor (VEGF). This is known to improve penile blood flow. Observations of an age-related decrease of this growth factor in the rat penis suggested that this approach may be beneficial in aging men (Monga and Rajasekaran, 2003). VEGF and its receptor Flt-1 in penile cells suggests an autocrine role for this growth factor in the penile cavernosal smooth muscle. Hence, further research towards the development of specific agonists for VEGF receptors will be valuable for the future pharmacotherapy of ED. The presence of VEGF and its receptor in rabbit clitoral cells indicates that the use of this growth factor in female sexual dysfunction merits further exploration.

CHAPTER 12

The prostate in health and disease

FUNCTIONAL ULTRASTRUCTURE AND SECRETORY ACTIVITY OF THE PROSTATE

The prostate, partly glandular and partly muscular, is situated immediately below the internal urethral orifice, around the commencement of the urethra. It is located in the pelvic cavity, below the caudal part of the symphysis pubis, cranial to the deep layer of the urogenital diaphragm. It is ventral to the rectum, through which it may be distinctly felt, especially when enlarged. The human prostate is 4 cm transversely at the base, 2 cm in anteroposterior diameter and 3 cm in vertical diameter, and weighs 20 g. It is held by puboprostatic ligaments, by the deep layer of the urogenital diaphragm, which invests the prostate and the commencement of the membranous portion of the urethra, and by the anterior portions of the levatores ani, which pass dorsal from the pubis and embrace the sides of the prostate. These portions of levatores ani, levatores prostatae, support the prostate. The prostate is enveloped by a thin but firm fibrous capsule distinct from that derived from the subserous fascia, and is separated from it by a plexus of veins. This capsule adheres firmly to the prostate and is structurally continuous with the stroma of the gland, being composed of the same tissues: non-striped muscle and fibrous tissue (Figure 12.1).

The prostate is present in all domestic animals. It is prominent in the dog. Its enlargement can cause obstruction of urine flow through the urethra; this condition is more common in older dogs. Multiple ducts from this gland empty directly into the urethra. The equine prostate is a nodular gland with two narrow lobes (each $7 \times 4 \times 1$ cm) connected by a thin transverse isthmus (about 3 cm long).

The prostate secretes a thin, milky fluid containing calcium, citrate ions, phosphate ions, a clotting enzyme and a profibrinolysin. During emission, the prostatic capsule contracts simultaneously with the contraction of the vas deferens so that the milky fluid of the prostate adds further to the bulk of semen. A slightly alkaline characteristic of the prostatic fluid may be quite important for successful fertilization, since the fluid of the vas deferens is relatively acidic, owing to the presence of citric acid and metabolic end-products of sperm, consequently helping to inhibit sperm fertility. Also, the vaginal secretions of the female are acidic (pH of 3.5–4.0). Sperm do not become optimally motile until the pH of the surrounding fluids rises to 6.0–6.5. The slightly alkaline prostatic fluid seems to neutralize the acidity of other seminal fluids during ejaculation to enhance sperm motility and fertilizability. The clotting enzyme from the prostatic fluid causes the fibrinogen of the seminal vesicle fluid to form a weak fibrin coagulum that holds the semen in deeper regions of the vagina at the cervix. The coagulum then dissolves within 15–30 minutes because of lysis by fibrinolysin of the prostate. The sperm remain immobile, owing to the viscosity of the coagulum. As the coagulum dissolves, the sperm become highly motile, and upon reaching the follicular fluid in the oviduct they undergo 'hyperactivation', a motility pattern necessary for ovum penetration and fertilization.

The prostate absorbs testosterone from the blood stream. Testosterone, trapped in the prostate, is

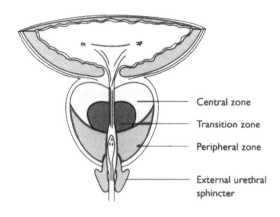

Figure 12.1 Anatomical zones of the prostate. (Reproduced with permission from Lunenfeld, 2002)

converted into dihydrotestosterone (DHT), which stimulates prostate growth. With increasing DHT levels the prostate enlarges. Finasteride (Proscar®) inhibits a critical enzyme, 5α-reductase, which changes into DHT. In men taking finasteride, blood DHT levels fall drastically. Shrinkage of the prostate alleviates pressure on the bladder, providing relief from obstructive symptoms associated with benign prostatic hyperplasia (BPH). A possible side-effect, in a few cases, is erectile dysfunction (ED).

ENDOCRINOLOGY OF THE PROSTATE

The prostate gland is sensitive to many hormones, the most important being androgen. In fetal development androgens regulate differentiation, but in neonatal development androgens function in prostatic growth and imprinting. Once at puberty, androgens trigger body and sexual maturation and maintain the accessory sex glands throughout life. Androgens function both actively and permissively to regulate prostatic growth and, therefore, are the target for research concerning treatment of prostate cancer.

Androgens are stimulated by the hypothalamic–pituitary–gonadal axis. The hypothalamus secretes gonadotropin releasing hormone (GnRH) in pulses approximately once every 70–90 min. This is transported to the anterior lobe of the pituitary gland via the portal venous system in order to stimulate follicle

stimulating hormone (FSH) and luteinizing hormone (LH) production. FSH stimulates the Sertoli cells in the testis to produce inhibin, which regulates the release of FSH and LH by the pituitary gland. LH is carried to the testis, where it attaches to the LH receptor found in the cytoplasm of Leydig cells, scattered in groups in the testicular stroma. This results in the production of cyclic adenosine monophosphate (cAMP) stimulating androgen synthesis. Testosterone is one of many androgens produced by the testes and has the largest impact on prostatic growth. Through a closed negative-feedback loop, androgens also act as a regulatory mechanism for the production of LH as well as FSH and ultimately its own production (Figure 12.2).

Androgens cause an increase in mainly prostatic epithelial mitotic activity as well as in connective tissue stroma and vasculature. In the absence of androgens, cell death is initiated by lysis, reducing the size of the prostate. Androgen deprivation by either orchidectomy or GnRH analogs, with alteration of the androgenic affect on the prostate, still remains the mainstay of treatment for managing patients with prostate cancer.

Testosterone is produced by the crystalloids of Reinke in the Leydig cells as well as by the adrenal cortex. The pathways are similar and both synthesize testosterone using cholesterol. The adrenal cortex forms androstenedione, which can be converted to other androgens such as testosterone and dehydroepiandrosterone (DHEA). However, this conversion process does not occur very readily. The testis produces 95% of the total body testosterone, while only 5% is produced from the extragonadal source. The plasma testosterone is composed of 2% free testosterone and 98% protein-bound testosterone. Free testosterone can either be converted to DHT by the enzyme 5α-reductase within the prostate, or undergo peripheral aromatization to estrogens or be inactived by hepatic conjugation. Although testosterone is the principal androgen, DHT also plays an active role in prostatic morphogenesis. DHT appears to be about two-fold more potent than testosterone. DHT has an important function in causing epithelial hyperplasia, embryogenesis and sexual differentiation, but its role is still not fully understood.

Androgens interact with androgen receptors, found in target tissues. Hormone homeostasis in normal and malignant prostate cells is obtained via the androgen receptors. The responsiveness of prostate tissue to

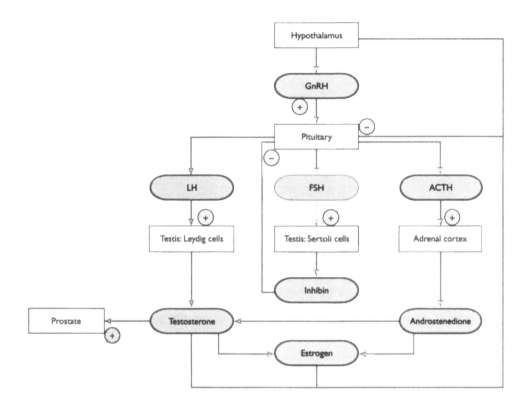

Figure 12.2 The hypothalamic–pituitary–gonadal axis and its regulation. GnRH, gonadotropin releasing hormone; LH, luteinizing hormone; FSH, follicle stimulating hormone; ACTH, adrenocorticotropic hormone

Adrenal steroids in the prostate

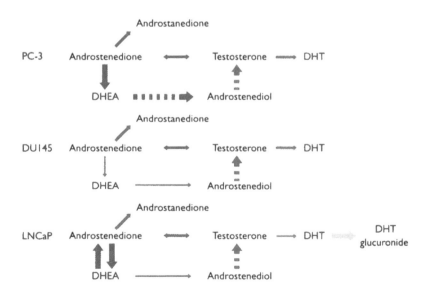

Figure 12.3 Metabolism of adrenal androgens in prostatic cancer cell lines. Arrow width indicates the relatively high activity. Dashed arrow indicates the relatively low activity. DHEA, dehydroepiandrosterone; DHT dihydrotestosterone. (Reproduced with permission from Koh *et al.* 2001 *Arch Androl*, 46:117–25. www.tandf.co.uk/journals)

androgens is partially regulated by the number of androgen receptors available for binding with the hormone. Other hormones such as estrogen, prolactin and retinoic acid also affect androgen receptor levels. Once an androgen binds to the receptor, a complex series of events is initiated which ultimately leads to the alteration of transcriptional activity of a particular gene. Initiation and evolution from being an androgen-dependent to an androgen-independent tumor may result from alterations in androgen receptors.

Adrenal steroids

Humans are a unique animal species in that they have adrenals that secrete large amounts of the inactive precursor DHEA and its sulfate (DHEAS) (Labrie *et al.* 1993). Adrenal precursors DHEA, DHEAS and androstenedione are taken up by the prostate cells and locally transformed into the active androgen DHT by 5α-reductase (Labrie *et al.* 1998). On the other hand, about 95% of testosterone is produced in the testis. This is also taken up from the circulation by the prostate, where it is converted to the most active androgen, DHT. Plasma DHEAS levels in adult men are 100–500 times higher than those of testosterone (Bartsch *et al.* 1990). These active androgens made locally in the prostate then exert their action by interacting with the androgen receptors in the same cells where their synthesis took place, without being released into the extracellular environment.

Androgen-independent cell lines PC-3 and DU145 and the androgen-dependent cell line LNCaP were investigated by Koh *et al.* (2001) (Figure 12.3). The effect of glucuronide and sulfate conjugates was also investigated. There was a strong tendency in the PC-3 and DU145 cells to convert androstenedione to DHEA or the DHEAS reservoir. On the other hand, LNCaP cells were capable of converting DHEA into androstenedione and subsequently into DHT. Androgens were converted into a glucuronide conjugate in LNCaP, but not in PC-3 or DU145 cells. The metabolism of the adrenal precursor shifted to androgen formation in LNCaP cells. The adrenal precursor pool has the potential to contribute to the regulation of prostatic cells. The presence of UGT activities in LNCaP cells may have a regulatory effect on the active androgen level in the intracellular environment.

PROSTATE CANCER

Incidence

Prostate cancer is an important public health problem with over a quarter of a million new cases diagnosed worldwide in the single year 1985 (Parkin *et al.* 1993). It varies markedly in incidence among various countries and racial groups (Figure 12.4). In much of East Asia, including China and Japan, the incidence is extremely low. However, the incidence of prostate cancer has been increasing and is becoming one of the leading ten cancers in males in these countries (Sasagawa and Nakada, 2002). Prostate cancer has become one of the most common malignancies in the world. In Japan, the age-adjusted death rates due to prostate cancer rose from 4.4 to 8.6 per 100 000 between 1980 and 1998.

Epidemiology

Prostate cancer is the most commonly diagnosed male cancer in the USA (317 000 new cases in 1996) and the second leading cause of all male cancer deaths (41 400 patients in 1996). The pattern of prostate cancer parallels that of breast cancer in the female and colon and pancreatic cancer in both sexes (Fahmy and Bissada, 2003).

Worldwide the incidence of mortality is unequally distributed, occurring more frequently in North America and northern Europe and much lower in Asia. Although the rate of prostate cancer in Japan is much lower than that in the USA, it is increasing continuously. This may be due to the increasing Westernized diet, widespread environmental contamination and improved screening techniques such as prostate-specific antigen (PSA).

Incidence data in the USA indicate that rates were highest in African-American men (188 per 100 000) per year, intermediate in Whites and lowest in Asians (Japanese and Chinese; 39 and 28 persons/100 000, respectively).

Regarding the mortality rates, in the years 1995–98 African-American men had double the prostate cancer mortality compared to Whites, and they had 1.6% higher mortality from non-prostate cancer causes of death. It was noted that African-American men usually have a later stage at diagnosis, higher grade of disease, more co-morbid conditions and less aggressive therapy.

This is related to screening, environmental, social and biological factors. The difference in screening was first noted in the year 1994 when the incidence of prostate cancer declined in Caucasians but continued to rise in African-Americans, although a recent report noted that the response of African-American men to radical prostatectomy was no less than that of Caucasian American men when the stage and grade were taken into consideration. However, the results are preliminary and may indicate a change in the current trend.

The difference in incidence rates may be explained by the increased fat intake in the diet of African-Americans, increased level of serum testosterone and reduced ability to produce vitamin D. Between the years 1973 and 1998 prostate cancer diagnosis increased more rapidly among Caucasian Americans compared to African-Americans. This may represent the differences in the access to early detection and treatment practices.

Although the geographic variation in the USA in prostate cancer is more limited than for most cancers, a distinct geographic pattern was seen among White males with the concentration of elevated mortality rates in the Northwest, Rocky Mountain areas and the North Central areas of the USA and the low mortality rates in the South Central areas. An inverse urban and rural gradient was also suggested, with the high rates in the less populated areas of New England and the Midwest, north plains, mountain states and the West.

The age distribution of the population greatly influences the burden of disease and disability, including cancer incidence and mortality. The likelihood of prostate cancer death increases by stage and grade and is strongly influenced by age. The incidence of prostate cancer increases with age much more than any other major cancer. The median age of diagnosis of prostate cancer is 71 years in White males and 69 years in African-American males. The probability of developing clinically significant prostate cancer in men younger than 39 years of age is less than 1 in 100 000, one in 78 for men aged 40–59 years of age, and one in six in men aged 60–79 years. The use of PSA as a screening tool for prostate cancer has resulted in improvement in the detection at an earlier stage, resulting in a decrease in the rate of distant metastasis at diagnosis by 50%. There was a substantial increase in the numbers of prostate cancers found after the introduction of PSA as a screening test in the late 1980s.

Multiple risk factors have been correlated with the occurrence of prostate cancer. These include race, family history of prostate cancer, oncogenes, some endogenous factors such as hormones, BPH, vasectomy, sexual activity, increased fat intake in diet, vitamins, physical activity, body habitus, smoking, some medications, infectious agents, education, socioeconomic status, occupation and the environment. Unfortunately, many reports lack convincing supportive data. In addition there are many conflicting data.

First-degree relatives of men with prostate cancer have a two- to three-fold increase in the risk of developing cancer. The risk increases for relatives of patients diagnosed at a lower age. In a study performed in southern Sweden, the risk of hereditary prostate cancer was 7.2% if the patient was diagnosed before the age of 60 years compared to 2.2% if diagnosed at an older age. The total amount and type of fat consumed was found to increase the risk for development of prostate cancer. Data from Japan and South Africa indicate that the incidence of prostate cancer increased with increased fat content in the diet.

Vasectomy increased the incidence of prostate cancer 1.2- to two-fold. These findings were debated, as they lacked scientific explanation. In a case–control study in 1636 subjects, there was no increased risk of prostate cancer in patients who underwent vasectomy. The normal growth and development of prostate cancer is under the hormonal control of androgens. Prostate cancer is rare in eunuchs castrated before puberty. Hormonal treatment is used for palliative treatment in men with advanced prostate cancer. Accordingly, hormonal influences were implicated as a causative factor for prostate cancer. Several investigators have tried to show differences in testosterone levels between patients with prostate cancer and controls, but the data were conflicting. In 2000, there were 180 000 cases diagnosed with prostate cancer. This represents a decline in the disease incidence from a peak of 334 000 in 1997. The rapid increase in the incidence of prostate cancer and the decline that followed is due to early detection attributed to the use of PSA as a screening test. The increase in the prostate cancer rates in the past decade reflects in part the prevalence of the disease rather than the incidence (Fahmy and Bissada, 2003).

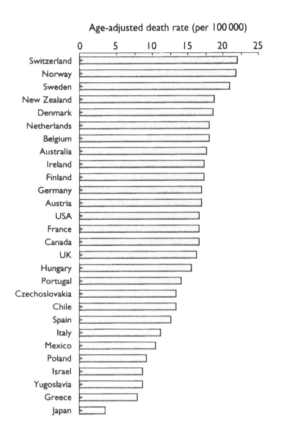

Age-adjusted death rate (per 100 000)

Figure 12.4 Age-adjusted death rates from prostate cancer per 100 000 males, standardized to the world population

Risk factors

Age

The prevalence of prostate cancer increases with age, and over age 60, both incidence and mortality rates due to prostate cancer increase strikingly. In Japan in 1994, the incidence of prostate cancer increased from 6.7 to 314 per 100 000 between the ages of 55 years and 80 years (Figure 12.5). Since prostate cancer increases faster with age than any other major cancers, the burden of prostate cancer will increase in the future with lengthening longevity.

Race

The incidence and mortality rates of prostate cancer vary widely among different ethnic groups. Both

incidence and death rates from prostate cancer are high in Scandinavian males and lower in East Asians. However, Japanese-Americans show higher mortality rates when compared with the mortality rates in Japan. Thus, immigrants tend to take on the risk of their host country. The risk of prostate cancer is influenced environmentally and cultural change accompanying migration may alter the risk.

Family history

Prostate cancer incidence in male relatives of patients with prostate cancer is increased. Families with a high incidence of clinically significant prostate cancer may be at higher risk because of shared environmental exposures or owing to a similar genetic makeup. Patients with prostate cancer are divided into three groups: 'hereditary', 'familial' and 'sporadic'. The 'hereditary' group is defined as a cluster of three or more affected relatives within any nuclear family; the occurrence of prostate cancer in each of three generations in either the proband's paternal or maternal lineage; or a cluster of two relatives affected at 55 years of age or less. The 'familial' group is described as those having a possible family history but not fitting the criteria for the hereditary group. The 'sporadic' group includes those without any family history of prostate cancer. A man with one first-degree relative with prostate cancer is estimated to have a 2.1- to 2.8-fold greater risk of being diagnosed with prostate cancer than the general population. Having a first-degree relative with prostate cancer may increase one's risk by a factor of six above that of the general population.

Genetics

Prostate cancer has been reported in excess in families with mutations of *BRCA1*, located on chromosome 17, and *BRCA2*, located on chromosome 13. In a study of Ashkenazi Jewish carriers of certain *BRCA1* and *BRCA2* germline mutations, they had an increased risk of prostate cancer that manifested after the age of 50 years. However, no studies assessing the effect of specific *BRCA1* and *BRCA2* mutations on prostate cancer risk have been carried out in Blacks or other non-White populations. A major prostate susceptibility locus was recently discovered on chromosome 1

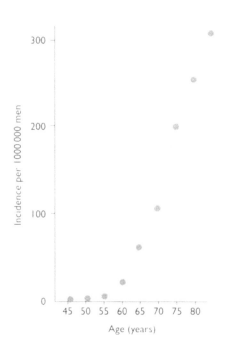

Figure 12.5 Age-specific incidence of prostate cancer per 100 000 males in Japan in 1994

(1q24-25), called HPC1, in a group of high-risk families with multiple males with prostate cancer.

Hormones

Testosterone is necessary for normal growth of the prostate epithelium, and early prostate cancer is endocrine dependent. However, no difference in baseline circulating testosterone level was found in prostate cancer patients compared with controls. Similarly, no significant association was found between serum estrone, estradiol, DHEA or DHEAS and prostate cancer risk. Young Black men have serum testosterone levels 15% higher than their White counterparts, and this difference may explain the increased risk of prostate cancer in Black men. American men were found to have different levels of testosterone-metabolizing enzymes than their Japanese counterparts. Although hormones play an important role in normal and cancerous prostate physiology, their relationship to the risk of prostate cancer remains undefined.

Diet

The dietary differences between ethnicities provide an interesting possible explanation for differences in the incidence and mortality from prostate cancer. The diet of Japanese males is low in animal fat and high in fiber content. This diet may relate to the lower incidence of prostate cancer in East Asia compared with Western countries. The traditional Asian diet has a high legume content, including beans, soybeans, lentils and chick peas. These vegetables are considered as the major source of fiber. As the fat content of the Japanese diet has increased toward Westernized levels, the incidence of prostate cancer in Japan has started to rise. Studies on the migration of Japanese and Chinese to Hawaii and then to the mainland of the USA support the concept that dietary factors influence disease etiology and that the mortality rate for prostate cancer will increase towards that of Americans within a few generations.

DIAGNOSIS

Prostate cancer is diagnozed by ultrasonography of the prostate (Figure 12.6) and/or by PSA measurements.

Prostate-specific antigen

PSA is a 33-kDa single-chain glycoprotein produced in the secretory epithelium of the prostate gland. The use of serum PSA for early detection and staging of prostate cancer as well as to monitor response to surgical, hormonal and radiation therapy is well established (Staney et al. 1989; Catalona et al. 1991). Since PSA gene expression is hormonally sensitive, the conversion of a hypogonadal patient to eugonadal status through parenteral testosterone substitution is expected to be associated with an increase in PSA level (Hanash and Mostofi, 1992).

Hormonal therapy

Yearly 40 000 men die of prostate cancer in the USA. Charles B. Huggins first published the effects of bilateral orchidectomies in prostate cancer in 1939. The prostate, seminal vesicles and Cowper's glands are secondary sex organs. Thus, prostate growth and function are hormone dependent and are governed by the hypothalmic–pituitary–gonadal axis.

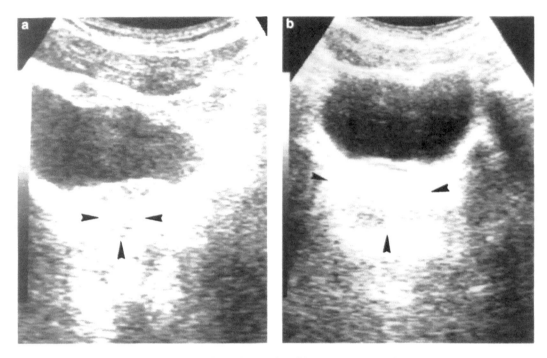

Figure 12.6 Ultrasonography of the prostate before (a) and after (b) testosterone replacement therapy in Klinefelter's syndrome. Arrowheads indicate the margin of the prostate. (Reproduced with permission from Shibasaki et al. 2001, Arch Androl, 47;173–6. www.tandf.co.uk/journals)

Almost all (98%) of testosterone in plasma is bound to protein as the testosterone binding globulin. Testosterone in the prostate is converted to DHT by the enzyme 5α-reductase. There is no evidence that prostate cancer is seen in the absence or deficiency of 5α-reductase. The 5α-reductase inhibitor Procar® inhibits the growth of BPH.

Of men with metastatic prostate cancer on hormonal therapy, 10% will live 10 years or more. Those patients with metastases and lower PSA levels will do better on hormonal therapy. Statistics and long-term follow-up favors early initiation of hormonal therapy in conditions of rising PSA levels. Owing to complications of hormonal therapy, the merits of intermittent hormonal therapy have been questioned; long-term results are unknown. On hormonal therapy after initial remission, ultimately hormone-resistant cancer cells develop, owing to genetic heterogeneity and disease progression. Hormone therapy has been used as neoadjuvant or adjuvant therapy in radiation therapy of prostate cancer with apparently good results (Table 12.1). Complications of long-term hormonal therapy include hot flushes, gynecomastia, loss of libido, impotence, weight gain, osteoporosis, memory loss and behavioral changes.

Several GnRH antagonists are currently most advanced in development (Table 12.2). Metabolism of [^{14}C]androstenedione formed by porostatic cancer cell lines is shown in Table 12.3.

The role of testosterone in prostate growth and the management of prostate cancer by androgen deprivation was initiated by the Nobel Lureate Charles Huggins and his colleagues in 1941. After androgen deprivation, the prostate rapidly decreases in size. Apoptotic death of androgen-independent cells occurs after androgen deprivation (Bissada, 2001).

Surgical castration

Since the testicles produce approximately 95% of testosterone in men, bilateral orchidectomy results in significant reduction in plasma testosterone levels. For decades, bilateral orchidectomy has remained the gold standard for androgen deprivation in patients with prostate cancer.

Medical castration

Continuous administration of an LH releasing hormone (LHRH) agonist results in downregulation of pituitary receptors with a loss of normal pituitary LH and follicle stimulating hormone (FSH) secretion. Accordingly, after a temporary period of a rise in testosterone levels (testosterone surge) castrate levels of testosterone are achieved in about 4–6 weeks. Antiandrogens may have a defined role during the initial use of LHRH agonists to counter this testosterone surge. LHRH agonists include leuprolide and goserelin.

Role of antiandrogens

About 5% of circulating androgens in men are accounted for by the adrenal glands. This is the rationale for utilization of antiandrogens in addition to surgical or medical castration to accomplish complete androgen blockade. However, surgical castration by bilateral orchidectomy has equivalent effectiveness with or without additional antiandrogens. Antiandrogens have a small role in patients undergoing medical castration by the use of GnRH agonists.

Non-steroidal antiandrogens

These include flutamide, bicalutamide and nilutamide. They have been used for long- or short-term combined androgen blockade (in conjunction with LHRH agonists) as well as single agents. Currently antiandrogen monotherapy is not considered as effective as surgical or medical castration in the initial management of advanced prostate cancer. However, they may have a role in combined androgen blockade. Additionally, they are used during the transitional phase of hormone refractory prostate cancer, at which time patients may still respond to secondary hormonal management, e.g. by use of high-dose bicalutamide, estrogen therapy or other steroidal antiandrogens such as ketoconazole. Timing of androgen withdrawal is not strictly defined. All symptomatic patients and those with evidence of skeletal metastases clearly benefit from androgen deprivation. Additionally, patients with pelvic lymph node metastases also benefit from early androgen deprivation. Patients with residual disease after definitive radiation therapy or cryosurgical ablation of the prostate are now detected early by a rising PSA level. The timing of androgen deprivation in those patients is not well defined. Based on recent data demonstrating that immediate treatment improved overall survival and prostate cancer-specific survival, androgen deprivation should be initiated before the development of metastatic symptoms.

Table 12.1 Selected chemotherapy regimens used in advanced prostate cancer

Treatment	n	Response (%)
Vinblastine + estramustine	25	33
Etoposide + estramustine	42	57
Paclitaxel + estramustine	32	58
Docetaxel + estramustine	34	63
Ketoconazole + doxorubicin	38	55

Neoadjuvant hormonal therapy

Adenocarcinoma of the prostate is the most common malignancy in men, and accounts for nearly 30% of all new cancers in men. Treatment decisions are based on the clinical stage of disease, histological grade of tumor and pretreatment PSA level. Radical prostatectomy is often recommended in men with long life expectancies and clinically confined prostate cancer.

Unfortunately, up to two-thirds of clinically confined tumors are understaged, and positive margin rates from 30 to 60% are reported after radical prostatectomy.

There are three possibilities for the patient with a positive resection margin: residual viable tumor resulting in local recurrence and/or systemic recurrence; residual tumor not surviving, because it is within the zone of tissue destruction created by the surgical knife, or it is destroyed by the ensuing inflammatory reaction; and the tumor meeting the pathological resection margin but not extending beyond it, a possibility that must be rare.

Radical prostatectomy has become the standard therapy for apparently localized prostate cancer. However, its usefulness is limited by a relatively high incidence of positive surgical margins, with consequent risk of recurrence and cause-specific morbidity. The relationship between resection margin status and rate of disease progression has not been specifically determined. Previous studies have shown an increased frequency of progression with increased tumor size and poor tumor differentiation. The goal of neoadjuvant hormonal therapy before radical prostatectomy is to reduce positive margins and biochemical disease recurrence rate, and not to down-stage the disease.

Several questions may be asked about this practice. Does it cause shrinkage of the prostate gland and/or tumor? Does it affect the technical aspects of surgery, for example blood loss or difficulty of dissection? Does it decrease the pathological stage of the tumor, particularly

Table 12.2 Gonadotropin releasing hormone (GnRH) antagonists currently most advanced in development. (Reproduced with permission from Zlotta, 2001)

Generic name	Brand name	Company	Phase of development
Abarelix (PPI-149)	Plenaxis®	Praecis/Sanofi–Synthelabo/Amgen	filed with USA Food and Drug Administration
A 84861		Abbott & TAP holdings	phase I
A 76154		Abbott & TAP holdings	pre-clinical
Cetrorelix (SB-75)	Cetrotide®	Asta Medica AG	marketed in 1999 for ovarian stimulation in assisted reproduction; phase II for prostate cancer
FE 200486 [4]		Peptide Biology/La Jolla–Ferring AG	phase I
Ganirelix (ORG-37462)	Orgalutran® Antagon®	NV Organon	marketed in 1999 for ovarian stimulation in assisted reproduction
GnRH pharmaccine (GnRH vaccine)		Aphton Corporation-SB	phase I-II
Ramorelix		Aventis	phase II
Teverelix	Antarelix®	Asta Medica AG	phase I

Table 12.3 Metabolism of [^{14}C]androstenedione formed by the prostatic cancer cell lines PC-3, DU145 and LNCaP. (Reproduced with permission from Koh et al. 2001, Arch Androl, 46: 117–26. www.tandf.co.uk/-journals)

Substrate and metabolites	PC-3 (%)	DU145 (%)	LNCaP (%)
[^{14}C]Androstenedione	5.2 ± 0.10	3.8 ± 0.04	24 ± 0.62
Metabolites			
DHEA	21 ± 0.33	16 ± 0.21	12 ± 0.21
androstenediol	2.2 ± 0.03	4.8 ± 0.12	ND
testosterone	4.2 ± 0.07	4.97 ± 0.08	6.4 ± 0.07
DHT	26 ± 0.31	17 ± 0.09	9.7 ± 0.13
androstanedione	22 ± 0.48	19 ± 0.15	18 ± 0.29

DHEA, dehydroepiandrosterone; DHT, dihydrotestosterone

the frequency and interval to local recurrence or metastases? Does it result in prolonged survival?

Reasons to consider neoadjuvent androgen deprivation treatment are as follows:

(1) Regression of prostate cancer following castration was documented more than 50 years ago.

(2) Apoptosis, or programmed cell death, can be induced in normal, benign hyperplastic and malignant prostatic epithelial cells by any procedure that decreases the intracellular concentration of DHT by 80% or more.

(3) Apoptotic cell death appears be a genetic suicide process that requires activation of a series of genes, and is characterized morphologically by shrunken cells with condensed and fragmented nuclei (apoptotic bodies), and biochemically by preferential intra-nucleosomal DNA digestion.

Neoadjuvant androgen withdrawal has many attractive theoretical features, and research in this area is justified and important. However, continued caution is required in interpreting studies using a pathological stage as an endpoint despite apparently encouraging results. It remains possible that pathological understaging occurs following neoadjuvant therapy and leads to a spurious decrease in positive margin rates. Accordingly, the role of neoadjuvant hormonal therapy before radical prostatectomy remains controversial. Many argue that apparent downstaging results in difficulty with pathological evaluation of neoadjuvant-treated prostatectomy specimens.

Several clinical trials have demonstrated a decrease in positive margin rates up to 50% after 3 months of neoadjuvant therapy. In another study biochemical and pathological effects of 8 months of neoadjuvant androgen withdrawal therapy before radical prostatectomy in a patient with clinically confined prostate cancer revealed low positive margin rates and PSA nadir levels. The initial rapid decrease in PSA level results from cessation of androgen-regulated PSA synthesis and apoptosis, while the subsequent slower decrease reflects decreasing tumor volume. In another randomized prospective clinical trial comparing radical prostatectomy alone versus radical prostatectomy preceded by androgen blockade in clinical stage B2 (T2bNxM0) prostate cancer revealed that patients who received androgen deprivation preoperatively had significantly lower rates of capsular penetration, positive margins and tumor at the uretheral margin (reviewed by Bissada, 2001; Bissada, personal communication).

In another study comparing the biochemical and pathological findings in 3-month versus 8-month neoadjuvant hormonal therapy before radical prostatectomy concluded that the optimal duration of neoadjuvant therapy is longer than 3 months. However, continued caution is justified in interpreting studies with pathological stage as an endpoint.

Several studies compared the result of radiation therapy alone versus neoadjuvant and neoadjuvant androgen deprivation with radiation therapy in the management of localized or locally advanced prostate cancer. The radiation therapy group randomized patients with locally advanced disease to radiation alone versus radiation therapy combined with total androgen blockade. The total androgen blockade began 8 weeks before the radiotherapy and continued for a total of 16 weeks. The combined therapy arm demonstrated an increase in local control and disease-free survival. Compelling data that androgen ablation with radiation therapy is superior to radiation alone was recently published (reviewed by Bissada, 2001; Bissada, personal communication).

Another trial for studying biochemical outcome following external beam radiation therapy with or without androgen suppression therapy for clinically localized prostate cancer showed significant benefit in 5-year PSA outcomes for men with clinically localized prostate cancer in intermediate and high-risk groups treated with radiation therapy plus 6 months of androgen suppression therapy versus those treated with radiation therapy alone (reviewed by Bissada, 2001; Bissada, personal communication).

Management of hormone-refractory prostate cancer

Prostate cancer that is progressive despite the maintenance of castrate levels of testosterone is generally referred to as hormone-refractory or androgen-independent prostate cancer. These terms, however, are misnomers,

as most progressive cancers remain sensitive to androgens and some may respond to alternative hormonal manipulations. Development of hormone-refractory prostate cancer is a significant clinical finding, with median survival of usually 9–12 months.

Hormone-refractory prostate cancer is a heterogeneous disease; prognosis may vary among different subgroups of patients. Patients may present only with a rising PSA level without significant disease-related symptoms, in contrast to patients with multiple osseous metastases, a declining performance status and severe pain. Mechanisms implicated in the development of androgen independence may include mutations in androgen receptor genes and expression of the anti-apoptotic protein, BCL-2. Assessing disease response to treatment has been a barrier in the development of new treatments, as about 60% of patients will have disease confined to bone, which is not amenable to classic response criteria. There is now evidence that suggests that patients with a decline in PSA level of 50% or more after cytotoxic therapy may have improved survival. Currently available treatments are palliative, and therefore measures of improvement in quality of life status and performance are often incorporated in clinical trials.

Most patients with advanced prostate cancer will be treated with a combination of medical or surgical castration and an antiandrogen. Discontinuation of antiandrogen is generally the first maneuver in patients with progressive hormone-refractory prostate cancer. Antiandrogen withdrawal is seen in about 15–30% of patients and the median duration of response is about 4 months. In addition, several other secondary hormonal manipulations can be performed, including use of a second antiandrogen, inhibition of adrenal steroidogenesis and treatment with alternative steroids. PSA responses in 23–38% of patients have been reported with the use of bicalutamide after flutamide failure. Duration of response is usually short, lasting about 4 months. Ketoconazole can effectively inhibit adrenal androgen synthesis, and a PSA response of 63% has been reported. Glucocorticoids and megestrol acetate can be used as palliative treatments, and a PSA response has been seen in a minority of patients. PC-SPEC, an extract of eight different Chinese herbs, has been shown to produce PSA responses in 54% of patients with androgen-independent prostate cancer. PC-SPEC can now also be considered a secondary hormonal maneuver.

Chemotherapy has been extensively evaluated in the management of patients with hormone-refractory prostate cancer. The combination of mitoxantrone and prednisone was shown in a randomized trial to be superior to prednisone, primarily with regards to palliation of symptoms. There has been renewed interest in the use of cytotoxic chemotherapy, as clinical trials in the past few years have documented PSA response of 30–60% (see Table 12.1). Recent data suggest that antimicrotubular agents such as estramustine, taxotere, etoposide and vinblastine may inhibit tumor growth and improve quality of life. Taxotere *in vitro* has been shown to be highly potent in inhibiting Bcl-2 and, as a single agent, has produced a PSA response of about 30–50%. The combination of estramustine with taxotere has been particularly attractive, with a PSA response in the range of 60 to 70%.

Many patients with hormone-refractory prostate cancer have bone pain or functional impairments adversely affecting quality of life. Bone-seeking radiopharmaceutical agents offer yet another approach to patients with widespread bone disease not controlled with analgesics. Glucocorticoids and radiation therapy are useful for treatment of painful bone metastases. Currently a wide variety of approaches are being investigated including differentiating agents, monoclonal antibodies directed at growth factor receptors, anti-angiogenic agents, matrix metalloproteinase inhibitors, signal transduction inhibitors, gene therapy, and bisphosphonates.

Treatment of hormone-refractory prostate cancer has changed dramatically over the past decade. However, despite therapeutic advances, treatment largely remains palliative. Enhanced understanding of the molecular mechanisms leading to androgen independence is critical for making further improvements. Well-designed randomized clinical trials are crucial to help elucidate improvements in quality of life and survival in patients with hormone-refractory prostate cancer.

Brachytherapy for localized prostate cancer

Brachytherapy is the placement of radioactive sources into or near tumors for therapeutic purposes. Prostate brachytherapy was first reported in 1913 and involved the temporary placement of radium sources into the prostate via the urethra. At the Memorial Sloan-Kettering Cancer Center, radioactive iodine (^{125}I)

implants were used with an open retropubic approach. Dosimetry, seed placement and outcomes were suboptimal and thus brachytherapy was note widely utilized until the transperineal ultrasound-guided approach was introduced in the 1980s. This largely initiated the current era of transrectal ultrasound-guided transperineal interstitial seeding for the treatment of prostate cancer. Currently, several techniques are employed to ensure proper seed placement. All modern techniques involve imaging of the prostate for planning and guidance in seed placement. Ultrasound is the most commonly utilized imaging modality, although computerized tomography (CT) and magnetic resonance imaging (MRI) have been used. Along with imaging modalities, several techniques have been proposed to determine the number and location of radioactive seeds.

Isotopes

Initial isotopes utilized for prostate brachytherapy include radium needles and ^{198}Au. With improved understanding of radiation physics, the use of these isotopes has given way to ^{125}I and palladium (^{103}Pd). ^{125}I is the most commonly used isotope at this time. It has a half-life of 59.6 days and a low X-ray energy of 27 keV. ^{103}Pd is the second most commonly utilized isotope for prostate brachytherapy. The energy spectrum is similar to that of ^{125}I with a 21 keV X-ray energy, but it has a significantly shorter half-life (17 days). Owing to the shorter half-life of ^{103}Pd, higher activity per seed is utilized to obtain similar tumoricidal dosages. While no clinical data exist to compare outcomes, ^{103}Pd has traditionally been used for patients with higher grades of disease. Some studies have suggested less long-term toxicity with ^{103}Pd.

Outcomes

The long natural history of prostate cancer and the patient population affected combine to make outcome analysis difficult. The use of disease-specific death rates as an endpoint is not feasible. PSA measurements are now widely utilized as a surrogate endpoint. Owing to the difficulties with comparisons of PSA failure from surgery or from radiotherapy, outcome analysis, which includes PSA levels as a surrogate endpoint, remain difficult. Post-radiation biopsy has been advocated, but this is not widely utilized, because of sampling errors and difficulties with interpretation. At this time, the definition for failure related to brachytherapy remains elusive. The definition of the American Society of Therapeutic Radiation and Oncology requires three consecutive rising PSA values, each obtained at least 3 months apart.

Concluding remarks

Interstitial radioactive seed implantation for prostate cancer offers another viable treatment for patients with prostate cancer. The advantages over surgery are the avoidance of a major surgical procedure, a lower incidence of significant complications such as incontinence, and the rapidity with which normal functions can begin. ED continues to be a concern. The true rate of ED after brachytherapy is approximately 50%. The major advantages over external beam radiotherapy involve the time commitment by the patient. Modern external beam radiotherapy is a weekly treatment, whilst brachytherapy is largely an out patient procedure. Longer follow-up is needed for adequate evaluation of how successful brachytherapy will be for the treatment of localized prostate cancer.

External beam management with high-dose conformal radiotherapy

External beam radiotherapy has been used for the curative treatment of prostate cancer for many years. The problems with traditional means of treating prostate cancer with radiotherapy has been a less than optimal cure rate and an unacceptable frequency of unpleasant adverse effects, most notably intestinal problems. Since 1995, external beam three-dimensional conformal radiotherapy was introduced in South Carolina with the dual aims of increasing the dose to the prostate and decreasing complications. The standard target to restrict high-dose treatment was altered to the prostate gland and seminal vesicles when indicated. Doses ranged between 72 and 80 Gy to the target point within the prostate.

Protocol

Patients were treated with the aid of CT-defined targets to encompass the prostate and seminal vesicles. Postoperative, metastatic and recurrent cases were not included. All patients were treated using immobilization devices custom made for each patient prior to CT scanning in the treatment position. A common five-field technique was employed in most cases; however, this treatment was part of clinical care. The targets (prostate and seminal vesicles) were defined by the treating physicians and the normal structures by trained dosimetry personnel. Treatment plans were intended to cover the targets with an isodose cloud that approximated 95% of the target dose. No specific restrictions were applied to any normal tissues, but the directions and intent were to minimize the dose to the rectum and bladder. The technique, commonly using five fields – opposed lateral (two), an anterior and two (right and left) posterior obliques. Patients were followed every 3 months for the first 2 years after treatment, and then every 6 months. A standard toxicity scoring system, the RTOG acute morbidity score, was used to assess toxicity.

The important issues monitored related to urinary and rectal toxicities. Grades 3 and 4 are important issues regarding function of these systems, such as bleeding, hospitalization and strictures. The grading system reports: grade 0, no toxicity; grade 1, symptoms, no treatment; grade 2, symptoms requiring treatment. These criteria were a means of assessing toxicity; however, grade-1 and -2 events are often subjective on the part of patients and examiners.

Results

A total of 64 patients were treated: 30 with doses of 69–73 Gy and 34 with doses of 75–80 Gy to the International Commission on Radiological Units and Measurements (ICRU)-50 point, usually the center of the gland. There were no grade-3, -4 or -5 (deaths) urinary or rectal toxicities. Rectal/intestinal complaints of tenesmus and diarrhea were scored. These occurred infrequently, regardless of dose. No patient had tenesmus in the low-dose group and only one in the high-dose group. An episode of diarrhea occurred in three patients treated in the lower dose group and in the higher dose group. Of six episodes of late bleeding, detected by guaiac or patient report, there was no case of rectal injury. Investigation disclosed polyps in two and hemorrhoidal causes in three, with only one unexplained. More than 75% of patients had no rectal or intestinal complaint through 2 years of follow-up.

Urinary symptoms are much more common in this age and disease population. Frequency was the most likely event to track. While there are more patients with no symptoms in the lower dose group, there were no differences in grade 2 toxicities. The higher dose produced complaints treated with medication in one-third of the patients. Importantly, no long-term exacerbation of urinary problems occurred. There was some correlation between volume of rectal irradiation and symptoms.

Concluding remarks

The reason to conform radiotherapy is to increase the dose and decrease the toxicity. CT technology provides a more precise means to identify targets, to treat and to protect. The risk of CT is that higher dose treatment might cause more toxicity and impair control if regional nodes are no longer part of the target. Wise targeting and delivery of therapy is not associated with a significant increase in normal tissue toxicity, at least to levels of 80 Gy. The relapse in nodes remains an infrequent event. The hypothesis that the prostate dose might be compromised if larger volumes are used for even a portion of the treatment leaves the door open for a dual approach. Nodal involvement may be the harbinger of distant metastasis; those at risk for distant disease may require systemic therapy.

The paucity of bowel toxicity despite a higher dose can be explained by volume. If the bowels are not irradiated, there should be less risk of diarrhea and late bowel effects. There is no clear relationship between volume of the bladder or dose or irradiation and symptoms. It is clear that the population begins with certain voiding issues before therapy, and one observation that is difficult to quantify or document is that treatment magnifies underlying pre-existing complaints. Pelvic radiotherapy is recommended by some authors, whereas others prefer categorically to refer high-risk patients for systemic management with hormones and increasingly with chemotherapy in the neoadjuvant setting.

Molecular oncology of prostate cancer

Cancer is a multiple-step disease resulting from a series of genetic and epigenetic changes that abrogate normal cellular controls, progressing through initiation, promotion and metastatic growth (Sementchenko and Watson. personal communication). In general terms, cancer can be viewed as a loss of control of cellular homeostasis. Cell homeostasis (steady state number of cells) is caused by a balance between proliferation and cell death. Cellular transformation can be viewed as a loss of the proper relationship between these events. Oncogenes and tumor suppressor genes act as modulators of cell proliferation, while the balance of apoptosis and anti-apotosis genes controls cell death. In addition to alterations that affect the function of single genes, mutations in some loci lead to alterations of multiple genes. While this concept has been best exemplified by defects in the mismatch repair genes that lead to increased genomic instability, it is likely that genes that affect mRNA processing, stability and translation also affect the function of many genes. Collectively, genetic and epigenetic alterations contribute to the multiple events that occur during cancer development. Molecular studies to elucidate genetic alterations that lead to cancer provide new possibilities for: earlier detection, as well as better diagnosis and staging of disease; detection of minimal residual disease recurrences and evaluation of response to therapy; and novel treatment strategies.

Prostate cancer is the most prevalent cancer in American males and the second leading cause of their cancer death. Several factors contribute to its etiology: age, race, diet, androgens, environment and genetic factors. The development of many tumor types progresses from normal dysplasia to carcinoma *in situ* to localized primary tumor to tumor with metastases. The progression of prostate cancer varies considerably among patients. Indolent prostate cancers may remain localized for decades, while aggressive cancers can metastasize rapidly to lymph nodes and/or by hematogenous routes. Human prostate cancer is heterogeneous in appearance and genetically unstable. Multiple genotypes from the same primary prostate tumor in phenotypically similar foci are frequently identified. A better understanding of the molecular controls that regulate prostate cancer growth and transformation is needed to develop more effective therapeutic approaches for aggressive prostate cancer. Furthermore, such understanding may allow insight into new markers for patient stratification, allowing those patients most likely to progress to clinical prostate cancer to be treated aggressively. Based upon these observations, genetic and epigenetic studies of prostate cancer have been directed towards elucidation of possible mechanisms that could account for the rapid progression in some patients.

Molecular progression

Despite recent advances in molecular genetics of prostate cancer, the molecular pathogenesis of this disease remains largely unknown. Several events may lead to aberrant gene expression in the prostate. Somatic mutations that occur in the coding or regulatory sequences may lead to activation of oncogenes, silencing of tumor suppressor genes or creation of mutant protein products unable to carry out normal function. Loss of DNA on the chromosomal level is called loss of heterozygosity (LOH). Several chromosomal loci vulnerable and frequently affected in prostate cancer, and candidate genes identified through LOH studies are potential tumor suppressor genes. In addition to LOH, microsatellite instability and DNA methylation may also contribute to inactivation of tumor suppressor genes in prostate cancer.

Methylation on demethylation of specific promoters may also lead to abnormal gene expression. Differential action of a multitude of transcription factors in normal and neoplastic tissue may result in the abnormal expression of many target genes, contributing to cellular transformation. Genes that have been implicated in prostate cancer progression can be subdivided by function into several groups. These include genes that encode products required for:

(1) Maintenance of intracellular homeostasis. An example is GST-π, which is ubiquitously expressed in the normal prostate and believed to be responsible for detoxification of free radicals and other compounds that damage the cell; it is reduced in prostate cancer following promoter methylation.

(2) Cell signaling molecules. PTEN, a lipid phosphatase that dephosphorylates PIP-3, is lost in prostate cancer, resulting in activation of the PKB-AKT pathway leading to increased cell survival.

(3) Cell cycle regulatory proteins. p27^{kip1}, a CDK4 inhibitor, is lost and is correlated with the tumor grade.

(4) Transcription factors. Ets2 is abnormally expressed in prostate cancer.

(5) Cell adhesion molecules. E-cadherin, a transmembrane glycoprotein, is deleted or mutated in prostate cancer.

(6) Apoptosis-related proteins. Bcl-2, an anti-apoptotic protein, is overexpressed late in prostate cancer progression, including androgen-refractory metastases.

(7) Mismatch repair proteins. These are lost or are present at a reduced level in prostate cancer and prostate cancer cell lines.

It is hypothesized that alterations in transcriptional control and repair offer two mechanisms leading to rapid changes in the transcriptome of the prostate cancer cell. Ets2 transcription factor is expressed at elevated levels in prostate cancer and is necessary for some of the transformed phenotypes of prostate cancer cells. There are defects in mismatch repair genes in prostate cancer likely to contribute to genomic instability. In addition to transcriptional changes, alterations in mRNA stability are expected to contribute to the mutator phenotype in prostate cancer.

Benign prostatic hyperplasia

BPH is the most common benign human neoplasm. Most men will live to an age where they have an 88% chance of developing histological BPH and a more than 50% chance of being symptomatic from benign prostatic obstruction. BPH seldom reduces the duration of a man's life, but it may impact heavily on his quality of life and on those closest to him (Bott and Kirby, 2001).

Genetic basis of cancer

Regardless of whether a cancer occurs sporadically in an individual or repeatedly in many individuals in a family as a hereditary trait, cancer is a genetic disease (Nussbaum *et al.* 2002).

Different kinds of genes have been implicated in initiating the cancer process. These include genes encoding:

(1) Proteins in signaling pathways for cell proliferation;

(2) Cytoskeletal components involved in maintenance of contact inhibition;

(3) Regulators of the mitotic cycle;

(4) Components of programmed cell death machinery;

(5) Proteins responsible for detecting and repairing mutations.

Different types of mutation are responsible for causing cancer. These include mutations such as:

(1) Activating gain-of-function mutations of one allele of a proto-oncogene;

(2) Loss of function of both alleles or dominant negative mutation of one allele of a tumor-suppressor gene;

(3) Chromosomal translocations that cause misexpression of genes or create chimeric genes encoding proteins that have gained novel functional properties.

Once initiated, a cancer evolves by accumulating additional genetic damage through mutations or epigenetic silencing of the genes that encode the cellular machinery that repairs damaged DNA and maintains cytogenetic normality.

FUTURE RESEARCH

Multicenter/multidisciplinary future research should include cancer biology, functional genetics and basic and preclinical therapeutics using several techniques: histopathology, microscopy, atomic force microscopy, molecular imaging lipidomics and combinatorial chemistry. This includes definition of signaling pathways involved in cell growth, metastasis, angiogenesis, enhanced tumorigenesis, tumor suppression and cell apoptosis. The roles should be defined of growth factors/G protein-coupled receptor signaling, lipid mediators of cell signaling, intracellular effectors and protein–protein interactions regulating signaling pathways, protein kinases and regulatory molecules in controlling cellular proliferation. Further definition is required of cell regulation by transforming growth factor-β_2, insulin-like growth factor-mediated tumorigenesis, proliferative signaling, signaling for cell apoptosis, lipid second messengers, reactive oxygen species and xenobiotics.

Future research in prostate cancer should include molecular markers, genetic mechanisms, tele-medicine and target genes for cancer gene therapy and inhibition of oncogene function. Functional genetics should be focused on the pathophysiological mechanisms by which either the gain or the loss of function of specific genes upsets critical pathways. Functional gene alterations leading to changes in cellular proliferation, differentiation or apoptosis are critical events for cancer progression. The role of genes whose normal expression is critical for maintenance of cellular homeostasis should be defined. This will provide several targets for therapeutic intervention that will probably be applicable to many cancers.

Rodent tumor models are applied to evaluate new anti-cancer drugs and therapeutic strategies. Data obtained from animal experiments are essential for optimizing study design for human clinical trials. The development of transgenic or human tumor xenograft mouse models allows the evaluation of various anti-cancer treatments in a more clinically relevant approach in terms of specificity of the targeted molecules, pathways, or effects on specific tumor types.

Several topics require further research, as follows: EAP1/Daxx interacts with ETS1 and represses transcriptional activation of ETS1 target genes, Ets transcription factors cooperate with Spl to activate human tenascin-C promoter, regulating Ets function by protein–protein interactions. ETS2, as required, maintains the transformed state of prostate cancer cells CaSm as an Sm-like protein that contributes to the transformed state in cancer cells. Cancer-associated Sm-like (Casm)gene antisense gene therapy is a novel approach for the treatment of pancreatic cancer. Targeting is allowed of the oncogenic transcription factor ETS2 with a triple helix-forming oligonucleotide in prostate cancer cells or mouse models in the study of the Ets family of transcription factors, hemorrhage, hematocytopenia and lethality in mouse embryos carrying a targeted disruption of the Flil transcription factor.

CHAPTER 13

Assisted reproductive technology

MICROMANIPULATION OF GAMETES AND EMBRYOS

Assisted reproductive technology includes a variety of techniques: *in vitro* fertilization (IVF) and embryo transfer (ET), gamete intra-Fallopian transfer (GIFT), zygote intra-Fallopian transfer (ZIFT), pronuclear-stage tubal transfer (PROST), tubal embryo-stage transfer (TEST), embryo banking, zona pellucida drilling, partial zona drilling (PZD), subzonal injection (SUZI), intracyloplasmic sperm injection (ICSI), semen manipulation, and cryopreservation of semen and embryos (Figures 13.1 and 13.2). The biological contribution of parents to offspring acquired by these techniques varies with respect to maternal effect, paternal effect and maternal–neonatal interaction (Table 13.1). Micromanipulation of embryos has shown that the embryos, in spite of a great reduction on their cell number, can develop through early cleavage and to blastocyst formation. The simple bisection of fully compacted late morulae or early blastocysts allows the production of identical twins in routine embryo transplantation procedures in animals.

ZONA PELLUCIDA

The zona pellucida is an extracellular glycoprotein matrix. These glycoprotein deposits are assembled during the growth phase. The zona does not attain the full ability to be recognized and penetrated until the final stages of oocyte maturation. Throughout the maturation stage of the oocyte, the zona pellucida undergoes various ultrastructural changes. During the

period from germinal vesicle breakdown until metaphase I, the oocyte secretes proteoglycan-type molecules into the developing zona pellucida. During subsequent phases of meiotic maturation (between metaphases I and II) the zona becomes more penetrable by sperm, owing to the presence of proteoglycan-filled pores that develop in its structure. The zona pellucida serves various important functions:

(1) During the induction of the sperm acrosome reaction, which is stimulated upon exposure of sperm to intact or digested zonae;

(2) Species-specific fertilization;

(3) During cleavage;

(4) Hatching of the blastocyst.

Release (hatching) of the blastocyst from the zona pellucida occurs in the uterus 4–8 days after ovulation according to the species. Dramatic functional ultrastructural changes take place in the zona pellucida during oocyte maturation, sperm binding, fertilization and polyspermy. Various methods are used in micromanipulation of the zona pellucida: assisted hatching drilling, blastocyst biopsy, blastomere transfer and nuclear substitution (Table 13.2).

In the rabbit, zona removal occurs through an enzymatic (termed blastomase) dissolution of the zona layer by cells of the underlying trophoblast. Zona layer removal by the mouse may involve rhythmic expansions and contractions of the blastocyst aided by production of zona lysin from the estrogen-sensitized

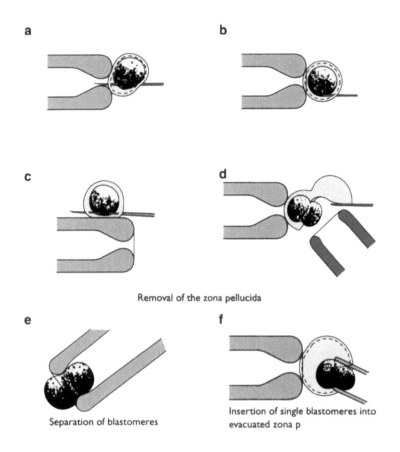

Removal of the zona pellucida

Separation of blastomeres

Insertion of single blastomeres into evacuated zona p

Figure 13.1 (a, b, c, d) Micromanipulation of the ovum, with removal of the zona pellucida. (e) Separation of blastomeres. (f) Insertion of single blastomere into evacuated zona pellucida

uterine epithelium. Changes in zona integrity that are due to enzymatic factors produced by the uterus or embryo have been implicated in the hatching of pig blastocysts.

Exposure to the estrogen-stimulated uterine environment may cause a softening of the zona pellucida. The blastocyst appears to play the major role in hatching, as the zona becomes torn by distension of the blastocyst to squeeze between the two edges of the opening. Expansion of the blastocyst involves both cellular hyperplasia and fluid accumulation in the blastocele. Fluid accumulation within the blastocele appears to assist the hatching process, since prostaglandin antagonists prevent both blastocyst expansion and hatching.

Extensive investigations have been carried out on surface properties of the zona pellucida, on the specificity of sperm–egg interactions and on the mechanics of fertilization. The transfer of pronuclei between eggs has been employed to assess changes induced in the development of embryos following an unusual pronuclear history. Eggs with two female pronuclei can result from various forms of parthenogenetic activation, or from the use of micromanipulation to remove and insert specific pronuclei into the oocytes. Gynogenetic embryos (those containing two female pronuclei) develop abnormally; this is especially evident in their extraembryonic tissues. Micromanipulation is also used to establish mammalian eggs containing two male pronuclei.

Several techniques of embryo micromanipulation have been used to produce identical twins in cattle, sheep and pigs. The success of the technique depends on the use of agar gel to seal incisions made in the zona pellucida during micromanipulation . The agar protects the blastomeres from damage by uterine secretion and leukocytes until the embryo has developed sufficiently to survive *in utero* without a zona.

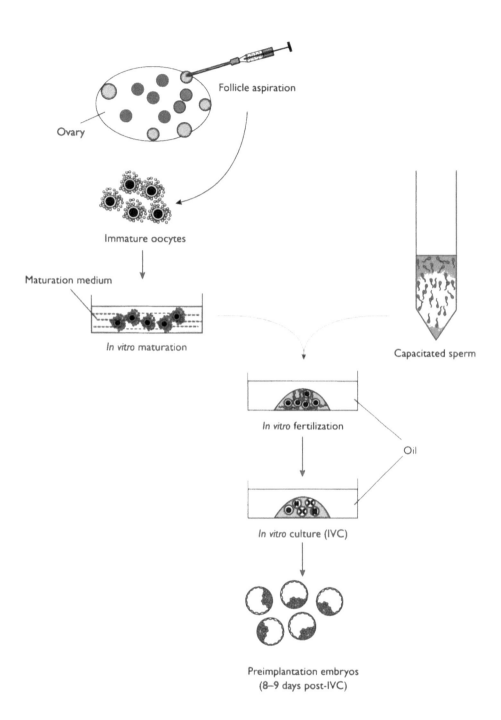

Figure 13.2 Basic steps in the *in vitro* production of embryos. Oocytes are aspirated from ovarian follicles and matured (*in vitro* maturation), fertilized with capacitated sperm (*in vitro* fertilization) and zygotes cultured (*in vitro* culture) for 8 to 9 days to obtain blastocysts for transfer to the uterus

Protocol

(1) Eggs are obtained by superovulation and denuded of cumulus cells with 0.1% hyaluronidase;

(2) Zona pellucidae are then isolated when eggs are drawn into a micropipette with an inner diameter of about 60 μm and the contents expelled;

(3) The zonae are separated from the vitelli and washed several times;

(4) The blastomeres of two-cell to eight-cell horse embryos recovered surgically 1 to 3 days after ovulation from pony mares were mechanically

separated and inserted, in various combinations, into evacuated pig zona pellucidae to make 'half' (demi) and 'quarter' micromanipulated embryos;

(5) The embryos are then embedded in agar and cultured *in vivo* in ligated oviducts of ewes for 3.5–5 days to allow development to the late morula–early blastocyst stage;

(6) Subsequent surgical or non-surgical transfer of 'half' and 'quarter' embryos to mares resulted in pregnancies, including monozygotic pairs.

INTRACYTOPLASMIC SPERM INJECTION

Various methods of assisted reproductive technology have been applied for different types of male and female infertility. The most popular method is ICSI. The micromanipulation techniques used to enhance fertilization in both animals and humans are reviewed. Using knowledge derived from the human research, direct sperm injection into the oocytes of domestic species was reinvestigated. Exogenous oocyte activation was not mandatory for fertilization. The birth of a lamb indicates that normal development can occur subsequent to sperm injection. The lamb was produced from sperm that had been sorted on a flow cytometer and was of the predicted sex. There are several potential uses of sperm injection for domestic and exotic species.

As the minimum number of human sperm required for ICSI is relatively small (determined by the number

Table 13.1 Biological contribution of parents to offspring acquired by various techniques. (Reproduced with permission from McLaren, 1970, p. 101)

	Paternal genome	Maternal genome	Maternal neonatal interaction
Normal conception	+	+	+
Artificial insemination (semen from husband)	+	+	+
Artificial insemination (semen from donor man)	–	+	+
Egg transfer (egg from wife)	+	+	+
Egg transfer (egg from donor woman; semen from husband)	+	–	+
Artificial insemination and egg transfer (sperm from donor man; egg from donor woman)	–	–	+
Adoption	–	–	–

Table 13.2 Manipulation/micromanipulation of eggs/morulae

	Description
Micromanipulation of zona pellucida and related techniques	'zona drilling' by mechanical force
	'puncture' with acid Tryod, pronase, or trypsin solution with micropipette
	'cracking' using two fine glass hooks controlled by a micromanipulator
	'PZD' partial opening using mechanical force only, followed by microinsemination
Transfer of early germ cells	transfer of male germ cells in PVS, chromosomes of male or female gametes undergo characteristics of species
Nuclear, cell or blastomere transfer	transfer of part of a cell, especially nucleus or whole cell (fusion of cytoblast/karyoplasts with host cells is inhibited by electrofusion)
Blastocyst biopsy	one or two blastomeres are removed (for preimplantation diagnosis of sex genetic anomalies) allowing remaining embryos to develop into an individual
Cloning (nuclear substitution)	nuclear transplant into enucleated egg, to enable continual propagation of particular gene, trait or species
Transgenic animals	cloned genes introduced into somatic cells or embryos

PZD, partial zona drilling; PVS, perivitelline space

of oocytes available for injection), a reliable preparation to yield a sufficient concentration of very motile cells would be of significant importance (Chen *et al.* 1995; Palermo *et al.* 1996). Variations of fertilization after ICSI include the following cytological parameters:

(1) Two pronuclei, two polar bodies;

(2) Three pronuclei, one polar body;

(3) One pronucleus, two polar bodies;

(4) No pronuclei, one polar body;

(5) Early cleavage.

The major technical problem that has arisen with the use of immotile sperm for ICSI has been differentiating between live and dead sperm. In this sense, fluorochromasia in a living cell is well characterized and some dyes are known to function in live or dead cells.

EMBRYO SEXING, NUCLEAR TRANSFER AND CLONING

Embryo sexing involves various techniques: detection of sex chromatin mass, fluorescent *in situ* hybridization, detection of H-Y antigen, use of Y-specific probes and chromosome analysis. Various factors are involved in nuclear transfer: use of a particle gun, sperm-mediated gene transfer, injection of the pronuclei, retroviral-mediated gene transfer, injection of cytoplasm of the oocyte and germinal vesicle gene injection.

Cloning, organ transplant and knockout genes

Organ failure is a major cause of death and disability and – except for the kidney – the only treatment is transplantation. Because of the shortage of human organs, a fraction of people who need transplants get them, and many die while waiting. In the USA, more than 80 000 people are awaiting an organ transplant. During 2001 some 24 000 transplants were performed, while 6000 people died waiting for their operation. Developing another source of organs would have a profound impact on society. In 2002 PPL Therapeutics and their competitor Immerge Bio Therapeutics both created pigs that lacked one of the two copies of the critical gene, called the GGTA1 gene. The GGTA1 gene makes a sugar called α1-galactose, which lines pig

blood vessels. Because it is nearly identical to a bacterial sugar, the human immune system attacks it.

The prospect of pigs providing humans with an endless supply of compatible organs for transplant is one step closer. Researchers have cloned piglets lacking both copies of the gene that makes the human immune system reject pig tissue. The Scottish company helped make Dolly the sheep, the first mammal cloned from adult cells. Four healthy piglets with both copies of the gene 'knocked out' were born in 2002 at the company's US subsidiary in Blacksburg, VA. A fifth piglet died shortly after birth, from unknown causes.

It is believed that the difference between the human heart, which does not have the sugar, and the pig's heart, which does, is an evolutionary process. Current studies are underway in which pig organs are transplanted into other mammals (baboon) to investigate whether the organs can survive in the primates for at least 3 months. This has to be established before Federal agencies authorize future studies in man. In making the cloned piglets, PPL started with cells taken from pig fetuses. The cells were manipulated to find and knock out the GGTTA1 genes.

SPERM TECHNOLOGY AND ARTIFICIAL INSEMINATION

Sperm retrieval

Since the introduction of ICSI it has been possible for azoospermic men to father a child by using epididymal or testicular sperm obtained by aspiration or surgery. Sperm retrieval may cause testicular or epididymal damage, including inflammation or hematoma, scars or calcifications. To avoid such side-effects and to increase the chance of obtaining pregnancy, a minimum interval of 6 months between two successive sperm retrieval procedures has been recommended. Schlegel and Su (1997) obtained sperm from only one to four men with non-obstructive azoospermia undergoing testicular sperm extraction (TESE) 2–4 months after the initial procedure, and compared them with 12 of 15 men with non-obstructive azoospermia with a repeat TESE performed more than 6 months after the initial procedure. Sperm motility and pregnancy rate were not increased by increasing the interval between two successive sperm retrievals from less from 90 days to more than 180 days. The pregnancy rate declined from 50% with a less than

90-day interval to 25% with a more than 180-day interval. The trend did not quite reach significance. Sperm retrieval procedures in men with obstructive azoospermia can be carried out with time intervals of only 3 months to obtain an optimal pregnancy rate, and it might be suggested that an epididymal aspiration procedure should be preferred to a TESE (Fedder, personal communication).

Schlegel (1999) developed a new microdissection procedure. In contrast to 'traditional' TESE carried out blindly, spermatogenetically active regions of the testicle are identified by direct examination with this new technique. Thus, seminiferous tubules containing many developing germ cells are likely to be larger and more opaque than tubules without sperm production. With this microdissection procedure it seems possible to improve sperm yield with minimal tissue excision (Schlegel and Su, 1997). The potential risks for damage to the male genitalia give good reasons for cryopreserving sperm in excess after microinsemination of oocytes with sperm retrieved from the testis or epididymis (Friedler *et al.* 1997), to reduce the need for further sperm retrievals. In addition to evaluation of pregnancy rates, further studies should include ultrasonography (including flow), and endocrine and immunological evaluations of the possible consequences of repeat sperm retrievals for the male.

Various methods have been applied for *in vitro* manipulation of sperm: swim up, swim down, and the acrosome reaction test to evaluate the physiological integrity of the acrosome reaction by fluorescent microscopy (acrosome intact, incomplete acrosome reaction, complete acrosome reaction, dead sperm, abnormal sperm) (Figure 13.3). The effect of biochemical and biophysical properties of storage media on primary motility of sperm: glucose-phosphate, skimmed milk–egg yolk, egg yolk–citrate and blood serum solutions are shown in Figure 13.4.

Successful pregnancy with testicular round spermatid

Testicular round spermatid injection (T-ROSI) is an option in cases of unexpected absence of elongated spermatid or sperm in the biopsy samples. T-ROSI has already resulted in a number of live healthy births. This is a gleam of hope for couples whose infertility does not seem to be treatable, because sperm cannot be obtained

through biopsies. The application of round spermatids is limited, owing to technical problems. The main difficulties with the application of this method may relate to incomplete nuclear protein maturation of spermatids, causing a low fertilization rate, as well as lack of appropriate methodology for identification, isolation, purification with minimum loss of viability, culturing and cryopreservation of these cells. Saremi *et al.* (2002) achieved the first successful testicular round spermatid conception, with a 40-year-old man with non-obstructive azoospermia and his 29-year-old healthy wife referred to an IVF center. The husband's testicular biopsy revealed only round spermatids. Ovarian superovulation was performed. Follicular aspiration was carried out by vaginal ultrasound-guided sonography 36 h after injection of human chorionic gonadotropin (hCG). At 4–6 h after follicular aspiration, oocytes were evaluated for their quality and maturity, and kept in 20-μl drops of culture medium layered with mineral oil prior to injection.

The round spermatids were distinguished by their small size, round nucleus with a clearly defined cytoplasmic zone around them and the possible presence of proacrosomal granules. Round spermatids are also spherical cells. Before injection, the tube containing the testicular tissue suspension was centrifuged at 1500–2000 rpm for 10 min and the pellet resuspended in culture medium. A drop of 10% polyvinylpyrrolidone (PVP) was placed in the center of the inner surface of a Petri dish cap, and eight drops of 5 μl of Ham's F-10 medium supplemented with 10% human serum were arranged around it, layered with mineral oil. Seven mature oocytes (M II) were placed within each drop. Two microliters of the suspension prepared above was transferred into the central drop (PVP). Using an injection needle (6 μm internal diameter, 8 μm outer diameter), T-ROSI were injected into the cytoplasm. The viability of the spermatid was evaluated by its survival after aspiration into the injection needle. The cell was considered alive in absence of lysis. Oocytes were repeatedly washed in culture medium, and returned to their own special culture medium with control for any possible damage. Sixteen hours after T-ROSI, the oocytes were examined for the presence of two pronuclei (2PN) and transferred to new culture medium. Three good-quality embryos, (grade B) were transferred. The patient received a single dose of 5000 IU hCG on

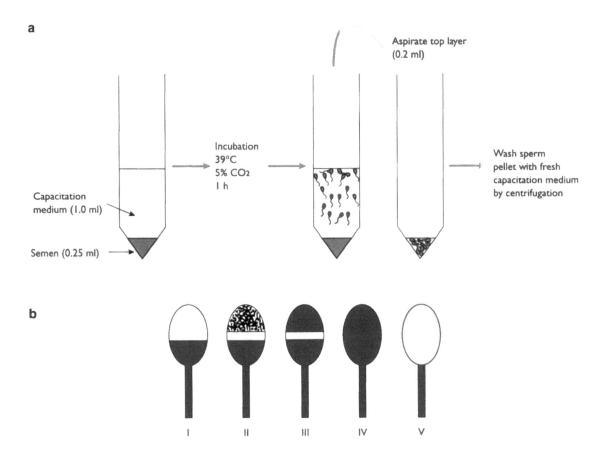

Figure 13.3 (a) The 'swim up' technique for the production of hypermotile sperm for *in vitro* fertilization. (b) The ARIC test. A population of spermatozoa are exposed to the calcium ionophore A23187 and then labeled with fluorescent lectins for specific surface sugars. The white area indicates fluorescence. I, acrosome intact; II, incomplete acrosome reaction; III, complete acrosome reaction; IV, dead sperm; V, abnormal sperm

the day of transfer for luteal phase support. One hundred milligrams of progesterone in an oil ampule was also administrated daily. Two weeks following the embryo transfer, chemical pregnancy was confirmed by levels of serum hCG. Clinical pregnancy was determined by the presence of a gestational sac 5 weeks after embryo transfer. Cesarean section was performed at the end of the 38th week of pregnancy, and a healthy girl with no congenital abnormality was delivered.

Artifical insemination

In farm mammals, artificial insemination (AI), multiple ovulation and embryo transfer (MOET), and *in vitro* embryo production (IVEP) can produce substantial increases in the rate of genetic improvement, with acceptable rates of inbreeding. In contrast, semen sexing, embryo sexing, and embryo cloning can produce only limited increases in the rate of genetic improvement. However, embryo cloning can produce a once-only substantial boost in the average genetic merit of commercial stock, and can revolutionize breed structure. Extensive investigations have been conducted on the micromanipulation techniques used to enhance fertilization and successful pregnancy with special emphasis on direct sperm injection into oocytes. Exogenous oocyte activation was not mandatory for fertilization and subsequent normal fetal development. Lambs were produced from sperm that had been sorted on a flow cytometer and was of the predicted sex. Several

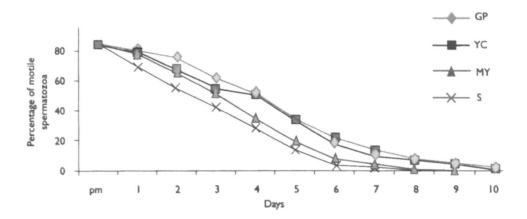

Figure 13.4 Daily percentage of motile spermatozoa during storage at 5 °C in different diluents. pm, Primary motility (prior to storage at 5 °C the first motility estimation values); GP, diluted with glucose-phosphate solutions; MY, diluted with skimmed milk–egg yolk solutions; YC, diluted with egg yolk–citrate solutions; S, diluted with blood serum. (Reproduced with permission form Güdoğan et al. 2002, Arch Androl, 49:69–75. www.tandf.co.uk/journals)

techniques have been applied for domestic and exotic mammalian species. By making possible the creation of large numbers of identical individuals, embryo cloning has the potential to greatly increase the accuracy of selection, because each potential candidate can be evaluated on the average performance of many copies of itself. However, if total testing capacity is fixed, as it usually is in practice, testing of clones can be achieved only at the expense of a reduction in the testing of families of full-sibs or half-sibs.

Microinsemination techniques include SUZI, ICSI, zona drilling (ZD) and PZD.

ASSISTED REPRODUCTION TECHNIQUES

Semen is usually diluted with egg yolk–citrate solution, homogenized whole milk, fresh and dried skimmed milk, coconut milk, seawater, blood sera or lactose solution. Skimmed milk is preferable to citrate diluents for semen. Both egg yolk and milk are used to protect against cold shock of the sperm cells as they are cooled from body temperature to 5°C. Primary motility of sperm and motility percentage before storing positively correlate with motility percentage after storing. Irrespective of the diluent, dilution rate, temperature or

conditions of storage, spermatozoa deteriorate with time of storage. The decrease in motility of spermatozoa occurs during 24 h of storage at 5°C. There is a significant effect of diluent type and storage times on the conservation rates after cooling for primary motility. The glucose phosphate diluent achieved greater values than blood serum and skimmed milk–egg yolk, while egg yolk–citrate had an intermediate value. In relation to time of storage, glucose phosphate and egg yolk–citrate diluents showed primary motility values up to day 10, but these values were 8 and 7 days for skimmed milk–egg yolk and blood serum, respectively. The glucose phosphate and egg yolk–citrate extenders maintained a primary motility of > 50% up to day 4, while skimmed milk–egg yolk showed more than 50% up to day 3 and blood serum to day 2.

Superovulation and cryopreservation of gametes

Several gonadotropin releasing hormone (GnRH) agonists and antagonists are used to superovulate fertile and infertile females (Table 13.3). There is an association between number of ovarian follicles during superovulation with human menopausal gonadotropin (hMG) versus clomiphene citrate + hMG and the

Table 13.3 Gonadotropin releasing hormone agonists available as approved drugs. (Reproduced with permission from Felberbaum et al. 2001)

Name	Structure	Route of administration
Leuprolide	pGlu-His-Trp-Ser-Tyr-DLeu-Leu-Arg-Pro-NHEt	sc, depot, 2- and 3-month depot
Buserelin	pGlu-His-Trp-Ser-Tyr-DSer(O'Bu)-Leu-Arg-Pro-NHEt	sc, nasal, depot, 3-month depot
Nafarelin	pGlu-His-Trp-Ser-Tyr-D2Nal-Leu-Arg-Pro-GlyNH$_2$	sc, nasal
Goserelin	pGlu-His-Trp-Ser-Tyr-DScr(O'Bu)-Leu-Arg-Pro-AzaglyNH$_2$	sc, depot
Histrelin	pGlu-His-Trp-Ser-Tyr-DHis(Bzl)-Leu-Arg-Pro-AzaglyNH$_2$	sc
Triptorelin	pGlu-His-Trp-Ser-Tyr-DTrp-Leu-Arg-Pro-GlyNH$_2$	sc, depot

sc, subcutaneous

percentage of implantations per follicle in different age groups of women (28–44 years) (Figure 13.5). Various methods are used for cryopreservation of mammalian embryos: in straws stored in liquid nitrogen tanks or by the use of programmable embryo freezers (Figure 13.6).

Follicle number, estradiol level and implantation

The relationship of follicle number to the outcome of IVF is universally acknowledged. Attempts to relate the number of preovulatory follicles to outcome in ovulation induction for intrauterine insemination (IUI) cycles have produced mixed results. Follicle numbers are related to pregnancy and multiple births. There is an association between estradiol level and pregnancy or multiple births in hMG–IUI cycles. There is concern about multiple births following ovulation induction with clomiphene citrate (CC) and hMG. Recommendations for preventing multiple births have included withholding hCG administration when more than six follicles are ≥ 12 mm, when more than three follicles are ≥ 14 mm or ≥ 16 mm, when more than two or three follicles are ≥ 18 mm, and when estradiol level exceeds 400 pg/ml, 600 pg/ml, 1000 pg/ml, or 2000 pg/ml. Dickey et al. (2002) evaluated the relationship between the number of preovulatory follicles or estradiol levels and multiple implantations, in patients treated with CC, hMG or CC + hMG. Inclusion of only hCG in timed IUI cycles insured that adequate sperm were present for fertilization at the time of ovulation. In hMG and CC + hMG cycles, triplet and higher-order implantations, but not twin implantations, were related to age, estradiol levels and number of follicles ≥ 12 mm and ≥ 15 mm, but not number of follicles ≥ 18 mm. In patients aged ≤ 35 years, the incidence of ≥ 3 implantations in hMG and CC + hMG cycles tripled when estradiol level was ≥ pg/ml, when ≥ 6 follicles were ≥ 12 mm or ≥ 4 follicles were ≥ 15 mm. In patients aged ≥ 35 years, pregnancy rated in hMG and CC + hMG cycles doubled when estradiol levels were ≥ 1000 pg/ml or ≥ 6 follicles were ≥ 12 mm, but ≥ 3 implantations were not significantly increased. In CC cycles, ≥ 3 twin implantations occurred in 15% of pregnancies when ≥ 6 follicles of ≥ 12 mm were present. Withholding hCG or IUI in CC, hMG and CC + hMG cycles when ≥ 6 follicles are ≥ 12 mm and in hMG and CC + hMG cycles when estradiol levels are ≥ 1000 pg/ml may reduce triplet and higher-order implantations by 67% without significantly reducing pregnancy in hMG or CC + hmG patients aged ≤ 35 years, but would reduce pregnancy rates in those aged ≥ 35 years and in CC cycles.

Retrograde ejaculation

Retrograde ejaculation is defined as absent or intermittent emission of ejaculates, orgasm without ejaculation, an ability to empty the bladder during an erection, and the presence of spermatozoa and fructose in post-coital specimens of urine. Although retrograde ejaculation is the most common cause for ejaculatory dysfunction, it is an uncommon cause of male infertility. Neurological abnormalities, bladder neck surgery, drug therapy, androgen deficiency, or retroperitoneal surgery may account for retrograde ejaculation. In addition, psychological disturbances associated with an inability to obtain orgasm present with similar findings (Ichiyanagi et al. 2003). Medical treatment for the correction of retrograde ejaculation is based either on increasing sympathetic tone at the bladder neck or on

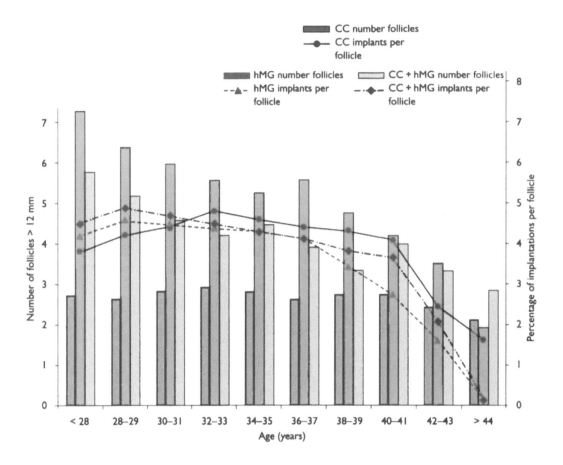

Figure 13.5 Association between number of ovarian follicles during superovulation with human menopausal gonadotropin (hMG) versus clomiphene citrate (CC) + hMG and percentage of implantations per follicle in different age groups (28–44 years). (Reproduced with permission from Dickey *et al.* 2002)

decreasing parasympathetic activity, and was conducted with α-agonistic or anticholinergic and antihistaminic drugs. At given doses, side-effects of drugs given for the reversal of retrograde ejaculation include various degrees of dizziness, sleep disturbances, weakness, restlessness, dry mouth, nausea or sweating during the medical treatment (Ichiyanagi *et al.* 2003).

Amezinium (4-amino-6-methoxy-1-phenylpyridazinium methyl-sulfate), a new type of antihypotensive agent, is a selective reversible inhibitor of intraneuronal monoamine oxidase and also shows only a moderately potent inhibition of extraneuronal monoamine oxidase. In the rabbit, amezinium shows a direct contractile response in the urethra.

Ichiyanagi *et al.* (2003) evaluated a new type of antihypotensive agent in three patients with retrograde ejaculation. They were orally administered with 10 mg amezinium once a day. All patients achieved antegrade ejaculation. Semen analyses revealed $6–50 \times 10^6$ /ml (mean 28.7×10^6/ml) spermatozoa with the motility of 20–50% (mean 36.7%). The wives of two patients became pregnant within 6 months of the initial treatment. None of the patients had any side-effects.

Equipment and accessories for gamete cryopreservation

The necessary equipment, glassware and accessories for cryopreservation include the following:

a

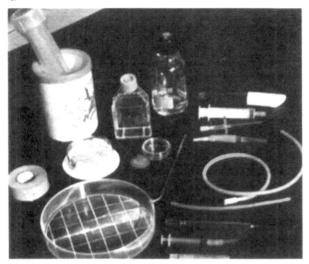

b

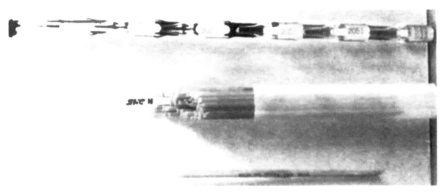

c

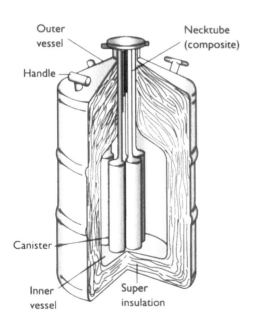

Outer
vessel

Necktube
(composite)

Handle

Canister

Inner
vessel

Super
insulation

Figure 13.6 (a) Glassware used for cryopreservation of embryos. (b) A 0.5 ml straw and goblet holding 36 straws in comparison with a 1.0-ml ampule on a six-ampule cane. (c) Liquid nitrogen container showing inner construction, including storage area, absorbent, vacuum and insulation. The high-strength aluminum shell is durable and lightweight

(1) Programmable freezer for cryopreservation of the embryo;

(2) Refrigerator for media, solutions and hormones;

(3) Liquid nitrogen tank with aluminum canes;

(4) Microscope and stereoscope;

(5) Laminar flow hood;

(6) Quantitative pipettes for preparation of cryoprotectant solutions;

(7) Catheters and pipettes for manipulation of embryos;

(8) Culture dishes of various sizes;

(9) Straws and ampules and selective sealer to seal ampules.

CHAPTER 14

Genetic engineering in mammals

Fertilization involves the union of the DNA of the nucleus in the sperm head with the DNA in the nucleus of the ovum. The egg undergoes complex maturational changes known as meiosis before it is ready for fertilization. These changes begin during fetal life and are completed only after ovulation and sperm penetration.

GENETIC MANIPULATIONS

Fundamental basic research, initiated on the regulation and function of specific genes, forged the way to *in vivo* genetic modifications that resulted in either the gain-of-function of a transferred gene or the ablation of an endogenous gene product (Pinkert, 2000). Extensive investigations have been conducted on embryonic stem (ES) cell physiology and transgenic animal technology (Palmiter *et al.* 1982; Matsui *et al.* 1992; Brinster, 1993; Wood *et al.* 1993; Pinkert, 1994a,b, 1997, 2000; Rexroad and Hawk, 1994; Houdebine, 1997; Wilmut *et al.* 1997).

The milestone of development of transgenic technology is summarized in Table 14.1. The definition and application of transgenic animal models and gene transfer methodology are shown below (Pinkert, 2000).

Application and use of transgenic animal models

Transgenic animals have provided models in biomedical, veterinary, agricultural and biotechnology disciplines in the study of gene expression and developmental biology, as well as for modeling:

Table 14.1 Transgenic animal milestones

Year	Milestone
0	Genetic selection to improve animal productivity
1880	Mammalian embryo cultivation attempted
1891	First successful embryo transfer
early 1900s	*In vitro* embryo culture develops
1961	Mouse embryo aggregation to produce chimeras
1966	Zygote microinjection technology established
1973	Foreign genes function after cell transfection
1974	Development of teratocarcinoma cell transfer
1977	mRNA and DNA transferred into *Xenopus* eggs
1980	mRNA transferred into mammalian embryos
1980–1981	Transgenic mice first documented
1981	Transfer of embryonic stem (ES) cells derived from mouse embryos
1982	Transgenic mice demonstrate an enhanced growth (GH) phenotype
1983	Tissue-specific gene expression in transgenic mice
1985	Transgenic domestic animals produced
1987	Chimeric 'knockout' mice described
1989	Targeted DNA integration and germ-line chimeric mice
1993	Germ-line chimeric mice produced using co-culture
1994	Spermatogonia cell transplantation
1997	Nuclear transfer using ES and adult cell nuclei in sheep

(1) In many fields including, embryology, endocrinology, genetics, immunology, neurology, oncology, pathology, physiology, toxicology and virology.

(2) Genetic bases of human and animal disease and the design and testing of strategies for therapy.

(3) Gene therapy.

(4) Disease resistance in man and animals.

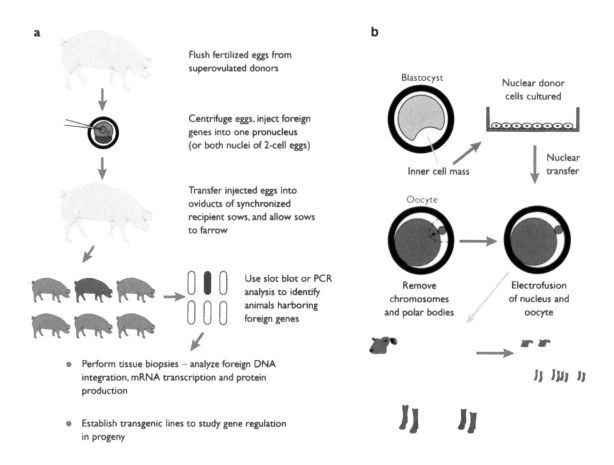

Figure 14.1 (a) The methodology used in the production and evaluation of trangenic pigs by DNA microinjection. Note that for microinjection into zygotes (or later-stage ova), visualization of the pronuclei (or nuclei) is necessary. This is accomplished by centrifugation of the ova to stratify the opaque (lipid) material, making pronuclei or nuclei readily visible (from Pinkert, 1994b). (b) Nuclear transfer and cloning. Cells from blastocysts (e.g. inner cell mass cells) or other somatic tissues are obtained and grown in culture. These cells are used as nucleus donors for transfer into enucleated oocytes. In contrast to DNA microinjection, this genetic-engineering process includes an electrofusion step to fuse the transferred nuclei and enucleated oocytes. The fused 'couplets' transferred nucleus + oocytes) are transferred to recipients and liveborn offspring are then evaluated for the genetic modification. (Reproduced with permission from Pinkert, 2000)

(5) Drug and product efficacy testing/screening. Toxicological screening protocols can now incorporate transgenic technology.

(6) Novel or improved products ('molecular farming'), ultimately targeting products or productivity of domestic animals. Models range from enhancing production traits of interest to 'foreign' protein production and human organ replacement (xenotransplantation).

Definitions

DNA microinjection is a gene transfer technique in which DNA constructs (transgenes) are directly injected (or microinjected) into pronuclei or nuclei of fertilized ova (Figure 14.1). DNA microinjection is the most commonly used gene transfer technique for creating transgenic mammals.

ES cell transfer involves transfer of pluripotent ES cells into a developing embryo.

Gene transfer is defined as one of a set of techniques directed toward manipulating biological function via the introduction of foreign DNA sequences (genes) into living cells.

A transgenic animal can be an animal either integrating foreign DNA segments into its genome following gene transfer, or an animal resulting from molecular manipulation of endogenous genomic DNA.

A transgenic line is a direct familial lineage derived from one or more transgenic founders, characterized by passing on of the transgene(s) to successive generations as a stable genetic element. The line includes the founder and any subsequent offspring inheriting the specific germ-line element.

Gene transfer methodology

Mouse modeling techniques evolved from procedures for non-specific (whole genome) transfer to the transfer of discrete genes and the modification of endogenous genes:

(1) Blastomere/embryo aggregation;

(2) Teratocarcinoma cell transfer;

(3) Retroviral infection;

(4) Microinjection;

(5) Electrofusion;

(6) Nuclear transplantation;

(7) ES cell transfer;

(8) Spermatozoa-mediated transfer and spermatogonial-cell-mediated transfer;

(9) Particle bombardment and jet injection.

There are advantages and disadvantages of the DNA microinjection technique (Table 14.2).

EMBRYONIC STEM CELL TECHNOLOGY

Gene transfer has been used to produce both random and targeted insertion or ablation of discrete DNA fragments into the mouse genome. For targeted insertions, where the integration of foreign genes is based on a recombinant gene insertion with a specific homology to cellular sequences (termed homologous recombination), the efficiency of DNA microinjection is

Table 14.2 Advantages and disadvantages of DNA microinjection. (Reproduced with permission from Pinkert, 2000)

Advantages

Relatively high frequency of generating transgenic animals (20–30% of liveborn offspring)

High probability of germ-line transmission of the transgene

Relative lack of constraints on the size or type of DNA construct used

Relative stability of the transgene as it is transmitted from generation to generation

Low frequency of mosaicism or double integration (combined estimate of 10–30% of founders)

Disadvantages

Random and potentially significant influence that the site of integration may exert on transgene expression (positional effects)

Potential for undesired insertional mutagenesis

Occasional production of mosaic founders

Occasional lack of germ-line incorporation

Time and expense required to obtain micromanipulation and microinjection skills

extremely low (Cappechi, 1989; Pinkert *et al.* 1997; Pinkert and Murray, 1998). The application of ES cells into mice embryos is a powerful tool to preselect a specific genetic modification, via homologous recombination, at a precise chromosomal position. Such a preselection provides an opportunity to produce mice with the following traits:

(1) Incorporation of a novel foreign gene into their genome;

(2) Carrying a modified endogenous gene;

(3) Lacking a specific endogenous gene following gene deletion;

(4) 'Knockout' procedures (Pinkert, 2000).

Pluripotential ES cells are derived from early pre-implantation embryos and maintained in culture for a sufficient period to perform various *in vitro* manipulations. The cells may be injected directly into a host blastocyst or incubated in association with a zona-free morula. The host embryos are then transferred into intermediate hosts or surrogate females for subsequent development. Chimeric animals are produced by the use of ES cells to provide transgenic animals. Also, the genome of ES cells can be manipulated *in vitro* by introducing foreign genes or foreign DNA sequences by techniques including electroporation and microinjection.

QUESTIONS ABOUT THE USE OF ADULT STEM CELLS

Adult blood stem cells are unable to transform themselves into other types of tissue. This raises new doubts about whether they could be used to reinvigorate ailing organs. The finding supports the view that ES cells offer the most promise for treating such conditions as heart disease, spinal injury, diabetes and Parkinson's disease. The American and other governments oppose using human ES cells in medical research because it involves the death of an embryo. Some researchers have attempted to trace the evolution of blood stem cells after placing them singly into mice whose bone marrow had been destroyed. The hope was that the study would show how a single blood-making cell could grow into millions of cells, including, perhaps, cells in other tissues of the body. The blood stem cells replenished the bone marrow but made almost no other types of tissue cell. It would appear that blood stem cells make only one thing – blood. Making skin, neurons, muscle or liver cells, from such stem cells, is an extremely rare event, reducing its value for the treatment of disease. There is a new field of study directed toward regenerative medicine, which would cure or control diseases by replacing worn out cells with new cells grown from stem cells. Eventually, stem cells may be cultured into new tissue that would be used to replace or repair ailing or diseased organs. Current research is focused on two basic types of stem cell. Somatic, or adult, stem cells come from mature tissue. ES cells come form embryos that have been allowed to grow to a certain point and are then killed to extract the cells. Some researchers argue that ES cell studies are not needed, because of growing evidence that adult stem cells, when properly cultured, could grow into other tissue cells for medical treatment. However, adult stem cells offer only an uncertain promise of ever being medically useful. The debate is still continuing about which type of stem cell will be the most medically useful.

DNA MICROINJECTION

Pinkert and associates conducted extensive investigations on DNA microinjection in a variety of mammalian species. Microinjected gene constructs integrate randomly throughout the host's genome, but usually only in a single chromosomal location (the integration site). This fact can be exploited to co-inject more than one DNA construct simultaneously into a zygote. The constructs will then co-integrate together at a single, randomly located integration site. During integration, a single copy or multiple copies of a tansgene are incorporated into the genomic DNA, predominantly as a number of copies in head-to-tail concatamers. Regulatory elements in the host DNA near the site of integration, and the general availability of this region for transcription, affect the level of transgene expression. Host DNA near the site of integration undergoes sequence duplication, deletion, or rearrangement as a result of transgene incorporation.

APPLICATION OF TRANSGENIC ANIMALS

There are several techniques for gene transfer in mammals. Transgenic technology has also been applied to several species: rabbits, rodents, farm animal ruminants, poultry and fish. Gene transfer technology is valuable for dissecting gene regulation and developmental pathways *in vivo*. Gene function is influenced by *cis*-acting elements and *trans*-acting factors. In a transgenic pig program, the pregnancy rate was 25% and 1.3 piglets were born per ovum transferred. When more than 41 ova were transferred per recipient, the pregnancy rate was 47% and 2.0 piglets were born per transfer.

GENE MAPPING: APPLICATIONS IN MALARIA

Malaria is the third most lethal infectious disease, just behind HIV/AIDS and tuberculosis. Malaria kills some three million people a year. The disease is gaining strength in Africa. Up to 1800 African children under 5 years of age die each day of its shivering chills and brutal fever. Researchers have mapped the genes of the parasite that causes malaria and the mosquito that spreads it, breakthroughs that may lead to better insecticides and repellents against the insect and new ways to combat the disease. A total of 160 researchers in ten countries mapped the genes for *Plasmodium falciparum*, the deadliest form of malaria, and for *Anopheles gambiae*, a mosquito that prefers human prey and spreads malaria to millions with its blood-sucking bite.

The enormous power of modern technology is penetrating the mysteries of an ancient disease. The gene map provides new molecular targets for vaccines and drugs. New drugs are desperately needed. All of the major drugs now in use are very old and their effectiveness is fading rapidly. The drugs used to treat malaria were introduced 50–2000 years ago. German researchers are developing a drug they first tested after spotting a genetic vulnerability in one chromosome of the parasite. Studies of the *Anopheles gambiae* genome have revealed genes that may explain why the mosquitoes favor human beings above all other prey for their blood meal. Genes linked to the insect's sense of smell may be exploited to develop new repellants, while other genes may lead to novel insecticides.

Completing the gene mapping of malaria and the mosquito comes at a critical time in international public health. Malaria is becoming increasingly resistant to chloroquine, a drug that has held the line on the disease for decades. At the same time, the mosquito has become tougher to control with current insecticides. The advances also come in a era when a warming climate will let the resistant malaria parasite move into areas where it has been rare or unknown. Officials have reported that malaria, though of a different strain, was recently detected in both humans and mosquitoes in Virginia, the first time in two decades that a wild reservoir of malaria has been found in the USA. Sequencing of the two genomes opens a door to a new era of scientific opportunity in combating a terrible scourge.

FUTURE RESEARCH

Future research in nuclear and DNA transfer is critical for developing pluripotential ES cell technology. In view of the complexity of the mammalian genome, the determination of appropriate genes to engineer and transfer is quite challenging. What are the appropriate genetic targets in different species and how will gene targeting manipulations influence mammalian development? Emphasis should be placed on several mammalian genomes. Accumulating data will prove informative and adaptable to different species, as conserved linkage groups are highly exploitable. Transgenic animal models can be effectively used in scientific discoveries. The application of nuclear transfer procedures or related methodologies to provide efficient and targeted *in vivo* genetic manipulations offers the prospects of creating profoundly useful animal models for agricultural and biomedical applications (Pinkert, 2000).

Transgene animal models

In 1981, Gordon and Ruddle and five other groups reported success at gene transfer for developing transgenic mice, animals receiving new genes (foreign DNA sequences integrated into their genome). These transgenic animals are recognized as specific strains or even species variants, following the introduction and integration of new gene(s), or transgenes, into their genome. This term has been extended to include 'knockout' mice of ES cell technology. Transgenic mice are an elegant tool to explore the regulation of gene expression as well as the regulation of cellular and physiological processes.

Pinkert (2000) outlined several areas of future research in ES cells and DNA microinjection:

(1) Development of alternative DNA delivery systems (e.g. liposome-mediated gene transfer, or targeted somatic cell techniques);

(2) Identification of optimal conditions for a given gene transfer procedure and identification of breeds best suited to the specific technologies;

(3) Complete animal genome mapping and identification of homologies to human genes;

(4) Establishment of routine and efficient germplasm culture and preservation systems (from preservation of gonadal tissue to culture and cryostorage of gametes);

(5) Development of a means to reduce the number of animals and embryos required (e.g. use of polymerase chain reaction amplification of blastomere DNA, or fluorescence-activated cell sorter analyses and gating of genetically modified germplasm);

(6) Ethical considerations and regulatory requirements associated with genetic engineering experimentation.

Genetic engineering

Extensive investigations have been conducted on microinjection of eggs, egg cytoplasm and gene control in development, translation of globulin messenger RNA by the ovum, transgenic animal technology, xenotransplantation and altering the genome by homologous recombination (Lin, 1966; Brinster *et al.* 1980; Cappechi, 1989; Hogan *et al.* 1994; Pinkert, 1994a, 2000; Monastersky and Robl, 1995; Houdebine, 1997; Pinkert *et al.* 1997; Pinkert and Murray, 1998).

Novel technologies to enhance experimental gene transfer in different species are needed. Detailed information on genetic manipulation and gene transfer have great application in surgical manipulation and embryo handling, tissue and cell culture and molecular andrology.

CHAPTER 15

Molecular andrology

Normal male sexual differentiation, testicular descent and spermatogenesis require androgens. Androgens display their biological activities by binding to the androgen receptor (AR). Therefore, attention has been focused on abnormalities in the AR as a possible cause of male genital anomalies, such as cryptorchidism, hypospadias, micropenis and impaired spermatogenesis in patients with idiopathic male infertility. The AR gene has been cloned and is localized at chromosome Xq12 (Lubahn *et al.* 1988). Its protein coding region comprises eight exons with code for various functional domains: exon 1 encodes the transactivation domain, exons 2 and 3 encode the DNA binding domain, the 5′ portion of exon 4 encodes the hinge domain and the 3′ portion of exon 4 and exons 5–8 encode the ligand-biding domain (Qungley *et al.* 1995).

The AR contains a polymorphic CAG repeat sequence for the polyglutamine tract in exon 1. Progressive expansion of the CAG repeat in the human AR results in a linear decrease in transactivation function (Chamberlan *et al.* 1994). Consistent with this fact, expansion of the CAG repeat tract results in spinal bulbar muscular atrophy, a fatal neuromuscular disease characterized by low masculinization, oligozoospermia or azoospermia, testicular atrophy and reduced fertility (La Spada *et al.* 1991). Mild but statistically significant expansion of the CAG repeat tract is often associated with azoospermia (Dowsing *et al.* 1999) and ambiguous genitalia in genetic males (Yong *et al.* 1998).

Recent advances in molecular andrology have included:

(1) Mechanisms of action of luteinizing hormone (LH), which binds to a specific receptor and activates adenylcyclase, resulting in an increase in intracellular cyclic-AMP (Figure 15.1);

(2) The amino acid sequence of gonadotropic-releasing hormone (GnRH);

(3) GnRH signaling in hypothalamic neurons (Figure 15.2);

(4) Sodium dodecyl sulfate (SDS)–polyacrylamide gel electrophoresis (PAGE) analysis of peptides obtained by digestion of human serum albumin (HSA) by peptidase (Figure 15.3);

(5) Regulation of adult Leydig cell differentiations in the postnatal testis;

(6) Immunohistochemical analysis of cytokeratin and vimetin;

(7) Major metabolic pathways involved in the biosynthesis of sex steroids;

(8) Generation of cell-mediated immune response for activation of native T-helper (Th) and cytotoxic T lymphocytes (CTLs);

(9) Mechanisms of action of sex steroids;

(10) Results of multiplex polymerase chain reaction (PCR) for screening for microdeletions and genomic DNA in infertile men;

(11) The neuroendocrinology of embryonic sex differentiation;

(12) The pathophysiology of spermatogenesis;

(13) Leydig cells and Sertoli cells;

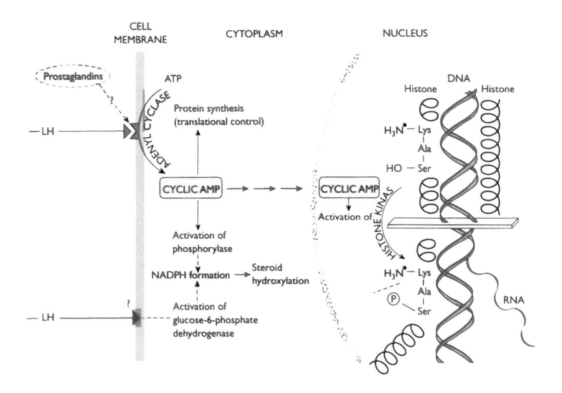

Figure 15.1 Diagrammatic representation of postulated mechanisms for the action of luteinizing hormone (LH). LH binds to a specific receptor and activates adenylcyclase, resulting in an increase in intracellular cyclic-AMP. The latter may act at the cytoplasmic level, probably by stimulating protein kinase(s), to effect control of protein synthesis at the translational level. Cyclic-AMP may also enter the nucleus and effect phosphorylation of nuclear proteins responsible for regulating DNA-dependent RNA synthesis. Newly synthesized RNA would be expected to initiate synthesis of protein, possibly a rate-limiting enzyme involved in steroid synthesis. The possibility that LH might enter the cell and directly activate an enzyme, such as glucose-6-phosphate dehydrogenase, is also illustrated.

(14) Oligoasthenoteratozoospermia (OAT);

(15) Genetic male infertility;

(16) Stem cells;

(17) Reactive oxygen species (ROS);

(18) Clusterin andropause;

(19) Erectile dysfunction (ED).

SPERMATOZOA

The structure of sperm chromatin is related to infertility and abnormal pregnancy outcome. Despite normal morphology a sperm population might contain chromosomes with microdeletions, aneuploidy, DNA strand breaks and abnormal sperm chromatin structure. The sperm chromatin structure assay (SCSA), a flow cytometric parameter, provides reliable and repeatable data on the percentage of cells with denatured DNA. The occurrence of Y-chromosome deletions is an important factor in men undergoing intracytoplasmic sperm injection (ICSI) treatment. Microdeletion in the AZF regions of the Y-chromosome is a prevalent cause of male infertility.

Clusterin (SGP-2), is constitutively expressed in Sertoli cells. The putative molecular structure and its detergent-like properties suggest a functional role. Clusterin binds to hydrophobic molecules and complexes to promote their clearance and/or uptake into cells by association with several cell-surface receptors.

Spermatid/Sertoli cell interaction

When the nucleus, covered by the acrosome, moves towards the cell surface of the spermatids during

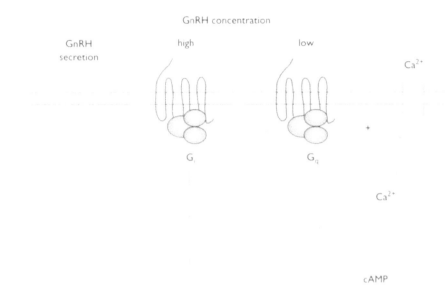

Figure 15.2 Gonadotropin releasing hormone (GnRH) signaling in hypothalamic neurons. Calcium- and cyclic AMP-dependent mechanisms are involved in the process of episodic GnRH secretion from hypothalamic neurons. Autocrine activation of GnRH receptors in GnRH neurons regulates Ca^{2+} and cAMP signaling and modulates the profile of neuropeptide secretion. Low GnRH concentrations activate cAMP signaling mechanisms via G-protein α_q. High GnRH concentrations inhibit cAMP production via G-protein α_q. (Reproduced with permission from Leung and Steele, 1992)

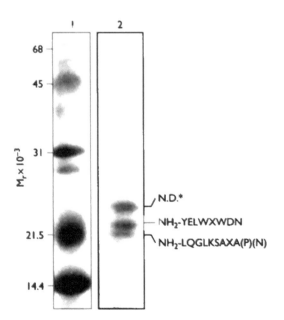

Figure 15.3 Analysis of peptides obtained by digestion of 80-kDa human serum albumin (HSA) with endoproteinase Glu-C and resolved by sodium dodecyl sulfate (SDS)–polyacrylamide gel electrophoresis (PAGE). The partial amino acid sequences of the two peptides were determined and shown against the individual bands. The sequences did not show homology with the protein in databanks. Lane 1: molecular weight markers; Lane 2: bands of the peptides obtained by the digestion of 80-kDa HSA; *N.D., not determined; X, amino acid that could not be unequivocally assigned. (Reproduced with permission from Bandivdekar et al. 2001)

mid-spermiogenesis, ectoplasmic specializations appear in the cytoplasm of Sertoli cells in apposition to the plasma membrane covering the acrosome. The ectoplasmic specialization is probably involved in attachment of the spermatids to the Sertoli cell, allowing for proper head–tail orientation of the spermatids, and remains apposed to the spermatid heads until spermiation.

There are complex interrelationships between Sertoli cells and each type of germ cell. Protein activation in response to several polypeptide ligands includes a variety of interferons, cytokines and growth factors. The testicular JAK-STAT pathway affects spermatogenesis at multiple levels, and is subserved by different intratesticular signaling molecules. Espin, an actin-bundling protein involved in the organization and function of the ectoplasmic specialization of Sertoli cells, anchors and positions spermatids with relation to the Sertoli cells. Espin binds actin with high affinity. Elegant mutational analysis has allowed identification of the actin-binding site of the protein.

Sperm–egg interactions

Gamete interaction involves the recognition between a sperm receptor located in the plasma membrane, and an oocyte receptor located in the zona pellucida (ZP). ZP3 induces the acrosome reaction. Closer interaction occurs between ZP2 and an inner acrosomal membrane receptor. Certain acrosomal proteins are needed for this process. The acrosome is necessary for the correct organization of plasma membrane proteins. Sperm–egg interaction involves several complex cell events:

(1) The acrosome reaction induced spontaneously through a variety of physiological mechanisms;

(2) The acrosome reaction induced by the cumulus cells and/or ZP;

(3) Mobilization of calcium ions;

(4) Response of some cell types to one stimulus whereas other cells respond to another stimulus;

(5) The physiological pathway utilized by the fertilizing sperm, depending on the cellular integrity of the sperm at any given time as well as the repertoire of signaling molecules within the penetrating sperm;

(6) The sperm–ZP binding interaction and subsequent acrosome reaction, with a high prognostic value of *in vitro* fertilization (IVF) outcome.

Acrosome reaction

The acrosome is a large vesicle localized on the sperm head. Fusion between the acrosomal membrane and the sperm plasma membrane results in the exocytotic release of acrosomal contents. This secretory event, known as the acrosome reaction, primes the sperm for zona penetration and sperm–egg binding and fusion (Yanagamachi, 1994; Breitbart and Spungin, 1997). The acrosome reaction is triggered by an intracellular calcium surge induced by signaling mechanisms that have been identified in some detail. The rab family of small GTPases are important regulators of intracellular membrane trafficking, and rab 3A, involved in synaptic vesicle exocytosis, has recently been detected on the acrosome of mature sperm, where it modulates the acrosome reaction (Lida *et al.* 1999; Ward *et al.* 1999; Michaut *et al.* 2000).

The final membrane merging step involves another large family of proteins, the SNAREs. A specific protein on a vesicular carrier (v-SNARE) interacts with a complementary protein on a target membrane (t-SNARE) to ensure proper docking (Rothman, 1994). SNAREs seem to be the final mediators of membrane fusion (Weber *et al.* 1998). An *N*-ethylmaleimide sensitive factor (the ATPase NSF) plays an important role in intracellular fusion. NSF was later found to exert its activity via the recruitment of soluble NSF attachment proteins (SNAPs) (Rothman, 1994; Pfeffer, 1999). NSF is an important regulator of membrane trafficking and fusion in somatic cells, and is present on bovine, murine and monkey sperm. The fact that NSF localizes mainly to the acrosome suggests that this protein, together with other factors such as rabs and SNAREs, may be a common feature in the triggering or regulating of membrane merging during the acrosome reaction (Ramalho-Santos and Schatten, 2002).

Several techniques have been applied to sperm/ acrosome morphology: acrosome assessment with prostate-specific antigen (PSA), and computer assessment of sperm morphology motility. Extensive investigations have been conducted on the ultrastructural characteristics of neurosecretory material of the hypothalamus in relation to gamete physiology.

Sperm DNA fragmentation

DNA fragmentation is a hallmark of apoptosis, and may be caused by abnormal endonuclease activity mediated by the plasma membrane protein Fas. Such apoptosis increases in the semen of infertile males, and in samples with abnormal sperm morphology or other pathologies (Hughes *et al.* 1996; Kodama *et al.* 1997; Shen *et al.* 2000; Zini *et al.* 2001a, 2001b). DNA fragmentation is also inversely correlated with IVF fertilization rates.

Spermicidal activity

Computer-assisted sperm analysis (CASA) has been applied to evaluate the spermicidal activity of several metallocene dihalides (vanadocene dichloride, VDC; titanocene dichloride, TDC; zirconocene dichloride, ZDC; molybdocene dichloride, MDC; hafnocene dichloride, HDC; vanadocene dibromide, VDB; and bis(methylcyclopentadienyl)vanadium dichloride, BVD.

METABOLIC AND ENZYMATIC PATHWAYS

Synthesis of glycosaminoglycans

The elevation in the level of dolichol may suggest the increased N-glycosylation of proteins. In Mg^{2+} deficiency, glycolysis, the citric acid cycle and oxidative phosphorylation are blocked and more glucose-6-phosphate is channeled for the synthesis of glycosaminoglycans (GAG) (Jaya and Kurup, 1986). Intracellular Mg^{2+} deficiency also results in defective ubiquitin-dependent proteolytic processing of glycoconjugates, as this requires Mg^{2+} for its function (Monia *et al.* 1990). The increase in the activity of glycohydrolases and GAG-degrading enzymes could be due to reduced lysosomal stability and consequent leakage of lysosomal enzymes into the serum (Kurup and Kurup, 2002). The increase in the concentration of carbohydrate components of glycoproteins and GAG in spite of increased activity of many glycohydrolases may be due to their possible resistance to cleavage by glycohydrolases because of a qualitative change in their structure.

Cytokines

Cytokines are secreted proteins that act as local immunological mediators, controlling the survival, development and differentiation of certain cell types, particularly those of the immune system. Growth

factors, interleukins, lymphokines, monokines, colony stimulating factors and interferon are all cytokines (Nicola, 1994). Cytokines are produced not only by somatic cells, but also by germ cells; sperm cells may use these factors in a paracrine manner to regulate spermatogenesis (Huleihel *et al.* 2000).

Isoprenoid pathway

The isoprenoid pathway is a key regulatory pathway in the cell. The important metabolites of the isoprenoid pathway are digoxin (endogenous membrane NA^+–K^+ ATPase inhibitor), dolichol (important in N-glycosylation of proteins), ubiquinone (important membrane antioxidant) and cholesterol (a component of cellular membranes) (Goldstein and Brown, 1990).

The hypothalamus (Haupert, 1989) produces the endogenous membrane Na^+–K^+ ATPase inhibitor digoxin. Digoxin, being a steroid, is synthesized by the isoprenoidal pathway (Ravikumar *et al.* 2001). Membrane Na^+–K^+ ATPase inhibition leads to hypomagnesemia (Haga, 1992). Another component of the isoprenoid pathway, ubiquinone, is a free radical scavenger and component of the mitochondrial electron transport mechanism. The alteration in mitochondrial function and qualitative changes in membrane glycoconjugates can alter sperm motility and function. The isoprenoidal pathway has been assessed in human male infertility. Systemic diseases are correlated with hemispheric dominance. Kurup and Kurup (2002) assessed individuals who were right hemispheric dominant, left hemispheric dominant and bihemispheric dominant to evaluate the role of hemispheric dominance in the genesis of infertility.

In men, the isoprenoid pathway produces three key metabolites: digoxin (membrane sodium–potassium ATPase inhibitor and regulator or neurotransmitter transport), dolichol (regulator of N-glycosylation of proteins) and ubiquinone (free radical scavenger).

Nuclear matrix-intermediate filaments

Extraction of soluble cell components is used to allow convenient observation of the cytoskeleton. A chemical dissection protocol described by Fey *et al.* (1984a, 1984b) has been designed to remove not only lipids and soluble proteins but also microtubules, microfilaments and chromatin, leaving only the nuclear matrix and the intermediate filaments (NM-IF). It includes three steps: removal of the soluble content using non-ionic detergent; high salt extraction of microtubules and microfilaments; and nuclease digestion of chromatin. The NM-IF scaffolds, easily observed by unembedded whole-mount transmission electron microscopy, preserve the essential cell architecture despite the presence of only a small fraction of the original protein content. NM-IF is composed predominantly of proteins with long, coiled coil domains. Extensive investigations have been conducted on NM-IF on several cell types: cervical epithelial cells (Odgen *et al.* 1996), breast cancer cells (Coutts *et al.* 1996), osteoblasts and osteosarcoma cells (Bidwell, *et al.* 1997) and prostatic normal and neoplastic cells (Alberti *et al.* 1996; Prasad *et al.* 1998). Markova (2001) isolated the NM-IF of sperm using sequential treatment with non-ionic detergent, high salt and nuclease. The cell membrane, acrosome and mitochondria were not present. The nucleas showed no apparent changes and revealed no details excepting pore complexes in the posterior part. Tissue-specific cytoskeletal elements (perforatorium, postacrosomal sheath, capitulum, segmented columns, outer dense fibers, submitochondrial reticulum, annulus and fibrous sheath) were retained, which permitted a parallel to be drawn between them and the intermediate filaments of somatic cells. The application of NM-IF extraction to mouse sperm revealed intermediate filament-like properties of their specific cytoskeletal elements, showed the relative stability of their microtubules and offered additional viewpoint to sperm ultrastructure (Markova, 2001).

Intracellular magnesium ion deficiency

An increase in intracellular Ca^{2+} can open the mitochondrial pore causing a collapse of the H^+ gradient across the inner membrane and uncoupling of the respiratory chain (Green and Reed, 1998). Intracellular Mg^{2+} deficiency can lead to a defect in the function of ATP synthase. All this leads to defects in mitochondrial oxidative phosphorylation, incomplete reduction of oxygen and generation of superoxide ion, which produces lipid peroxidation. Ubiquinone deficiency also leads to reduced free radical scavenging. The increase in intracellular calcium may lead to increased generation of nitric oxide (NO) by including the enzyme NO synthase (NOS)

which combines with the superoxide radical to form peroxynitrite (Olanow and Arendash, 1994). Increased calcium can activate phospholipase A_2, resulting in increased generation of arachidonic acid, which can undergo increased lipid peroxidation (Kurup and Kurup, 2002).

In infertile men there is an upregulated isoprenoid pathway with increased digoxin and dolichol and reduced ubiquinone, magnesium and red blood cell Na^+–K^+ ATPase activity (Kurup and Kurup, 2002). The increase in endogenous digoxin, a potent inhibitor of membrane Na^+–K^+ ATPase, can decrease this enzyme activity (Haupert, 1989). There is increased synthesis of digoxin as evidenced by increased human menopausal gonadotropin (hMG) CoA reductase activity. The inhibition of Na^+–K^+ ATPase by digoxin causes an increase in intracellular calcium resulting from increased Na^+–Ca^{2+} exchange, increased entry of Ca^{2+} via the voltage gated calcium channel and increased release of Ca^{2+} from intracellular endoplasmic reticulum Ca^{2+} stores (Haga, 1992). This increase in intracellular Ca^{2+} by displacing Mg^{2+} from its binding sites causes a decrease in the functional availability of Mg^{2+}. The decrease in the availability of Mg^{2+} can cause decreased mitochondrial ATP formation, which along with low Mg^{2+} can cause further inhibition of Na^+–K^+ ATPase. The Mg^{2+}-related mitochondrial dysfunction results in defective calcium extrusion from the cell. There is thus a progressive inhibition of Na^+–K^+ ATPase activity first triggered by digoxin (Haga, 1992).

Functional ultrastructure of Leydig cells

Testosterone is regulated by LH which binds to receptors of Leydig cells to activate G-protein and adenylate cyclase, which subsequently converts ATP into cyclicAMP (cAMP). This latter constituent functions as a secondary messenger to stimulate protein kinase A (PKA). PKA can phosphorylate some proteins, and those proteins can further phosphorylate other proteins or induce new protein synthesis, such as steroidogenic acute regulatory (StAR) protein. The function of StAR protein is to transfer free cholesterol from the cytoplasm into the inner membrane mitochondria; this is the rate-limiting step in steroidogenesis. An increase in StAR protein is concomitant with an increase in steroid production in steroidogenic cells stimulated with the cAMP in the MA-10 cells. After cholesterol enters the inner membrane of mitochondria, it is concerted to pregnenolone by the P450scc enzyme. Pregnenolone is transported to the smooth endoplasmic reticulum to be processed as a substrate for testosterone through various steroidogenic enzyme activities (Liu *et al.* 2002).

Nitric oxide

NO, a free radical free formed by NOS from L-arginine, functions as an intracellular messenger in various biological systems (Moncada *et al.* 1991; Nathan, 1992). NO has multiple functions in the male reproductive system. Low concentrations of NO in the sperm enhance capacitation and the ability to bind to the ZP (Zini *et al.* 1995). NO also reduces sperm motility at micromolar concentrations (Tamlinson *et al.* 1992) and both sperm motility and viability at millimolar concentrations (Weinberger *et al.* 1995). At nanomolar concentrations, NO can improve sperm motility and viability after thawing. The testosterone concentration in rat serum and testicular interstitial fluid is increased by administration of an NOS inhibitor (Adams *et al.* 1992) and suppressed by an NO donor (Adams *et al.* 1994).

Endogenous NO inhibits testosterone production, and inducible NOS mRNA expression in Leydig cells is increased by interleukin (IL)-1β (Noboris *et al.* 1997). The rate-limiting regulatory step in steroidogenesis is transport of cholesterol from the outer to the inner mitochondrial membrane. After transport the enzyme P450scc further regulates the synthesis of steroid hormones (Stocco and Clark, 1996). The transport step is mediated by StAR, which is rapidly synthesized in response to cAMP. StAR mRNA exists in Leydig cells as two major transcripts with lengths of 3.8 kb and 1.7 kb, and one minor transcript of 1.2 kb (Lin *et al.* 1998). Sodium nitroprusside, an NO generator, did not alter basal testosterone, but dose-dependently reduced testosterone production in the Leydig cells stimulated by LH at 3 h after addition of sodium nitroprusside. Induction of StAR mRNA transcripts could be detected as early as 1 h after the addition of LH (Dobashi *et al.* 2002).

Endorphin and substance P

Although the levels of both β-endorphin and substance P in the reproductive tract are several-fold higher than those found in blood serum, their role in sperm function is not clear. The seminal plasma level of β-endorphin in fertile and infertile men is not correlated with sperm concentration, motility or the egg penetration test. There is also no correlation between the concentration of β-endorphin and sperm motility parameters in *in vitro* experiments. Only Fraioli *et al.* (1984) reported that the percentage of motile sperm is reduced by human β-endorphin used at an extremely high concentration (140 000 ng/ml). An endogenous opioid peptide, β-endorphin is distributed widely in the central nervous system (CNS) and peripheral organs, including the reproductive organs.

Substance P, produced in the CNS, plays an inhibitory role in reproduction. The tachykinin reduces the GnRH-induced LH release (Battmann *et al.* 1991). Changes in concentration of substance P are correlated with the estrous cycle in rats (Parent *et al.* 1990) and with LH, follicle stimulating hormone (FSH) and estradiol levels in the human menstrual cycle (Jones, 1986). Simultaneously, the concentration of substance P in follicular fluid is similar to that of blood plasma. Several sperm functions can be modified at the time of ovulation by diverse components of the oocyte microenvironment. Thus, follicular fluid can accelerate capacitation, stimulate the acrosome reaction, induce sperm motility (Mbizvo *et al.* 1990) and attract the sperm chemotactically (Eisenbach and Ralt, 1992; Eisenbach and Tur-Kaspa, 1994). Only some substances are present in the follicular fluid; for example, heparin (Silwa, 1993) and hormones (Silwa, 1994, 1995a, 1995b) have been investigated as sperm hemoattractants.

The chemotactic effect of β-endorphin is not known in physiological conditions, but substance P stimulates chemotactic activity of different moving cells, such as eosinophils and microglia (Maeda *et al.* 1997).

N-Ethylmaleimide sensitive factor on the acrosome

Ramalho-Santos and Schatten (2002) conducted extensive and elegant investigations into NSF on the acrosome of mammalian sperm. Their initial studies in membrane trafficking identified an NSF (the ATPase NSF) as having an important role in intracellular fusion. NSF exerts its activity via the recruitment of SNAPs. However, these components were ubiquitous in many fusion events and could not, therefore, determine specificity. This paradox was partially resolved with the discovery of the membrane-bound SNAREs, the differential localization of which seems to ensure that a vesicle fuses with its appropriate target, and not with any other membrane. NSF and SNAPs act to disentangle SNARE interactions that may have formed within a single membrane, and thus free them to interact with SNAREs in another membrane. NSF may itself promote membrane fusion, although this has been immediately questioned. Similarly to both rabs and SNAREs, NSF was recently detected on both the mature and the developing acrosome. In conjunction with rab 3A there is moderate exocytosis during the acrosome reaction in human sperm. NSF is present not only in human, but also in several other types of mammalian sperm, notably on the acrosomal region. α- and β-SNAPs, the principal members of the SNAP family, although present in the developing acrosome, could not be detected in the mature organelle (Ramalho-Santos and Schatten, 2002).

Mutated mtDNA and transfection into isolated mitochondria by electroporation

There are several point mutations and rearrangements of the mitochondrial genome that cause various degenerative disorders. These mutations affect mainly tissues with high cellular energy requirements such as brain, optic nerve, cardiac muscle, skeletal muscle, kidney and endocrine organs. The ability to manipulate the mitochondrial genome in a directed fashion, followed by the introduction of modified mtDNA into functional mitochondria, represents a powerful technical breakthrough, enabling the creation of some of the first animal models to study mitochondrial dynamics and diseases of the mtDNA. When the introduction of a 7.2-kb plasmid into mitochondria by electroporation became possible, the optimum internalization was accomplished at 12 kV/cm field strength using low-range, high-fidelity PCR and standard molecular cloning protocols. Irwin *et al.* (2001) produced a 6.5-kb mouse mtDNA deletion construct, designated mt-del, and introduced this construct into isolated mitochondria by electroporation. The resultant transfected mitochondria are intact and coupled by closed-chamber respirometry, according to the functional parameters of the respiratory control ratio (RCR) and P/O ratio (ADP added/atomic oxygen consumed in state 3 respiration).

Irwin *et al.* (2001) observed alterations in mtDNA populations. Changes in cellular levels of heteroplasmy are indicative of important though relatively unexplored mechanisms in germline development and oogenesis. Therefore, the ability to introduce engineered mitochondrial genomes into viable mitochondria *in vitro* represents a significant step towards producing animal models of human development and disease related to mutations of the mtDNA. To produce a biomedically relevant mtDNA deletion, the investigators used long-range PCR and molecular cloning techniques to generate a 6.5-kb circular construct of mouse mtDNA that contained the origins of replication for both heavy and light strand synthesis.

Membrane receptors

Bolander (1994, 2000) conducted extensive investigations into membrane receptors.

Androgen-binding protein

Androgen-binding protein (ABP) is a testicular lipoprotein that binds androgens with high affinity and transports them to the epididymis. This protein, secreted by Sertoli cells, is similar to a plasma protein produced by the liver and bound dihydrotestosterone, testosterone and estradiol. The plasma protein is known by several names: sex hormone-binding globulin, sex steroid-binding protein and testosterone–estradiol-binding globulin. These are very similar physicochemically, sharing the same primary amino acid sequence, even though they differ in their carbohydrate content. The protein originates from the prostate and seminal vesicles and is present in blood serum and seminal plasma. There is a smaller protein with androgen-binding capacity in the seminal fluid. Like the nuclear receptors, receptors with intrinsic enzymatic activity are modular in structure: an aminoterminal extracellular domain binds the ligand and a carboxy-terminal intracellular domain possesses enzymatic activity. A single transmembrane α-helix connects these two regions. Three enzymatic activities are associated with these receptors. The largest group are receptor tyrosine kinases (RTKs), which mediate the effects of growth factors. The serine-threonine kinase bind only members of the transforming growth factor-β family. The last group are the guanylate cyclases.

Hormone stimulation of the RTKs is simple. These enzymes have a low basal activity; ligand binding induces receptor dimerization and mutual transphosphorylation of the activation loops of the kinases. This modification activates both enzymes, which undergo extensive autophosphorylation elesewhere.

Activation of the serine-threonine kinases is similar to that for RTKs, except that hormones induce the formation of tetramers and the transphosphorylation is unidirectional. The guanylate cyclases also form tetramers that are allosterically activated to synthesize the second messenger, cyclic GMP.

The overall structure of cytokine receptors is similar to that of RTKs, except that the carboxy terminus does not contain a kinase domain. Rather, a soluble tyrosine kinase (STK) is constitutively associated with it; i.e. the cytokine receptors can be envisioned as RTKs, whose carboxy-terminal kinase is now located on a separate subunit.

GTP-binding protein (G protein)-coupled receptors (GCRs) cross the plasma membrane via seven α-helices clustered together in a central binding pocket. The helices extend a short distance into the cytoplasm where they bind a G protein. G proteins are trimers: the β and γ subunits anchor the α subunit to the membrane and facilitate its interaction with the GCR.

The subunit is a molecular switch. When bound to GDP, it is 'off'; when bound to GTP, it is 'on' and can act as an effector for adenylyl cyclase, several ion channels and phospholipase C. Hormones bind in the pocket formed by transmembrane helices and cause them to rotate; this, in turn, alters the conformation of the α subunit, resulting in exchange of GDP for GTP, activation and dissociation of the α subunit from $\beta\alpha$ components (Figure 15.4).

There are two major families of ligand-gated ion channels. First, nicotinic acetylcholine forms pentamers having homologous subunits; each subunit contributes an α-helix to the channel wall. This α-helix has a proline that kinks the helix and narrows the lumen. A hydrophobic amino acid is located near this site and its projection into the channel further blocks the pore. Hormones bind between subunits and cause them to rotate. The kink and hydrophobic side-chain are moved to the side, thereby opening the channel like the diaphragm of a camera lens. The resulting flow of ions then mediates the biological effects of the hormone. This family includes receptors for acetylcholine, γ-aminoisobutyric acid (GABA), 5-hydroxytryptamine

and glycine. Second, are the glutamate receptors, which form tetramers having homologous subunits. Each channel consists of an eight-stranded β-barrel.

BIOMEDICAL DIAGNOSTIC TECHNOLOGY

Without medical diagnostic reagents, the practice of medicine would be difficult if not impossible. Medical reagents play an important role in maintaining and improving human wellness. Research in this area will continue unabated, and use of these reagents will ever increase. The gene chip will revolutionize the ability to fight diseases. There has been recent development of newer concepts and rapid advances in medical diagnostic reagents, immunodiagnostics, biosensors, new signals for analyte detection, newer diagnostic polymers and coatings, and enzyme stabilization (Law et al. 2002). A 'sandwich' scheme of immunoassay has been used. Iodine formed as the result of the enzymatic oxidation of iodide by a peroxidase label has been detected. The practical application of the immunoassay system has been demonstrated in the detection and quantification of IgG and IgM in human blood. The enhanced sensitivity and short assay time permit the application of the developed system to rapid detection of a wide range of analytes in medical diagnostics. The metric flow-through immunoassay system may be easily adapted for the detection of drugs and hormones. Implementation of other immunoassay schemes, such as displacement analysis and competitive schemes, is extremely valuable. The first response of the immune system to an invasion is a low-affinity (10^3/mol) interaction with antibody-coated cells in a system in which multiple interactions of low affinity produce reactivity while protecting from a spurious response. For detection or quantification of an analyte, immunological measurements can be effectively used. In immunological measurements, the enzyme-linked immunosorbent assay (ELISA) is widely used, because it can be applied easily with high sensitivity (Figure 15.5).

The use of an enzyme as a label has many advantages over the use of other kinds of label molecule in both immunohistochemistry and immunoassay. In immunohistochemistry, an enzyme–antibody conjugate permits localization and demonstration of cellular antigens in relation to tissue structures via optical microscope and electron microscope. However, in the

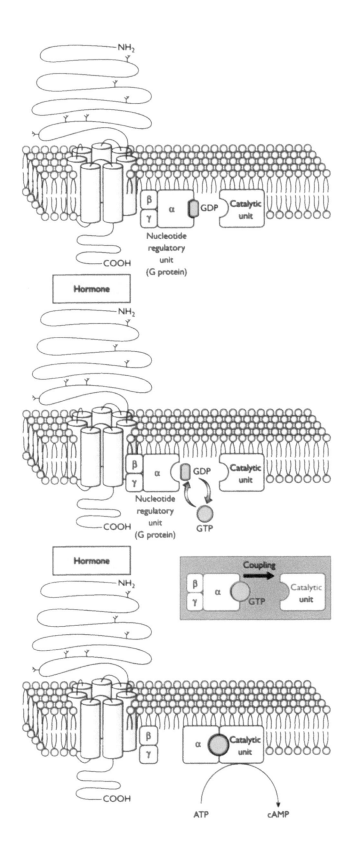

Figure 15.4 Hormone biosynthesis and metabolism. The G protein in its inactive state (top and middle) and in its active state (bottom). (From Gordon and Speroff, personal communication)

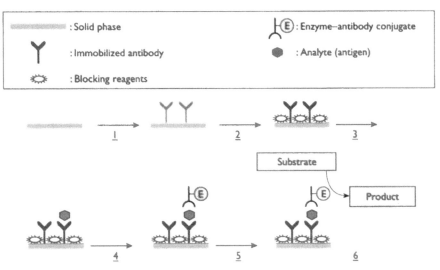

1. Add antibody solution to prepare immobilized antibody. Wash to remove non-immobilized antibody.
2. Add a blocking reagent solution to cover adsorption points of antibody and restrain non-specific adsorption.
3. Add an analyte solution for immobilized antibody–analyte reaction. Wash.
4. Add an enzyme–antibody conjugate solution for analyte–enzyme–antibody conjugate reaction. Wash to remove non-reacted enzyme–antibody conjugate.
5. Add a substrate solution for enzyme–substrate reaction. (Absorbance is increased in proportion to the amount of analyte.)
6. Measure absorbance.

Figure 15.5 Principle of the enzyme-linked immunosorbent assay (ELISA) method. (Reproduced with permission from Sakaki et al. 2002)

ELISA method, non-specific adsorption of the enzyme–antibody conjugate to the solid phase considerably decreases the reliability of the measurement. Extensive investigation has been conducted on the optical properties and applications of these bioconjugated polymers in molecular electronics and sensors.

The unique integration of a signal transduction component with biomolecular recognition may allow miniaturization of the device and eventually multichannel, simultaneous detection in a manner similar to that used in gene chip technology. There have been significant improvements in liposome formation and color development. The modified microdialysis probe will be applied to diagnostic devices used in medicine, pharmaceuticals and bioengineering.

Piezoelectric crystal surfaces were first modified by a glow-discharge treatment by using ethylenediaminetetraacetic acid plasma, in order chemically to immobilize antibody molecules to the surface. Changes of the crystal surfaces after each modification step were successfully followed by a novel technique, scanning tunneling microscopy. The piezoelectric immunosensor developed by the methodology may be utilized in the measurements of antigens in aqueous medium with high sensitivity and selectivity.

The present gene-sensing method, which is quick and convenient and provides high detection sensitivity, is applicable to practical gene diagnosis. The evanescent waveguide-based biosensor approach (EPW™) provides rapid, sensitive quantification of several important clinical analytes in whole blood directly, with little or no interference from common interfering substances (Abdel-Hamid *et al.* 2002; Ishihara *et al.* 2002; Katayama *et al.* 2002; Maeda *et al.* 2002; Mutlu *et al.* 2002; Sakaki *et al.* 2002).

CHAPTER 16

Technology and instrumentation in andrology

ENDOCRINOLOGY

Immunoassays

Estradiol and testosterone levels in blood and seminal plasma are measured by competitive immunoassay, for example with the Immulite analyzer (Diagnostic Products Corp., Los Angeles, CA, USA). With this analyzer, the sensitivities of the assays are 12 pg/ml for estradiol and 0.1 ng/ml for testosterone. Melatonin concentrations are assessed by radioimmunoassay (RIA), for example by the Buhlman Laboratory (Albschwell, Switzerland). The immunoassays used are validated for measurement of hormones in semen by the addition of standards as follows: melatonin 50 pg/ml, 17β-estradiol 62.9 pg/ml and testosterone 0.3 ng/ml. The same antisera are used for determination of hormones in blood plasma and seminal plasma. The antisera are highly specific for testosterone, estradiol and melatonin according to the manufacturer's instructions.

Tests for gonadotropin releasing hormone and human chorionic gonadotropin

In a study by Osuna et al. (2001), peripheral venous blood was obtained under fasting conditions; samples obtained at −30 and 0 h were pooled to measure luteinizing hormone (LH), follicle stimulating hormone (FSH), total testosterone, free testosterone and sex hormone binding globulin (SHBG). Blood was collected at 30, 60 and 90 min after the intravenous

injection of 100 µg of synthetic gonadotropin releasing hormone (GnRH) (Relisorn, Serono), to measure LH and FSH. Two weeks after the GnRH stimulation test was performed, serum total testosterone, estradiol and 17-hydroxyprogesterone (17-OHP) were determined, before and 2, 24, 48 and 72 h following the intramuscular injection of 2000 IU of human chorionic gonadotropin (hCG) (Profasi-Serono). Serum LH, FSH, testosterone, estradiol and SHBG were analyzed in duplicate by fluorometric assay (Delphia; Wallac, Helsingfors, Finland). Free testosterone and 17-OHP were analyzed in duplicate using a conventional RIA. LH and FSH values were expressed in mlU/ml; testosterone, 17-OHP and SHBG in ng/ml; and free testosterone and estradiol in pg/ml (Osuna et al. 2001).

Steroid metabolism in vitro

To determine the metabolic pathways of steroid systems in vitro, the cells are plated onto 30-mm cell culture dishes at a density of 10^6 and allowed to grow for 3–5 days until they reach approximately 80% confluence. At this stage, the culture medium is replaced with fresh medium containing 100 nmol/l of the radiolabeled substrates [^{14}C]androstenedione (0.1 mCi; 0.2–0.4 mol/l) and [^{14}C]dehydroepiandrosterone (DHEA) (0.1 mCi; 0.2–0.4 mmol/l) in 2 ml of the medium at 37 °C for 12 h (Koh et al. 2001).

At the end of the incubation, the medium is collected and transferred to extraction tubes. Each tube is vortexed for 30 s, followed by the addition of 2 ml of ethyl acetate, after which the second vortex is introduced and the phases are separated into organic and aqueous phases. The organic phase is transferred to a second tube and evaporated to dryness with nitrogen. The residue is taken up in 20 µl methanol and applied to a silica TLC plate (Whatman, Clifton, NJ, USA). The plates are developed once in chloroform/ethyl acetate 3 : 1 (v/v). With this solvent system, dihydrotestosterone (DHT) (R_f = 0.74) can be thoroughly separated from testosterone (R_f = 0.60), DHEA (R_f = 0.69) and androstenedione (R_f = 0.83). Quantitation of each radioactive product is performed by scanning autoradiographs with the bio-image analyzer (Koh *et al.* 2001).

Unconjugated and conjugated steroids

During incubation of cells with a labeled substrate, conjugated steroids are produced by uridine diphosphoglucuronosyltransferase (UGT). The aqueous phase is transferred to separate glass tubes and freeze-dired in an evaporator–concentrator. The dried extracts are solubilized with 1 ml of 0.1 mol/l phosphate buffer (pH 6.5) and incubated with either 200 U of β-glucuronidase type VIII or with 5 U of sulfatase type VIII at 37° C for 24 h to hydrolyze steroid conjugates. The released steroid is then extracted twice with ethyl acetate and the organic phase is evaporated with nitrogen. The residue is treated as previously described (Koh *et al.* 2001).

RNA extraction and reverse transcriptase-polymerase chain reaction

Total RNA from the cell lines is extracted by using a commercially available RNA extraction kit. cDNA is synthesized with a reverse transcription kit (Gibco BRL), using 1 µg of total RNA, 100 ng of 20-mer poly T primers and 200 U of SuperScript II for a total volume of 20 µl. cDNA is amplified by means of primers specific for the UGT2B15 gene, or with the β-actin gene, which is used as a control. Polymerase chain reaction (PCR) conditions consist of denaturation at 94 °C for 1 min, annealing at 55 °C for 1 min and extension at 72 °C for 2 min. Thirty cycles of PCR are performed. The following PCR primers for UGT2B15 are used: forward primer, 5′-CCTTGCCAGATCCCACAAA-3′ and reverse primer, 5′-TATCACAGTTGCCACGCAGG-3′,

according to the UBG2B15 gene structure (Guillemette *et al.* 1995). For β-actin, the forward primer is 5′-GAAAATCTGGCACCACACCTT-3′ and the reverse primer is 5′-TTGAAGGTAGTTTCGTGGAT-3′.

Hydroxy-steroid-receptor binding

Semen is processed (Zaneveld and Polakoski, 1979) and aliquots containing 25×10^7 sperm are centrifuged at 1000*g* for 2 min. Sperm pellets are resuspended in 2 ml of cold TETG-KCL buffer containing Tris-HCl 0.01 mol/l, ethylenediaminetetra-acetic acid (EDTA) 0.0015 mol/l, monothioglycerol 0.01 mol/l, glycerol 10% and KCl 0.8 mol/l at pH 8.5. This suspension is homogenized every 15 min with a glass–glass homogenizer (two pulses, each for 20 s at 80 rpm with intervals of 20 s). The homogenate is incubated at 4°C for 60 min and centrifuged at 105 000 *g* for 60 min, to obtain the nucleosol.

The estrogen receptors (ERs) are measured by incubating the nucleosol at various concentrations (0.125–5 nmol/l) of [^{3}H]estradiol during 18–20 h at 4°C. The non-specific is assayed using a 200-fold excess of diethylstilbestrol. Radioactive bound and free estradiol are separated using a dextran-coated charcoal separation method (Calzada *et al.* 1998). *In vitro* capacitation is induced by adding calcium 2.5 mmol/l and the ionophore to $20–40 \times 10^6$ washed sperm resuspended in 250–500 ml of BWW medium (Biggers *et al.* 1971; Parrish *et al.* 1993). The sperm suspension is incubated at 37°C for 50 and 120 min under a 5% CO_2 plus air atmosphere. The acrosome reaction induced in the sperm by the *in vitro* capacitation schedule is evaluated using the triple-stain (Talbot and Chacon, 1981).

Serum, inhibin A, inhibin B and inhibin pro αC assays

Inhibin A and B as well as pro αC are measured using a commercially available, double-antibody, enzyme-linked immunoassay (Serotec, Oxford, UK). For inhibin A, intra- and interassay coefficients of variation are each less than 10%. Intra- and interassay coefficients of variation for inhibin B are 6% and 15%, respectively. For pro αC, intra- and interassay coefficients of variation are 5% and 10%, respectively. The lowest detectable inhibin A, inhibin B and pro αC concentrations are 2 pg/ml, 20 pg/ml and 2 pg/ml, respectively.

Hemicastration

Male rats are hemicastrated according to the method of Mayorga and Bertini (1982). Briefly, under aseptic conditions the rats are anesthetized by injection of sodium pentrobarbital (15 mg/kg). The testis and epididymis of one side are exposed by scrotal incision and the testicular vascular supply is ligated before removal of the testis, without compromising the epididymal blood supply. As a control, the contralateral testis is manipulated similarly, although the testis is not excised. Rats are killed on day 4 after the hemicastration, and the epididymis removed and processed as desired.

Ovarian stimulation and intracytoplasmic sperm injection

Ovarian stimulation is performed using human menopausal gonadotropin (hMG) (Menogon, Ferring, Kiel, Germany) after GnRH densensitization (Decapeptyl, Ferring, Kiel, Germany). Oocytes are collected 36 h after hCG injection. After retrieval, oocytes are exposed to 80 IU/ml hyaluronidase (type VIII, Sigma Chemical Co., St Louis, MO, USA) to denude their cumulus–corona cells. Intracytoplasmic sperm injection (ICSI) is carried out in 20 µl of IVF 50 medium microdroplets under mineral oil. M II oocytes are injected with non-motile ejaculated sperm. M II oocytes of patient II are injected with non-motile sperm from testicular sperm extraction (TESE) after their tails have been crushed with the injection pipette in a 10% polyvinylpyrolidine (PVP) droplet (ICSI-100, Scandinavian IVF Science, Stockholm, Sweden) and cultured at 37°C in a humidified atmosphere with 5% CO_2. After 18–20 h of incubation, oocytes show two pronuclei in the ooplasm. Two embryos of grades 3 or 4 are transferred into the uterus. Embryo grading is assessed according to the usual criteria: blastomere number, size, shape, symmetry, cytoplasmic appearance and percentage fragmentation (Evirgen et al. 2003). Progesterone is administered during the luteal phase. Two weeks after embryo transfer, pregnancy can be detected by measuring β-hCG plasma levels.

SEMEN

Semen evaluation

For semen evaluation, semen is obtained masturbation following 2–5 days of abstinence. Samples with more than one million round cells are discarded. Semen quality is assessed in terms of sperm concentration, total sperm count, motility and morphology, using the guidelines laid down by the World Health Organization.

Semen samples are processed with a standard 45%/90% density gradient preparation (PureSperm®, Nidacon International AB, Gothenburg, Sweden) followed by semen analysis. Semen samples are also incubated in the Zech glass capillary dish (Astromedtec, Salzburg, Austria) consisting of two concentric wells overlaid by a U-ring and coverglass (Sills et al. 2000).

The functional integrity of sperm membranes can be evaluated by the hyposmotic swelling test (HOS). However, there are several varieties of HOS protocol and a serious controversy has arisen over which one of the HOS protocols should be used to obtain a high fertilization rate (Casper et al. 1996; Liu et al. 1997).

There are several assays to evaluate the kinematic characteristics of sperm: head lateral displacement, straight motility, sperm flagella beating and wave amplitude. All these parameters evaluate the sperm capacity to penetrate through the egg vestments. There are other techniques to evaluate the peroxidative capacity of the sperm membrane lipids as a membrane fluidity evaluation parameter, or even membrane damage, and to evaluate the zone pellucida receptor aggregation capacity, a prerequisite for the acrosomal reaction or the transduction signaling aspects due to correct establishment of the tyrosine kinase activity in sperm receptors. Fluorescein-labeled peanut agglutinin plus a fluorescein extender permit a simple evaluation of sperm membrane integrity. The acrosome reaction is affected when the zona pellucida is reduced.

Sperm viability

Cell viability of nucleons and sperm cells was determined with a simultaneous staining using fluorescein diacetate and propidium iodide (Jones and Senft, 1985). Fluorescein diacetate, a non-polar ester, is hydrolyzed by intracellular esterases to produce fluorescein, which exhibits green fluorescence when excited by blue light. Propidium iodide intercalates with DNA and RNA to form a bright red fluorescence seen in dead cells and/or those without metabolic activity. Stained cells were examined with a microscope (Nikon E-600) equipped with an epifluorescence attachment (Keyhani and Storey, 1973; Rotman and Papermaster, 1966).

Evaluation of the percentage of sperm cells that fluoresce bright green (intact membrane) or red (damaged membrane) is performed by counting 20 random high-magnification fields (400 × for 200–400 sperm) (Jones and Senft, 1985).

Cell viability of nucleons and sperm is determined with a simultaneous staining using fluorescein diacetate and propidium iodide. Stained cells are examined with a microscope (Nikon E-600) equipped with an epifluorescence attachment (Delgado *et al.* 1999).

Semen filtration *in vitro*

The cervical mucus selectively allows only progressively motile sperm of normal shape and size to penetrate and migrate through the cervix. The glass wool column filtration (GWCF) method for sperm processing selects such a sperm population *in vitro*. Sperm recovered from GWCF is higher in quality than the original ejaculate. GWCF processing is reliable and highly repeatable, when compared to other sperm processing techniques. Sperm penetration into denuded hamster oocytes improves with GWCF, while binding to human zona pellucida occurs in higher numbers. *In vitro* fertilization (IVF) outcome also improves as compared to that from other processing techniques (Jeyendran, 2003).

Flow cytometry

To prepare for flow cytometry, sperm are incubated with the primary antibody at 4 °C for 30 min. The samples are then washed with phosphate-buffered saline (PBS) and incubated with the secondary antibody in the same conditions. Labeled sperm are centrifuged at 600*g* for 5 min. The pellet is resuspended and fixed in 1% paraformaldehyde. The proportion of sperm that are labeled and the fluorescence intensity are measured using an EPICS XL flow cytometer (Epics Division, Coulter Corporation, Hialeah, FL, USA) (Fierro *et al.* 2002).

Sperm leukocyte count

Leukocytes are counted by using the peroxidase stain for polymorphonuclear granulocytes (Politch *et al.* 1993). The seminal vesicle function marker fructose is analyzed by the modified Roe method (Foreman *et al.*

1973). Seminal citric acid, the prostate function marker, is measured using the citric screen (Fertil Pro N.V., Belgium) and α-glucosidase, the epididymal marker, is measured using Episcreen (Fertile Pro N.V.).

In vitro manipulation of semen

Human periovulatory mucus is an effective barrier against semen containing decapacitating factors, non-motile or dead sperm, leukocytes, prostaglandin and various infectious agents. The cervical mucus is particularly selective in allowing only progressively motile sperm of normal shape and size to penetrate and migrate through the cervix. Sperm processing methods that mimic this periovulatory mucus selectivity may therefore favorably influence outcomes of oocyte fertilization and, thus, pregnancy. There are three techniques to recover a select population of normal motile sperm from a raw ejaculate:

(1) Sperm migration method (swim-up technique and sperm selection system: Select Medical Systems, Williston, VT, USA);

(2) Density gradient centrifugation method (colloidal silica isolation: Irvine Scientific, Santa Ana, CA, USA; PureSperm: Nidacon International AB, Goteborg, Sweden and Nycodenz and Accudenz: Accurate Chemical & Scientific Co., Westbury, NY, USA);

(3) Adherence column method (sephadex column filtration: SpermPrep, ZBL Inc., Lexington, KY, USA and Glass Wool Column Filtration: Cook Sperm Filter, Cook Ob/Gyn, Spencer, IN, USA) (Jeyendran, 2003).

In vitro processing of the ejaculate involves the separation of viable and potentially fertile sperm from the ejaculate, so that the processed sperm population has a higher fertilizing capacity than the original ejaculate. Sperm with functionally inactive or physically damaged membranes are non-viable, and tend to adhere to glass wool. Therefore, their migration through a column of glass wool is hindered or prevented, allowing greater facility for passage of viable sperm. Leukocytes and other deleterious agents adhere to glass wool, with their passage similarly hindered or prevented

(Jeyendran, 2003). Such processing should be effective in cases of oligozoospermia, asthenozoospermia and viscous ejaculate, and should consistently recover a significant proportion of viable and fertile spermatozoa. Many techniques have been developed to recover viable sperm from an ejaculate. However, many of these techniques yield poor sperm or produce inconsistent results, particularly when the ejaculate is oligozoospermic, asthenozoospermic, or viscous.

In vitro capacitation

In vitro capacitation has been induced by adding calcium 2.5 mmol/l and the ionophore A23187 µmol/l to 20–40 × 10^6 washed sperm, resuspended in 200–500 µl of BWW medium (Biggers *et al.* 1971) according to the reported methodology (Reyes *et al.* 1978). The sperm suspension was incubated at 37 °C for 60 and 120 min under a 5% CO_2 plus air atmosphere. The acrosome reaction induced in the spermatozoa by the *in vitro* capacitation schedule was evaluated using the triple-stain technique (Talbot and Chacon, 1981).

Electron microscopy

Major head shape and tail abnormalities can be detected simply with light microscopy (Figure 16.1). Detailed observations using a transmission electron microscope (TEM) can improve the evaluation of cytological details and should ideally be the method of choice for investigation of male factor infertility (Figure 16.2). An accurate clinical and morphological assesment of patients may reduce the incidence of cycles with only immotile sperm available for ICSI on the day of oocyte pick-up.

After liquefaction of ejaculates, samples are centrifuged at 1500 rpm for 10 min and the supernatant discharged. Semen pellets are fixed in a solution of 2.5% glutaraldehyde in 0.1 mol/l phosphate buffer. Pellets are post-fixed in 1% osmium tetroxide. Samples are dehydrated through a graded series of ethanol and propylene oxide and embedded in araldite. The blocks are cut in a Leica ultracut R ultramicrotome with glass and diamond knives. Semithin sections are stained with toluidin blue–azur II and examined on a Zeiss Axioscope photomicroscope. Ultrathin sections are double-stained with uranyl acetate and lead citrate and studied on a LEO 906 E transmission electron microscope (Zeiss).

Sperm chromatin condensation

Smears are prepared before and after semen processing by the swim-up technique, air dried and fixed for 30 min in 3% glutaraldehyde in PBS. Morphology and nuclear maturity is assessed by the aniline blue staining method (Terquem and Dadoune, 1983). The smear is stained for 5 min in 5% aqueous aniline blue solution (pH 3.5). Sperm heads containing immature nuclear chromatin stain blue (chromatin not condensed) and those with mature nuclei do not take up the stain (chromatin condensed). The percentage of sperm stained with aniline blue was determined by counting 200 sperm on a slide under bright-field illumination. Using 25% as the cut-off point, samples were classified into two categories: good quality (unstained, chromatin condensed) and bad quality (stained, chromatin uncondensed).

Nucleus decondensation kinetics

Decondensation kinetics of heparin–reduced glutathione (GSH) mixtures is studied by keeping constant the concentration of one of the reagents before adding the other. The range of concentrations used is kept below those normally required to induce decondensation. At predetermined times, aliquots containing 10^7 cells are extracted from the incubation mixtures, and nucleons and/or sperm are fixed by the addition of three volumes of 0.1 Mcacodylate buffer, pH 7.3, containing 1% paraformaldehyde plus 2.5% glutaraldehyde. Fixed cells are washed twice by centrifugation and resuspended in 0.1 mol/l cacodylate buffer. Nuclear decondensation is studied by phase microscopy. The number of swelled nuclei is evaluated by counting 20 random high-magnification fields (approximately 700–900 sperm). Nucleus decondensation is scored. The nucleon and/or sperm cells are considered positive from the moment in which the basal region of the nucleon head opens, or when slightly enlarged dark-phase nuclei are observed.

Chemotaxis assays of sperm

Semen samples from one patient were used to fill an experimental plate, as follows. Five wells, 10 mm in diameter and 5 mm deep, were prepared, one in the center and one at each corner, 15 mm apart, on non-toxic plastic plates (50 × 50 × 10 mm). The wells were

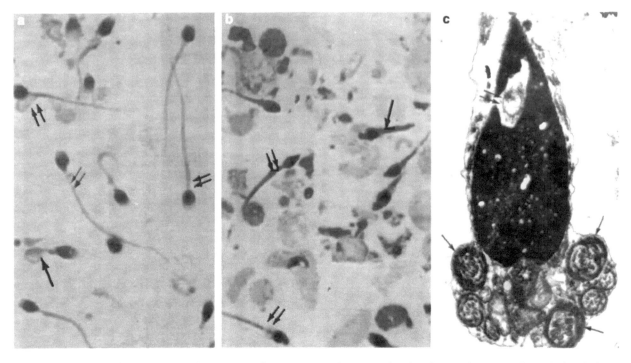

Figure 16.1 (a and b) Smear and semithin sections of spermatozoa, showing coiling, breaking, rudimentary, short thick tails (arrow), diameter variations and cytoplasmic droplets of midpiece (double arrows) with abnormal head shape. (a) Spermac stain kit, × 100; (b) toluidin blue–Azur II, × 100. (c) Longitudinal section of a short-tailed spermatozoon, showing multiple cross-sections of tail pieces with peri-axonemal and axonemal atterations tightly packed and surrounded by plasmalemma (arrows). Head region also shows vacuolated chromatin (double arrows). (Reproduced with permission from Evirgen *et al.* 2003, *Arch Androl*, 49:57–67. www.tandf. co.uk/journals)

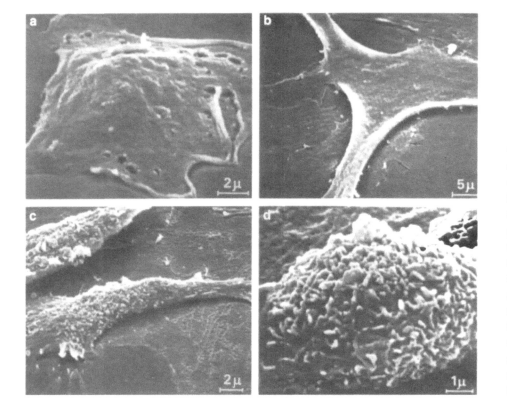

Figure 16.2 Scanning electron micrographs of peritubular cells (a and b), Leydig cells (c) and a fibroblast (d) cultured in MEM containing 10% calf serum. (a) A peritubular cell prepared from 20-day-old rats, after 8 h in culture. Note the smooth periphery and free surface. (b) Peritubular cell after 4 days in culture. Note the characteristic criss-crossing behavior, extremely attenuated cytoplasmic extensions (arrows) and smooth topography. (Reproduced with permission from Parvinen and Soderstrom, 1977)

connected by a groove (1 mm wide and 3 mm deep). The central (basal) well was filled with 250 µl PBS and supplemented with 200 µl of sperm samples. The corner wells were filled with 450 µl of the following fluids: PBS only (control well) and PBS containing the investigated substance (Sigma Chemical, St Louis, MO, USA) in three final pharmacological concentrations, respectively (experimental wells). The plates were incubated at 37°C (Silwa, 1993, 1995a,b, 2001).

Sperm chromatin decondensation *in vitro*

Semen was washed (by 5 min centrifugation at 250g) three times with Ham's F-10 medium in order to remove the seminal plasma. A 1-ml sample of follicular fluid obtained from patients who underwent oocyte retrieval for ICSI was added to the washed spermatozoa. The mixture was then incubated for a minimum of 24 h at 37°C, in 5% CO_2 in air and 99% humidity. Smears were made at several time intervals: directly within 1–10 min, after 30 min of incubation with follicular fluid, after 60 min, after 120 min and after 24 h. The reaction was immediately stopped by spraying of the smears with 3% glutaraldehyde in PBS. The chromatin decondensation was evaluated after staining with acridine orange according to the method of Tejada *et al.* (1984). The female partners underwent ovarian stimulation for ICSI therapy (Hammadeh *et al.* 1996). The percentage of chromatin decondensation was evaluated by analyzing 100–200 spermatozoa at each time period (30, 60, 160 min 24 h) and the results were correlated with fertilization rates using Sperman's rank correlation coefficient (Hammadeh *et al.* 2002).

TUNEL analysis of sperm DNA fragmentation

DNA fragmentation is evaluated using a commercially available kit for the TUNEL assay (Roche Molecular Biochemicals). Semen is smeared onto clean microscope slides, and fixed with paraformaldehyde. The sperm are permeabilized by incubation with 0.1% Triton X-100. The slide is incubated for 60 min with the TUNEL reaction mixture (fluorescein-labeled dUTP and terminal transferase) at 37°C. At least 200 sperm are evaluated to determine the percentage of TUNEL reactive sperm. Each microscopic field is first evaluated under phase contrast microscopy to determine the total number of sperm in the field, then under fluorescence microscopy to determine the number of reactive sperm. For quality control, a digital overlay is performed to assure that positive reactions are sperm cells (Carrell *et al.* 2002).

Sperm redox state

The alamarBlue assay incorporates a fluorometric/colorimetric indicator based on detection of metabolic activity. The system incorporates an oxidation–reduction (REDOX) indicator that both fluoresces and changes color in response to chemical reduction of culture medium resulting from cell activity. The specific (fluorometric/colorimetric) REDOX indicator incorporated into alamarBlue has been carefully selected based on several properties. The indicator exhibits both fluorescence and colorimetric change in the appropriate REDOX range relating to cellular metabolic reduction. The indicator is demonstrated to be minimally toxic to living cells. Finally, it produces a clear, stable distinct change that is easy to interpret, from the oxidized (non-fluorescent, blue) form to the reduced (fluorescent, red) form (Lancaster and Fields, 1996).

Sperm retrieval

Sperm retrievals are carried out in men with azoospermia due to vasectomy (and unsuccessful attempts at vaso-vasostomy), absence of the vas deferens, or sequelae of a genital infection. Testicular sperm are primarily obtained using TESE on the theory that, with an open biopsy, it is possible to identify testicular vessels. Sperm are retrieved in funicular blockade with 20 ml of lidocaine (20 mg/ml), injected high in the scrotum on both sides of the funicle with a 21-gauge needle. Percutaneous epididymal sperm aspiration (PESA) is carried out with a 21-guage butterfly needle and TESA with an 18-guage needle. Testis tissues are dissociated in Petri dishes using microscope slides and held at 37°C in 5% CO_2. ICSI is carried out using conventional procedures. Motile sperm are used for ICSI when available. When only immotile sperm are obtained, sperm are chosen for ICSI according to morphological criteria.

Repeat sperm retrieval procedures are primarily performed on the same side as the previous time unless it is considered more probable to find sperm on the other side. When no motile sperm are found on the first side, sperm retrieval is also performed on the other side. Sperm retrieval is carried out the same day or the day before oocyte aspiration to obtain more motile sperm (Hu *et al.* 1999). It is often more convenient for the couple and the clinic to perform the sperm retrieval procedure the day before oocyte retrieval.

Isolation of epididymal sperm and purification of DNA

Sperm heads are isolated and after a preliminary screening of the decondensing agents, complete decondensation of the head suspension is achieved with a combination 0.25 mol/l B-Me and 0.5 mg/ml pancreatic trypsin on incubation at 37°C for 24 h at a pH of 8.0. DNA is isolated from decondensed material by extraction with a chloroform–isoamyl alcohol mixture (24 : 1). The isolated DNA is free from impurities such as RNA and protein. The total content of isolated and purified DNA is around 3×10^{-9} mg/sperm. Sperm DNA is present in double-stranded super-coiled form with a G + C content of around 50–100 mol.

Postejaculatory urinalysis

Postejaculatory urinalysis is performed in patients with ejaculate volumes of less than 1 ml, unless they have bilateral vasal agenesis or clinical signs of hypogonadism. The presence of sperm in a postejaculatory urinalysis specimen from a patient with azoospermia (absence of sperm in the ejaculate) or aspermia (complete absence of semen during or immediately after ejaculation) suggests retrograde ejaculation. In addition to retrograde ejaculation, the ejaculate may be of low volume or absent, owing to complete lack of emission, ejaculatory duct obstruction, hypogonadism, or congenital bilateral absence of the vasa deferentia (CBAVD) (Sharlip *et al.* 2002).

Release of chromatin by decondensation of the sperm head

Sperm are highly resistant to conventional procedures for the extraction of DNA. There is a major difference between somatic and spermatozoal DNA: in somatic cells, the DNA is present in a complex with histones, while in mature spermatozoa the histones are replaced by proteins (called protamines) with extremely low molecular weight. The association between the DNA and protamines is unusually strong, resulting in the highly condensed state of the chromatin, causing difficulty in isolating the sperm DNA by existing methods.

Decondensation of the sperm heads is a prerequisite for the release of the DNA–protamine complex from which the DNA can be isolated in a pure state. The resistance to chemical treatments for decondensation is due to the presence of impervious membranes around the sperm head. Good results are obtained with a combination of a disulfide bond-reducing agent in conjunction with a detergent such as sodium dodecyl sulfate (SDS) for decondensation of the sperm head and subsequent extraction of DNA from the sperm chromatin. Reagents used for disulfide bond reduction and cleavage included chemicals such as dithiothreitol and β-mercaptoethanol. Human sperm can be decondensed at 28 °C effectively using a medium in which heparin is substituted for the polyanionic egg protein nucleoplasmin, and β-mercaptoethanol for egg-glutathione.

Extraction of DNA from released chromatin

Extraction of DNA decondensed sperm heads is challenging, because of the presence of very-low-molecular-weight, highly basic protamine molecules in close association with the DNA. Extraction with phenol is effective separating DNA from the complex, while another popular deproteinizing agent is the chloroform and isoamyl alcohol mixture. The basic function of phenol is to denature the proteins. When a suspension of the chromatin material in Tris–saline–EDTA solution is shaken with water/buffer saturated with phenol, the upper aqueous layer contains the DNA and protein is precipitated at the interface between the aqueous and organic layers. Chloroform–isoamyl alcohol acts similarly, removing protein contaminants and leaving the purified DNA in an aqueous solution.

Isolation of sperm protamines

The sponge-like networks of arginine-rich protein molecules that are cross-linked by several disulfide bonds hinder the isolation of nuclear proteins from sperm. Therefore, methods of isolation involve the reductive cleavage of the disulfide bonds in some suitable medium such as guanidine hydrochloride, which acts as a dissociating and denaturing agent. For optimal extraction, it is essential to block the once liberated sulfhydryl groups with either sulfur ethyl amine or sulfur methyl groups, depending on the nature of the amino acid sequence. Biochemical analyses of sperm from fertile and infertile men suggest that the relative proportion of protamine 1 or 2 bound to DNA is important for fertility. Sperm obtained from infertile individuals who produce only sperm with large, round heads (round-headed sperm syndrome) are deficient in protamine 2. Deficiencies in protamine content are observed in other cases of male infertility, with some individuals appearing to produce sperm lacking protamine 2 altogether.

Collection and isolation of sperm heads

Freshly ejaculated semen contains a mixed population of cells with dead, immotile and morphologically abnormal cells coexisting in varying numbers with the normal, highly motile cells. Special care is required to collect the sperm with high motility and normal morphology and to minimize the dead and immotile contaminants for a meaningful interpretation. The swim-up technique is used to collect motile sperm using BWW medium containing human serum albumin (HSA). Two major methods are used for the detachment and purification of the sperm heads from the tail and middle pieces: sonication followed by discontinuous sucrose density gradient centrifugation; and chemicals, e.g. *N*-butylamine and secondary butyl amine.

To remove lipoprotein membranes from the sperm, samples are treated with repeated washing with saline citrate solution without any special defatting agent, or washing with ethanol or ether–ethanol mixtures.

Granulocyte elastase in semen

The total concentrations of both extracellularly liberated elastase and the inactive elastase–α 1-Pl complexed form are measured by using an enzyme immunoassay (EIA) with a new reagent (ELASPEC, Sanwa Nagoya, Japan). Seminal plasma is diluted at a ratio of 1 : 100 with a solution containing sheep α 1-Pl, resulting in the conversion of free elastase to an inactive elastase–α 1-Pl complexed form. Intra-assay variability of the elastase kit is 1.6–3.0% and its interassay variability is 3.9–6.9%.

Seminal plasma

Assays of interleukin-6 and interleukin-10

Interleukin (IL)-6 and IL-10 are estimated by the use of an ultrasensitive enzyme-linked immunosorbent assay (ELISA), performed with a commercially available Cytoscreen immunoassay kit (Biosource International, Camarillo, CA, USA).

Prostaglandin E$_2$ measurement

Prostaglandin (PG) E$_2$ levels in seminal plasma are measured by the use of an ACE™ competitive EIA kit (Cayman Chemical, MI, USA). This assay is based on competition between PGE$_2$ and a PGE$_2$–acetylcholinesterase conjugate (PGE$_2$ tracer) for a limited amount of PGE$_2$ monoclonal antibody. The intra- and interassay coefficient of variation is 10%, with 100% specificity for PGE$_{2\alpha}$.

VARICOCELE

Testicular varicocele

Boys (6–16 years) are examined clinically by urology specialists to grade varicocele/genital development (Tanner system). Boys with stage 1 are grouped as prepubertal while those with stages 2–5 are grouped as pubertal. Height and weight are also recorded. Boys with varicocele are examined by ultrasound to determine testicular size, as this is the most accurate method. A 7.5-MHz probe is used to measure breadth, length and height, and the testicular volume is calculated (formula of Lambert). Multivariate analysis of covariance, χ^2 and paired t tests are used for statistical analysis of the results (Stavropoulos *et al.* 2002).

Ultrasonography of the prostate

Transabdominal ultrasonic examinations are performed with Bruel and Kjaer 3535 ultrasound equipment with a convex 3.5-MHz probe (Bruel & Kjaer, Copenhagen, Denmark). The probe gives the cross-sections of the prostate in transverse as well as sagittal scanning planes. The maximum transverse diameter, anteroposterior diameter and cephalocaudal distance were measured. The volume of the prostate was calculated from the formula for the volume of an ellipsoid (width × height × π/6) (Bangama *et al.* 1996).

Pediatric laparoscopic varicocelectomy

Pediatric varicoceles occur in 6% of those at age 10 years and in 15% by the age of 15 years, which is similar to the incidence among men. Varicocele may induce changes in testicular growth and histology that may ultimately affect spermatogenesis. Boys with testicular atrophy, a large varicocele, bilateral varicocele, or an abnormal GnRH stimulation test undergo varicele repair to prevent subsequent infertility. In parallel with the recent increase in urological laparoscopy, laparoscopic varicocelectomy has progressively improved.

Sasagawa *et al.* (2000b) performed laparoscopic varicocelectomy in adolescents using an ultrasonically activated scalpel to divide spermatic vessels. A 15-mm umbilical incision was made, and the fascia and peritoneum opened. A 10-mm trocar was placed into the peritoneal cavity and secured to prevent gas leakage. CO_2 was insufflated to produce pneumoperitoneum at a pressure of 10–12 mmHg. Two additional trocars were placed at midline. Suprapubic vessels were carefully freed from the underside of the peritoneum, which was split medially perpendicular to the initial incision. Blunt dissection was used to isolate the packet of spermatic vessels. This cutting instrument vibrates longitudinally at a frequency of 55 000 Hz. When activated, the ultrasonic scalpel is a precision cutting instrument that generates less smoke and less char than regular electrocautery.

Transrectal ultrasonography

Transrectal ultrasonography (TRUS) is indicated in azoospermic patients with palpable vasa and low ejaculate volumes to determine whether ejaculatory duct obstruction is present. Normal seminal vesicles are less than 1.5 cm in anteroposterior diameter. Dilated seminal vesicles, dilated ejaculatory ducts, or midline prostatic cystic structures on TRUS suggest, but are not diagnostic of, complete or partial ejaculatory duct obstruction. Some experts recommend performing TRUS in oligospermic patients with low-volume ejaculates, palpable vasa and normal testicular size (Sharlip *et al.* 2002).

Scrotal ultrasonography

Scrotal ultrasonography is indicated in patients with inconclusive findings on examination (as may occur in patients with testes that are in the upper scrotum), small scrotal sacs, or other anatomy that makes physical examination of the scrotum and spermatic cord difficult. Scrotal ultrasonography is also indicated in patients in whom a testicular mass is suspected. Most scrotal abnormalities, including varicoceles, spermatoceles, absence of the vasa, epididymal induration and testicular masses, are palpable on physical examination. Non-palpable varicoceles on scrotal ultrasonography have not been shown to be clinically significant (Sharlip *et al.* 2002).

Varicocelectomy

Three laparoscopic parts are used. The patient empties his bladder (to reduce the risk of bladder puncture) and is placed in the head-down position at 10°. A 5-mm subumbilical trocar is inserted by open laparotomy, and the abdominal cavity is insufflated by CO_2 to a maximum of 5 mmHg. The other two 5-mm ports are placed in the right and left lower quadrants under laparoscopic vision. The peritoneum overlying the internal spermatic vessels is incised longitudinally about 2–3 cm superior to the internal ring over a distance of about 3 cm. Blunt dissection is used to isolate the packet of spermatic vessels, which is divided by ultrasonically activated scalpels at level 2 (Harmonic Scalpel LCS15; Ethicon, Cincinnati, OH, USA). At the end of the procedure the fascia at the 5-mm ports and the skin are sutured with silk (Sasagawa *et al.* 2000b).

Patients are examined 6 weeks postoperatively for any complications, symptomatology, testicular size and presence of hydrocele. Recurrence is the most common complication after varicocelectomy, owing to persistence or missed small collateral veins at the time of ligation. Preservation of the testicular artery is associated with a higher recurrence rate of varicocele, and this could be related to incomplete ligation of venous concomitants adjacent to the preserved testicular artery (Katten, 1998). Collateral branches of the internal spermatic vein intimately associated with the internal spermatic artery are not functionally significant unless the main internal spermatic venous channels are ligated. When the artery is preserved these small venous channels become difficult to identify and interrupt (Kass and Marcol, 1992). After varicocelectomy, however, the increased venous pressure facilitates blood flow through these collaterals and subsequently produces operative failure (Itoh *et al.* 2002).

GENES AND DNA

Microarray analysis

Broad-scale gene expression is performed by Atlas glass mouse 1.0 microarrays (Clontech Laboratories, Inc., Palo Alto, CA, USA) that includes 1081 mouse DNA fragments. A list of these genes is available at the Clontech Website (http://www.clontech.com/atlas/genelists/index.shtml). Fluorescent labeling of mRNAs is performed by using an Atlas glass fluorescent labeling kit (Clontech Laboratories, Inc.) according to the manufacturer's protocols. Hybridization of the microarrays is carried out in a hybridization solution (supplied by Clontech Laboratories, Inc.) for 16 h at 50 °C. The microarrays are scanned in both Cy3 and Cy5 channels with a microarray scanner, Scanarray 4000 (GSI Lumonics, Bedford, MA, USA). QuantArray software (GSI Lumonics, Bedford, MA, USA) is used for image analysis (Ohta *et al.* 2002a, 2002b).

Separation of mRNA

mRNAs were extracted from the cells using a RNeasy Total RNA Extraction Kit (QIAGEN K.K., Tokyo, Japan) and an Oligotex-dT30 mRNA Purification Kit (Takara Shuzo Co., Kyoto, Japan).

Amino acid sequencing

The N-terminal amino acid sequencing of 80-kDa HSA and its peptides obtained by enzymatic digestion with endoproteinase Lys-C was performed using automated Edman degradation chemistry at the Protein/DNA Technology Center, Rockefeller University, New York (Fusigawa *et al.* 2002). Briefly, the purified protein was subjected to SDS-polyacrylamide gel electrophoresis (PAGE) and transferred onto a polyvenylidene difluoride membrane using 10 mmol/l CAPS buffer, pH 11.0, containing 10% methanol. The protein band is visualized by staining with 0.1% Ponceau S in 1% acetic acid followed by destaining with 5% acetic acid. The excised protein band is subjected to N-terminal sequencing. The protein is digested with endoproteinase Lys-C in the presence of hydrogenated Triton X-100. The peptides generated are purified by microbore reverse-phase chromatography on a Hewlett-Packard 1090 HPLC system. The four major peptides are subjected to amino acid sequencing.

Amino acid sequencing can also be performed by cleavage of 80-kDa HSA by endoproteinase Glu-C. Approximately 20–30 µg of purified 80-kDa HSA is resolved by 7.5% SDS-PAGE under reducing conditions and stained with Coomassie blue R-250. The protein band is excised from the gel, equilibrated in protease buffer (0.125 mol/l TRIS, pH 6.8, at 22 °C, containing 0.1% SDS and 1 mmol/l EDTA) and cleaved with endopeptidase Glu-C (*Staphylococous aureus* protease V8, Boehringer Mannheim) at an enzyme substrate ratio of 1 : 10 in protease buffer containing 15% glycerol and subjected to electrophoresis on a 15% SDS–PAGE gel. These resolved protein fragments are subsequently trasnferred onto a PVDF membrane using a buffer system consisting of 10 mmol/l 3-(cyclohexylamino)-1 propanesulfonic acid, pH 11.0, at 22 °C, containing 10% methanol. The membrane is then stained with Coomassie blue R-250 and fragments are subjected to microsequencing. Phenylthiohydantoin (PTH)-amino acids are identified and quantified by high performance liquid chromatography (HPLC) utilizing a Brownlee PTH-C18 (2.1 × 220 mm) column (Perkin-Elmer Applied Biosystems) in an Applied Biosystems 473A pulse-liquid phase protein sequencer.

Purification of 80-kDa human serum albumin

Sperm is separated from seminal plasma and washed three times with PBS, pH 7.4, and stored at –70 °C until used (Fusigawa *et al.* 2002). The proteins are solubilized from pooled sperm samples with 0.05% sodium deoxycholate in 0.01 mol/l TRIS–HCI, pH 8.0, containing 0.5 mol/l NaCI and 2 mm phenyl methyl sulfonyl fluoride. The solubilized proteins are extensively dialyzed against distilled water and fractionated with 40% saturated ammonium sulfate. The supernatant is dialyzed extensively against 0.1 mol/l ammonium acetate, pH 7.0, and lyophilized. Subsequently, 80-kDa HSA is purified to homogeneity by sequential anion exchange chromatography (MonoQ HR 10/10), using a fast protein liquid chromatography (FPLC) system and gel permeation chromatography (TSK G3000 SWG, 21.5 × 600 mm) on HPLC. The homogeneity of the protein is ascertained by SDS–PAGE. The homogeneous preparation is then subjected to amino acid sequence analysis.

Respirometry

Mitochondrial respiration rates are measured with a Clark-type oxygen electrode and a closed-chambered respirometer (Strathkelvin Instruments, Glasgow, UK). The mitochondrial pellet is resuspended with respiration buffer to a concentration of 2.5–13 mg/ml mitochondrial protein. Mitochondrial protein concentration is determined using the Bio-Rad Protein Assay with a bovine serum albumin (BSA) standard (Irwin *et al.* 2001). Resuspended mitochondria (0.1–1.3 mg protein) are added to a stirred (550 rpm), temperature-controlled (30 °C) aliquot of respiration buffer to a final volume of 1.25 ml (background oxygen depletion is measured for 5 min in the absence of mitochondria and subtracted from O_2 consumption of mitochondria in different respiratory states). Respiratory states, RCR and P/O ratios are determined in the presence of succinate as substrate. State 1 respiration is determined by adding mitochondria to the reaction chamber. O_2 consumption is stimulated upon addition of 5 mmol/l succinate. State 3 respiration is initiated by the addition of 150 nmol ADP. State 4 respiration follows upon exhaustion of ADP. The RCR is calculated by taking the quotient of state 3 divided by state 4 oxygen consumption rate. The P/O ratio is calculated as the amount of ADP added divided by the amount of atomic oxygen consumed during state 3 respiration.

Isolation of mitochondria

Mitochondria are isolated from liver by differential centrifugation (Irwin *et al.* 2001). Liver is minced in ice-cold isolation buffer (210 mmol/l mannitol, 70 mmol/l sucrose, 5 mmol/l HEPES, 1 mmol/l K-EGTA, 0.5% fatty acid-free BSA, pH 7.2, at 4 °C) and homogenized with a glass/Teflon homogenizer at 100 mg tissue/ml buffer. The crude homogenate is centrifuged for 10 min at 750*g*, and the pellet, containing nuclei and cell debris, is discarded. The supernatant is then centrifuged for 15 min at 9800*g* to sediment a crude mitochondrial pellet. The mitochondrial pellet is resuspended by dropwise addition of isolation buffer to the original volume, then centrifuged for 10 min at 750*g*. The resultant supernatant is centrifuged for 10 min at 9800*g*, and the mitochondrial pellet from this final centrifugation is resuspended in 200–300 μl respiration buffer (225 mmol/l mannitol, 75 mmol/l sucrose, 10 mmol/l KCl, 10 mmol/l Tris-HCl, 5 mmol/l KH_2PO_4, pH 7.2, at room temperature).

Electroporation

Freshly isolated mitchondria (12 mg/ml mitochondrial protein) in 80 μl respiration buffer and 50 ng of the 6.5-kb mitochondrial deletion construct in 20 μl water are added to a 0.1-cm electroporation cuvette and electroporated at 12 kV/cm field strength with 25 μF capacitance in a Bio-Rad Gene Pulser (Bio-Rad, Hercules, CA, USA). Respirometric measurements of mitochondria electroporated at 8, 9, 10, 11, 12, 13 and 14 kV/cm are obtained in pilot experiments to confirm the substantial decrease in mitochondrial coupling at field strengths above 12 kV/cm (Irwin *et al.* 2001).

Polymerase chain reaction amplification and cloning of the mitochondrial DNA deletion construct

The 6563 bp mtDNA deletion construct was amplified from *MUS musculus domesticus* mtDNA by long-range PCR using Elongase™ and PCRx™ buffer containing 1.5 mmol/l $MgCL_2$ and 0.5% enhancer (all PCR reagents and restriction enzymes were from Life Technologies, Inc., Gaithersburg, MD, USA). The amplification product extended from nucleotides 5393 to 15175 of the mouse mtDNA sequence (NCBI, assession no. J01420). Both 5′ and 3′ PCR primers included 5′ Sal I linkers and additional 6 bp spacers 5′ to the Sal I sites (forward primer: 5′-CATGCAGTC-GACTTGGGGGCCAACCAGTAGAACACCC-3′; reverse primer: 5′-CAGTAGGTCGACGTACCCAC-TATTCCCGCTCAGGCTCCG-3′). Thermal cycling parameters for amplification were: 94 °C for 2 min followed by 35 cycles of 94 °C for 1 min, 55 °C for 45S and 68 °C for 7 min; with a final extension step at 68 °C for 15 min. The amplification product was resolved on a 0.8% agarose gel and purified using the QiaEx II Gel Extraction Kit (Qiagen, Inc., Valencia, CA, USA). The purified amplification product was cloned into the PCR 2.1 vector and used to transform TOP 10F′ competent cells (TA Cloning Kit; Invitrogen, Carlsbad, CA, USA). Clones containing the insert were selected by blue–white screening on ampicillin plates containing X-Gal and IPTG. Automated nucleotide sequencing was used to confirm the identity of selected plasmids; plasmid 2.1 was used for all subsequent manipulations. The 6.5-kb insert was then excised from plasmid 2.1 by overnight Sal I digestion at 37 °C, and the digestion product was purified from a 0.8% agarose gel with QiaEx II. The 6.5-kb, Sal I digested fragment was then circularized by overnight ligation at 15 °C using T4 DNA ligase (Promega, Madison, WI, USA), and circular 6.5-kb monomers were extracted from 1.0% agarose gels with QiaEx II (Irwin *et al.* 2001).

Polymerase chain reaction analysis

The post-electroporation mitochondrial suspension is removed from the electroporation cuvette and placed in a 1.5-ml microcentrifuge tube (Irwin *et al.* 2001). Five units of RQ1 DNase (Life Technologies, Inc.) and 20 µl of 10× digestion buffer are added and the volume brought up to 200 µl with respiration buffer. The sample is incubated for 2 h at 4 °C to remove residual, non-internalized mitochondrial deletion construct. The mitochondria are then washed four times in 1.0 ml respiration buffer with centrifugation after each wash for 2 min in a refrigerated microcentrifuge. Supernatants from washes are heated to 100 °C for 2 min to destroy DNase activity prior to PCR analysis. Following the last wash, mitochondrial pellets are resuspended in 100 µl of lysis buffer (950 mmol/l NaCl, 1% SDS, 20 mmol/l EDTA in 10 mmol/l Tris-HCl, pH 8.0) at 55 °C for 10 min with frequent vortexing. The PCR analyses are run with 1 µl of each sample (wash supernatants and lysed mitochondria) in 50 µl reaction volumes using recombinant Taq DNA polymerase (LTI) and a standard buffer compostition (as recommended by the manufacturer) with 1.5 mmol/l $MgCl_2$. The diagnostic primer set used in the PCR amplified an 835-bp product which extended across the Sal I splice site (forward primer, complementary to nucleotides 5078–5097: 5′-TAAGACCTCAACTAGATTGG-3′; reverse primer, complementary to nucleotides 15, 619–15, 638: 5′-GAGTTTATGACTGTATGGTG-3′). Thermal cycling parameters for amplification were: 94 °C for 2 min, followed by 40 cycles of 94 °C for 45 s 54 °C for 45 and 72 °C for 1 min; with a final extension for 5 min at 72 °C. Positive control reactions contained approximately 10 pg of mitochondrial deletion construct. Samples from washes and lysed mitochondria were re-amplified for an additional 40 cycles by adding 1 µl of the first round PCR to 50 µl of fresh

PCR cocktail prepared as above. Amplification products were resolved on 1.0% agarose gels, stained with ethidium bromide and photographed with Polaroid 667 film.

Reverse transcription–polymerase chain reaction

First-strand complementary deoxyribonucleic acid (cDNA) is synthesized from total RNA using a GeneAmp RNA PCR kit (Perkin-Elmer, Branchburg, NJ, USA). For PCR of selenoprotein P transcripts, a sense primer (mouse, 541–560; rat, 443–462) 5′-TATGACAGATGTGGCCGTCT-3′ and an antisense primer (mouse, 949–968; rat, 866–885) 5′-CTTCGTCAGAGCTTCCTCTG-3′ are used to amplify a 428-bp (mouse) or a 443-bp (rat) fragment (Sharma and Agarwal, 1996). Thermal cycling is performed for 35 cycles at 94 °C for 2 min, 52 °C for 1 min and 72 °C for 2 min, followed by final extension at 72 °C for 5 min. As primers for B-actin, a sense primer (176–195) 5′-GTGGGGCGCCCCAGGCACCA-3′ and an antisense primer (692-715) 5′-GTCCTTAATGTCACGCACGATTTC-3′ are used to amplify a 539-bp fragment (Harada *et al.* 1999). Thermal cycling is performed for 35 cycles at 94 °C for 1 min, 60 °C for 1 min, 72 °C for 2 min, followed by final extension at 72 °C for 5 min. Amplification is performed using a DNA thermal cycler (TaKaRa Thermal cycler MP, TaKaRa Shuzo, Ohtsu, Japan). After amplification, PCR products are electrophoresed in 1.0% agarose gel and stained with ethidium bromide.

Northern analysis

Total RNA is isolated by the method of Chomczynski and Sacchi (1987). Samples of 20 µg RNA are electrophoresed through a 1.0% agarose gel containing formaldehyde. Membranes are incubated with a random-primed, [^{32}P]deoxy-CTP-labeled rat StAR cDNA probe containing two major StAR-specific transcripts of 3.8 kb and 1.7 kb. Non-specifically bound radioactive probe is removed by washing in 2 × SSPE (1 × SSPE : 150 mmol/l NaCl, 10 mmol/l NaH_2OP_4 and 1 mmol/l EDTA) for 30 min at room temperature, followed by 2 × SSPE-1% SDS for 90 min at 65 °C, and then 0.1 × SSPE for 30 min at room temperature. Membranes are then analyzed using a BAS 2000 Fujix Bioimaging system. Membranes are subsequently stripped and rehybridized with a random-primed [^{32}P]deoxy-CTP-labeled β-actin cDNA probe, containing a transcript of 2.2 kb as an internal control.

DNA disc chip assay

The DNA disc chip assay (Chan *et al.* 2002) consists of exposing SYBR Gold-stained (Molecular Probes, Inc., Eugene, OR, USA) single-stranded test DNA to bisbenzimide-stained (Hoechst 33342) single-stranded control DNA attached to a Nytran (Schleicher & Schuell, Inc., Keene, NH, USA) positively charged membrane paper disc, and analyzing the intensity of test (target) DNA attached to the complementary control DNA on the disc chip. The colloid or swim-up processed sperm cells are thawed at room temperature and pipetted into PCR tubes. Each set of negative control sperm (previously incubated at 37 °C for 4 h) is divided into two portions to serve as a matching internal quality control set. Tubes of negative control or test sperm (previously incubated at 40 °C for 4 h) are centrifuged at 3000*g* for 1 min to remove culture media. A third set of sperm is incubated in culture medium containing either 0, 100, 1000 or 10 000 μmol/l hydrogen peroxide at 37 °C for 1 h to serve as positive DNA-damaged controls. Tubes of positive controls are also centrifuged (3000*g* for 1 min). Each pellet is resuspended in 0.1 ml of TE buffer (10 mmol/l Tris chloride at pH 7.4 and 1 mmol/l EDTA at pH 8.0). DNA staining is carried out in a darkened room. One portion of the control sperm is added with 9 μmol/l bisbenzimide and hybridized to a second portion stained in 1 : 10 000 diluted SYBR Gold stock stain to serve as an internal quality control. Each tube of test sperm is added with the 1 : 10 000 diluted stock SYBR Gold stain. There is no need to adjust the sperm concentration in tubes, owing to the matched control-test design and saturation of the positively charged miniature disc.

Sperm are stained for 5 min and centrifuged to remove excess stain. Pellets are resuspended in TE and recentrifuged. The resultant pellet is resuspended in 4 °C alkaline lysis buffer (1% *N*-lauroylsarcosine, 1.0 mol/l Tris HCl at pH 7.5, 0.5 mol/l EDTA, 0.3 mol/l mercaptoethanol, and the pH adjusted to > 10 with sodium hydroxide pellets) for 20 min with occasional vortexing to release sperm DNA. Tubes of control and test DNA are placed in a PCR thermal cycler, and heated at 94 °C for 5 min to denature the DNA into single strands, similar to the 'hot start' PCR protocol. Tubes of single-stranded DNA are immediately placed in ice to retard renaturation similar to loading a sequencing gel.

The DNA disc chip is made by pressing a 2-mm Acupunch biopsy punch pen (Acuderm, Inc., Fort Lauderdale, FL, USA) into a Nytran membrane sheet. The size of the disc is chosen to fit the ×40 lens of the fluorescent microscope. Each disc is held using a pair of microforceps, which is first dipped into a tube of control DNA for a few seconds, blotting off the excess. The disc is dropped into the tube of test DNA still in the ice. This process is repeated several times to obtain replicated data points. Each tube with submerged discs is placed at room temperature for 10–20 s for annealing. The DNA disc chip is examined using an ultraviolet (UV) epifluorescent microscope at ×40. The florescent images are captured by placing an inexpensive QuickCam Pro camera (Logitech, Inc., Fremont, CA, USA) over the microscope eyepiece and saving 640- by-480 pixel images to hard-disk. For comparison purposes, the color images are computer-cut and pasted onto a photograph of a 50-well microtiter plate in a microarray design using the Microsoft Paint program. Images are converted to the gray-scale pixel intensity of each disc analyzed using Paint Shop Pro 6 software (Jasc Software, Inc., Eden Prairie, MN, USA). Greater fragmentation of sperm DNA is reflected in lower pixel intensity of the disc (for details see Chan *et al.* 2002).

CELL ISOLATION, CULTURE AND CO-CULTURE

Epididymides are cut into three segments corresponding to caput, corpus and cauda. A small piece of each segment is processed as a histological control. After removal of surrounding connective tissue, segments are separately incubated in culture medium containing 0.35% trypsin, 0.2% hyaluronidase, 0.1% BSA and 0.01% DNAse for 2–3 h at 35 °C, in a water bath. Segments are washed and separately incubated in culture medium containing 0.35% collagenase, 0.2% hyaluronidase, 0.1% BSA, 0.01% DNAse and 5% fetal bovine serum (FBS), for 8–10 h at 35 °C. Tubule fragments are cut into small pieces, washed and dispersed by gentle pipeting in the presence of 5% FBS, to obtain cell aggregates (20–30 cells). Aggregates of each segment are washed with culture medium without FBS and resuspended (approximately 10^6 cells/ml) in culture medium containing human transferrin 5 mg/l, insulin 2 mg/l, epidermal growth factor 10 µg/l, vitamins A and E 200 µg/l, hydrocortisone 10^{-8} mol/l, sodium selenite 2 µg/l and cytosine arabinoside 3 mg/l to prevent fibroblasts from growing. Depending on the experiment, 0, 10 or 100 nmol/l DHT is added to the culture medium. Aggregates are plated on Matrigel-coated multi-well culture plates (24-well) at an approximate density of 10^6 cells/ml (2 ml/well). Media are collected every 48 h, centrifuged at 3000g and stored at −25 °C until assayed. Cell homogenates are obtained by sonication after 8–10 days of culture. The percentage of epithelial cells is over 70%, as evaluated by immunocytochemical assay for cytokeratin (Immunotech, Marseille, France).

Culture and co-culture

Several culture/co-culture media are used for *in vitro* physiological maturation and subsequent cleavage at various degrees: modified Krebs-Ringer's bicarbonate, modified Dulbecco's, TCM199, modified Ham's F-10, Whitten medium, Eagle's basal medium with Hank's salts and modified minimum essential medium (MEM) with Earl's salts.

In human IVF centers, animal tissues are used in human co-culture systems to evaluate pregnancy rates after embryo replacement. Fetal cattle uterine fibroblast monolayers are used to evaluate *in vitro* development in implantation of human embryos. Fetal uterine endometrial linings, obtained from healthy bovine fetuses and cells after several subcultures, are used for co-culture. Human embryos co-cultured with cattle monolayers are transferred back to patients. The pregnancy rate is increased when human embryos co-cultured with human ampullary cells are replaced back into patients.

Enzymes and other metabolites

Plasma electrolytes

The Na^+-K^+ ATPase activity of the erythrocyte membrane is measured by the procedure of Wallach and Kamath (1966). Digoxin in the plasma is determined by the method of Arun *et al.* (1998a). Ubiquinone and dolichol in the plasma are measured by the procedure of Palmer *et al.* (1984).

Tryptophan is estimated by the method of Blioxam and Warren (1974) and tyrosine by the method of Wong *et al.* (1964). Serotonin is estimated by the method of Curzon and Green (1970) and catecholamines by the method of Well-Malherbe (1971). Quinolinic acid content of plasma is estimated by HPLC (C_{18} column micro Bondapak™ 4.6×150 mm), with solvent system 0.01 mol/l acetate buffer (pH 3.0) and methanol (6 : 4), flow rate 1.0 ml/min and detection with UV 250 nm). Morphine, strychnine and nicotine are estimated by the method of Arun *et al.* (1998b). Reduced glutathioine is estimated by the method of Beutler *et al.* (1963). Plasma nitric oxide (NO) is estimated by the method of Gabor and Allon (1994).

NADPH–diaphorase enzyme activity

The frozen tissues are homogenized in five volumes of homogenization buffer (Tris/HCl 50 mmol/l, pH 7.4) containing EDTA (0.1 mmol/l), EGTA (0.1 mmol/l), β-mercaptoethanol (12 mmol/l), leupeptin (1 µmol/l), pepstatin A (1 µmol/l) and phenylmethylsulfonyl fluoride (1 mmol/l) with a Polytron homogenizer. After centrifugation of the homogenates at 100 000g, for 1 h at 4 °C, the supernatant is treated with freshly prepared paraformaldehyde (4% w/v) for 30 min at 4 °C. NADPH– diaphorase activity is determined as the reduction of 0.5 mmol/l nitroblue tetrazolium with 1 mmol/l β-NADPH in 0.3 ml of 50 mmol/l Tris-chroride, pH 8.0, at 37 °C for 8 min. The reaction is stopped with 0.3 ml of 100 mmol/l sulfuric acid, and the absorbance of the formazan product is determined at 585 nm. Triplicate measurements for each sample should be performed.

NADPH–diaphorase staining

NADPH diaphorase activity is detected histochemically after the reduced form of NO synthase (NOS) is oxidized by nitroblue tetrazolium. A part of the tissue is immersed in O.C.T. compounds (Miles Inc., Elkhart, IN, USA), rapidly frozen in liquid nitrogen and stored at −80 °C. The frozen tissues with 6 µm thickness are sectioned using a cryostat. They are fixed on silan-coated glass slides with 4% formaldehyde/PBS, pH 7.4, for 15 min. The slides are incubated with 1 mmol/l β-NADPH/0.2 mmol/l nitroblue tetrazolium in 0.1 mol/l Tris-HCl, pH 8.0/0.2% Triton X-100 for 30 min at 37 °C.

Enzyme assays

GST activity is measured in 150 μl of conditioned media or cell homogenates in a mixture containing 0.1 mol/l potassium phosphate buffer, 1 mmol/l GSH and 1 mmol/l 1-Cl-2, 4-dinitrobenzene, pH 6.5. Change in optical density is monitored at 340 nm (Habig et al. 1974). Enzyme activity is expressed as μmol of substrate/min per mg of protein. GGT activity is measured in 150 μl of conditioned media or cell homogenates in a mixture containing 5 mmol/l γ-glutamyl-p-nitroanilide as a donor substrate and 20 mmol/l glycylglycine as acceptor (Orlowsky and Meister, 1963). Enzyme activity is expressed as nmol of product/min per mg of protein. GSH is measured in 150 μl of conditioned media or cell homogenates using 5, 5-dithiobis (2-nitrobenzoic) acid. The resultant color is measured at 412 nm (Ball, 1966).

Serum enzymes

Serum glycolipids are estimated (Lowenstein, 1969) and cholesterol is estimated by using commerical kits supplied by Sigma Chemicals, USA. Superoxide dismutase (Kakkar et al. 1984) and catalase activity are assayed. Glutathione peroxidase and glutathione reductase are estimated (Maehly and Chance, 1954; Paglia and Valentine, 1967; Bergmeyer, 1978). NO is estimated in the plasma by the method of Gabor and Allon (1994).

SEMEN IMMUNOLOGY

A microagglutination method (Friberg, 1974) and indirect immunofluorescence (Husted, 1975) reported sperm antibodies in 23% of men from infertile couples. However, with immunofluorescence, 18% of many blood donors were also positive. There is an association of decreased penetration of cervical mucus by sperm of men with serum titers of sperm agglutinating and immobilizing antibodies (Fjallbrant, 1968; Ansbacher et al. 1971; Ansbacher, 1973). Several techniques have been developed to evaluate semen immunology:

(1) Spermagglutination techniques

   (a) Gelatin agglutination (Kibrich et al. 1952)

(b) Tube-slide agglutination (Franklin and Dukes, 1964)

(c) Microtray agglutination (Friberg, 1974)

(2) Sperm cytotoxicity techniques

   (a) Sperm immobilization (Isojima et al. 1968)

   (b) Microtechniques for immobilization and cytotoxicity (Husted and Hjort, 1975)

(3) Cervical mucus penetration

   (a) Capillary mucus penetration methods (Fjallbrant, 1968)

   (b) Sperm cervical mucus contact method (Kremer and Jager, 1976)

(4) Labeled-antibody techniques

   (a) Indirect immunofluorescent method (Hjort and Hansen, 1971)

   (b) Indirect immunofluorescence on swollen sperm heads (Kolk et al. 1974)

(5) Antiglobulin method

   (a) Mixed-cell antiglobulin reaction (Coombs et al. 1973)

Production of monoclonal antibodies

The dodecamer YLPVGGLRRIGG, designated as YLP_{12}, is synthesized by solid-phase synthesis using Fmoc chemistry (Biosynthesis Inc., Lewisville, TX, USA), and purified by using reverse-phase HPLC. The peptide is water-soluble, and has > 95% purity level. The purified peptide is coupled to the binding subunit of recombinant cholera toxin (rCTB) (List Biological Labs, Inc., Campbell, CA, USA) by a two-step glutaraldehyde procedure as described elsewhere (McKenzie and Halsey, 1984). Virgin CD-1, 10–12-week-old female mice were immunized against the YLP_{12}–rCTB vaccine through intramuscular injections. Each animal received a total of four injections at 2-week intervals. Each injection consisted of 100 μg of the conjugate vaccine. The animals showing high antibody titers were boosted via intravenous injection of the vaccine, and spleen cells were harvested. Spleen cells were fused with NR 6 mouse myeloma cells using polyethyleneglycol (PEG) by the standard hybridoma technology (Kohler and Milstein, 1976; Naz *et al.* 1984). The hybridomas secreting monoclonal antibodies were identified by ELISA (Naz and Chauhan, 2001).

Antibodies and cytometry

Two mouse monoclonal antibodies are used: CD25, specific for the IL-2R α-chain (DAKO, Glostrup, Denmark) and CD122, specific for the IL-2R β-chain (Immunotech, Marseille, France). The secondary antibody used for flow cytometry is a fluorescein isothiocyanate (FITC)-conjugated anti-mouse IgG polyclonal antibody (DAKO). For electron microscopy, the secondary antibody used is a colloidal gold-conjugated anti-mouse IgG polyclonal antibody (Sigma Chemicals, St Louis, MO, USA).

HIV-1/HIV-2 antibody tests

The HIV-1/HIV-2 ELISA kit is developed to detect HIV-1 and/or HIV-2 antibody in serum (Cambridge Biotech, Ireland). It is a stationary-phase assay kit, and is based on recombinant antigens containing immunodominant regions of the env and gag gene products. The capillus HIV-1/HIV-2 assay kit is a mobile-phase kit (Cambridge Diagnostics, Ireland) that detects antibodies to both HIV-1 and HIV-2. In this test the major antigens from the envelope proteins of HIV bind to polystyrene latex beads, forming the basis of a direct latex aggregation assay for the detection of antibodies to HIV-1 and/or HIV-2. Using capillus and ELISA kits, it is possible to detect the HIV antibodies in both semen and blood with equal sensitivity. The capillus method is user-friendly and reliable, and does not require any special equipment for all preliminary investigations. Paired semen and blood sample tests are reported earlier, but those methods are time-consuming and expensive. The high prevalence of leukocytospermia in HIV-1 patients indicates the possibility that increased transudation of serum antibodies into semen occurs in men with genital tract inflammation. White blood cells in semen not only provide a vehicle for the presence of HIV-1, but may also play a role in the sexual transmission of HIV-1.

CHAPTER 17

Male contraception

Reversible male contraception is highly desirable for several considerations. In developing countries, there is an increasing demand from both men and women to share the responsibility and burden of family planning. A significant number of women are intolerant of female methods and most would prefer their male partners to be able to undergo reversible contraception over part of the reproductive life span. Continued growth of the world population, estimated to reach some eight billion by the year 2020, makes it indispensable to develop and make available reliable contraceptive choices for men. Men have four options: abstinence, withdrawal prior to ejaculation, condoms and vasectomy. Unfortunately, for those men who wish to father children at a later time, abstinence, withdrawal and condoms are the only options, because vasectomy is essentially irreversible.

There are several methods to interfere with the reproductive process in men (Table 17.1). The sequence of events in contraceptive drug development includes: chemical experimentation, application to experimental animals, procedural processes and clinical trials in men (Figure 17.1).

What is adequate contraceptive protection? Little is known about the clinical efficacy and feasibility of hormonal contraceptives. The World Health Organization (WHO) has conducted various clinical trials, which indicate that azoospermia (complete absence of sperm in the ejaculate) induced in 60% of men can provide adequate contraceptive protection (Pearl Index 0–1.6). However, documented contraceptive efficacy data in the other 35% of men who suppress sperm production

only to oligozoospermia (0.1–1 million/ml) is limited to a mere 39 man-years. The Pearl Index of 5 (0.6–19) for induced oligozoospermia is an imprecise estimate. Although oligozoospermia leads to significantly attenuated fertility, it remains uncertain whether 'severe' oligozoospermia (< 0.1 million/ml) at this level is an acceptable target for male contraception. It is possible that combined oral and injectable formulations might increase acceptability and compliance.

HORMONAL MALE CONTRACEPTION

For hormonal contraception for men, the term 'male fertility control' is better than 'male contraception', but the latter term is widely used in distinction from 'female contraception'. Unfortunately, the pharmaceutical companies do not have a significant interest in developing and marketing a male contraceptive. One major problem has been the lack of an effective but safe and acceptable method of testosterone delivery, essential for both combination and single-agent hormonal male contraception. The frequent injections of testosterone enanthate or 4-monthly testosterone pellet implants are unlikely candidates for development into practical methods for wide usage. This problem seemed to be solved with the availability of testosterone undecanoate for intramuscular injection. Testosterone enanthate was declared obsolete for further clinical trials. Fortunately, two pharmaceutical companies in Germany (Jenapharma and Schering) raised the hopes for a first realistic step into the development of a

Table 17.1 Summary of methods of interference with the reproductive process in men

Reproductive function	Possible method of interference	Research needed
Sperm formation	periodic injection of long-acting androgen encouragement of decapitation of spermatozoa in testes	development of methodology for separation of cellular components of seminiferous tubules effects of exogenous androgens administered acutely or chronically, on cellular activity in testes and endogenous androgens
Sperm maturation	oral tablet of synthetic (non-steroidal) spermatogenic inhibitor subdermal implant of progestin or anti-androgen (silastic capsules) interference with migration of kinoplasmic droplet of sperm interference with activation of enzyme systems responsible for sperm maturation	factors affecting sexual behavior role of the epididymis in sperm transport and maturation
Sperm transport in the male reproductive tract	reversible vas deferens occlusion with plugs, valve, vulcanizing liquid, polymers, clips, or intravascular thread	
Function of male duct system and accessory organs	interference with function using a hormonal or immunological approach	origin of constituents of seminal plasma and their relation to fertilizability of spermatozoa effects of exogenous androgens on structure and function of accessory organs

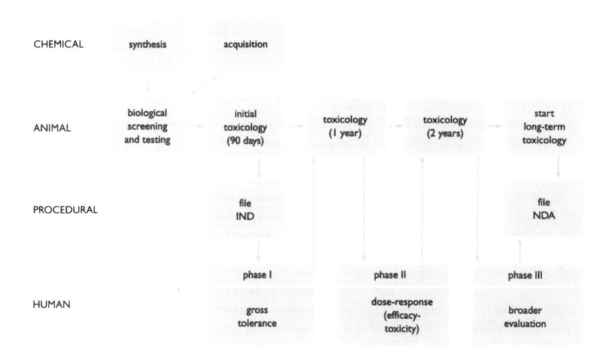

Figure 17.1 Sequence of events in contraceptive drug development

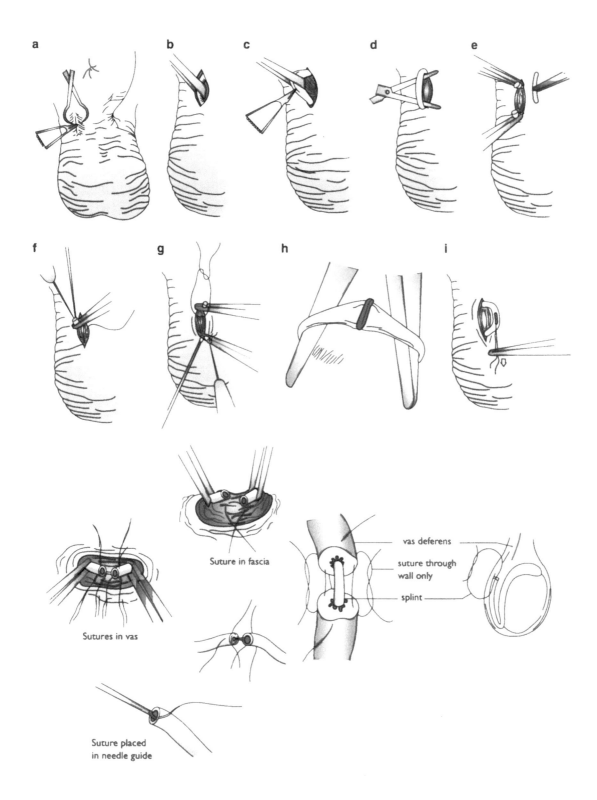

Figure 17.2 Top: (a) technique of vasectomy: skin incision under local anesthesia. (b) Identification and isolation of the vas and sheath. (c) Incision of sheath to expose the vas. (d) Isolation of the vas from within the sheath. (e) Removal of a segment of the vas after securing the stumps. (f) Electrocoagulation of the distal stump of the vas. (g) Closure of the sheath with externalization of the stumps of the vas. (h) Single tantalum clip applied to the vas without division. (Left) Application of tantalum clip prior to division of the vas; (middle) vasectomy between two tantalum clips on each stump; (right) postoperative view of two clips on each vas stump. (i) Insertion of a prosthetic device for vasocclusion. (Reproduced with permission from Hulka and Davis, 1973). Bottom: Method of vasovasostomy. (Reproduced with permission from Bunce, 1969)

hormonal male contraceptive. The morning androgen-only single-agent approach to male contraception is undoubtedly effective, but high doses yielding supraphysiological levels of testosterone are required. Employing testosterone-sparing agents, such as progestins, in combination is attractive, especially when improved efficacy of gonadotropin and spermatogenic suppression, presumably via an additional direct action on the testis or sperm function, can be achieved. Professors Oetell and Saad of Jenapharma/Schering are developing daily progestin pills in combination with an injectable androgen. Although these are potentially helpful for rapid suppression in an induction phase, they are unlikely candidates for development into practical methods for long-term use.

VASECTOMY

Extensive investigations have been conducted into the development of surgical and no-scalpel vasectomy, as well as the microsurgical techniques of vasovasotomy (Figures 17.2 and 17.3). The post-vasectomy ejaculation is a true biological emptying phenomenon, i.e. at ejaculation approximately 65% of the sperm remaining past the point of vasectomy are expelled from the vasa. Each succeeding ejaculate contains one-third the number of sperm of the previous ejaculate. Plasma testosterone levels before and after vasectomy are the same. There is no effect on prostatic or seminal vesicle secretion and there are few adverse sexual effects, except those that may be psychologically induced. Hematomas and infections may develop in the scrotum, because the blood supply to the scrotum is abundant and diffuse. Various layers of the scrotum do not contract readily and blood may diffuse within the layers. Between 30 and 50% of males undergoing elective vasectomy have circulating factors appearing in their serum that will cause agglutination of sperm under a number of experimental conditions.

Sasagawa *et al.* 2000b divided spermatic vessels using an ultrasonically activated scalpel. No bleeding from vessels was noted after the division.

CONTRACEPTIVE VACCINES

The development of a vaccine based on sperm antigens represents a promising approach to contraception. The utility of an antigen in contraceptive vaccine development is contingent upon its tissue (testis/sperm) specificity and its involvement in the fertilization process. Extensive investigations are being carried out to find testis/sperm-specific antigens that can be used for immunocontraception. Complementary DNA excoding a few sperm antigens has been cloned and sequenced, and the recombinant proteins or their peptides expressed by some of the cloned cDNAs are being examined for their effect on fertilization.

The acrosome reaction of the sperm is associated with the release of several proteolytic enzymes. There is also a sequence referred to by Naz and associates as YLP_{12} on human sperm that is involved in binding to the zona pellucida (ZP) of the human oocyte. This sequence is localized on the acrosomal region of the human sperm (Naz and Packianathan, 2000). The YLP_{12} sequence is expressed only in the human testis and not in other somatic cells or tissues. The synthetic 12-mer peptide based on this sequence and its monovalent Fab' antibodies specifically and significantly inhibit human sperm–ZP binding in the hemizona assay.

Naz and Packianathan (2000) conducted an elaborate investigation to evaluate whether or not the YLP_{12} sequence is also involved in human sperm capacitation and the acrosome reaction. This was investigated by examining the effects of the monovalent Fab' antibodies against the YLP_{12} peptide on capacitation and acrosome reaction *in vitro*. The long-term objective of the study was to examine the potential clinical applications of the YLP_{12} peptide in the diagnosis and treatment of male infertility, and in the development of a contraceptive vaccine (Figure 17.4). The YLP_{12} sequence is also involved in immunoinfertility in men (Naz and Chauhan, 2001). Naz *et al.* (2002) raised the monoclonal antibody against the YLP_{12} peptide to first, use this epitope-specific antibody to study its role in fertilization; Second, evaluate it as a probe for screening the testis expression library to obtain a full-length cDNA/gene; and third, examine its potential as a passive immunocontraceptive.

The monoclonal antibody against the YLP_{12} peptide was raised and its immunobiological properties were examined. In the Western blot procedure, the YLP_{12} monoclonal antibody recognized a specific protein band of 50 ± 5 kDa in a human sperm extract and $72 \pm$ kDa in a human testis extract. The myeloma immunoglobulin control did not recognize these specific protein bands. In the immunofluorescence studies, the YLP$_{12}$ monoclonal antibody showed a significant ($p < 0.001$) and a concentration-dependent inhibition of the acrosome reaction. The myeloma immunoglobulin did not affect the acrosome reaction. There was no apparent effect of antibodies on sperm motility. Thus, the monoclonal antibody, if humanized by genetic engineering technology, may provide a useful immunocontraceptive agent (Zhu and Naz, 1997; Naz *et al.* 2002).

SPERMICIDAL HERBS

There is increasing interest in the identification of safe herbal products with spermicidal properties that have a potential for being developed as vaginally delivered contraceptive formulations. Products that have antibacterial, antifungal and/or antiviral activities in addition to spermicidal properties would be preferable, as they would also be useful prophylatics for preventing vaginal infections. The seed oil of *Azadirecta indica* or neem has both spermicidal and antimicrobial activities. The medicinal properties of the seed oil of *Pongamia glabra* are well known in the traditional form of Indian medicine. It has antimicrobial activity against a variety of organisms. It is used in the treatment of herpes and scabies. Systemically, it is also used in the treatment of dyspepsia with sluggish liver.

THE EPIDIDYMIS AS A TARGET FOR CONTRACEPTION

There has been a recent burst in the study of the physiology and biochemistry of the epididymis. This was largely due to the recognition that contraceptive agents that interfere with sperm maturation in the epididymis have many advantages over those that suppress sperm production in the testis. The former agents are expected to have a quick onset of action, rapid reversibility upon withdrawal and reduced chance of mutagenic damage and endocrine impairment of libido. These advantages have been borne out by α-chlorohydrin and chlorinated sugars, which act by interfering with sperm metabolism in the epididymis. However, interest in these agents as potential male

contraceptives soon waned, owing to their neurotoxicity. The advent of molecular biology techniques has let to the identification and cloning of genes encoding sperm-coating or epididymal-specific proteins that can be targeted for immunocontraception. However, for these methods to be effective, organ-specific delivery systems of antisense oligonucleotides/antibodies will have to be developed. Reduction of the prominent constituents of the epididymal fluid, namely α-glucosidase and L-carnitine, or enhancement of sperm transport through the epididymis by pharmacological means have not led to infertility in animals. Despite the consensus held that the epididymis is indispensable for the full expression of male fertility, attempts to induce infertility via an epididymal approach remain elusive.

Future research is needed to generate new leads for effective contraception in the male. The functions of the epididymis by way of electrolyte and water transport can be exploited to develop new male contraceptives.

EXPERIMENTAL PROSTHESIS CONTRACEPTIVES

Experimental contraceptives have been made of prostheses: the plug, the vas clip, the intravas device and the vas valve. None of these devices have been tested in large clinical trials.

The plug

Injections of silastic and other non-reactive synthetic materials have been attempted in animals and men. These injections cause temporary occlusion but subsequent reappearance of the sperm, usually around a channel of recanalization between the foreign body and a side of the wall of the vas in which it has been placed.

Experimental approaches include the insertion of a 1–2-cm length of suture material into the lumen, to be withdrawn outward through a distal puncture and held in place with an external suture. Another approach is to thread one end of the vas with a filament of varying lengths, and anchor it externally.

Metal or plastic designs (microscopic sponges, valours, etc.) and have borrowed from similar studies in bone prostheses, arterial grafts and valvular prostheses.

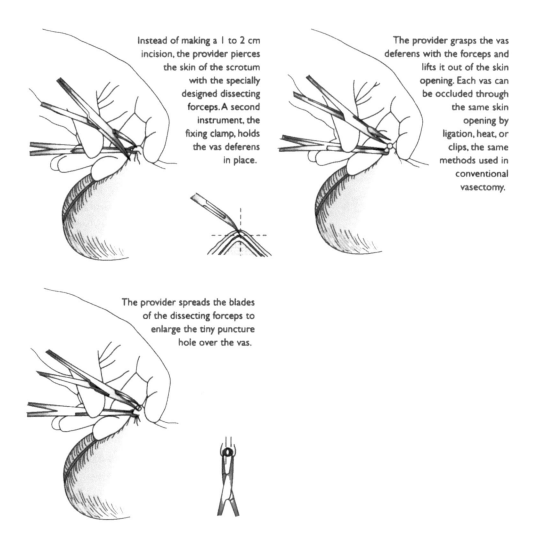

Instead of making a 1 to 2 cm incision, the provider pierces the skin of the scrotum with the specially designed dissecting forceps. A second instrument, the fixing clamp, holds the vas deferens in place.

The provider grasps the vas deferens with the forceps and lifts it out of the skin opening. Each vas can be occluded through the same skin opening by ligation, heat, or clips, the same methods used in conventional vasectomy.

The provider spreads the blades of the dissecting forceps to enlarge the tiny puncture hole over the vas.

Figure 17.3 Steps in no-scapel vasectomy as developed by Johns Hopkins University

Vasectomy was originally developed not as a sterilization procedure but as a means of preventing retrograde testicular infection following prostatic surgery.

The vas clip

The vas is occluded with the application of pressure from without by means of a clip. The initial attraction of this approach was its ease of application and the hope that it would be reversible by simply removing the clip.

Use of spring metal material to occlude the vas under constant pressure (as opposed to constant configuration in the case of the tantalum clip), use of hydrophilic plastic material to exert pressure by chemical means, and a combination of an internal vas occlusive device and an external clamp or clip to hold the internal device in place has been attempted to interfere with sperm migration by external pressure around the device.

Intravas device

Interfering with the function of the vas has been attempted by introducing an intravas device, which will not interfere with sperm flow. It is theorized that, as the sperm travels through the vas, it may be vulnerable to minute changes, which might be induced by the presence of a foreign body. This would not occlude the

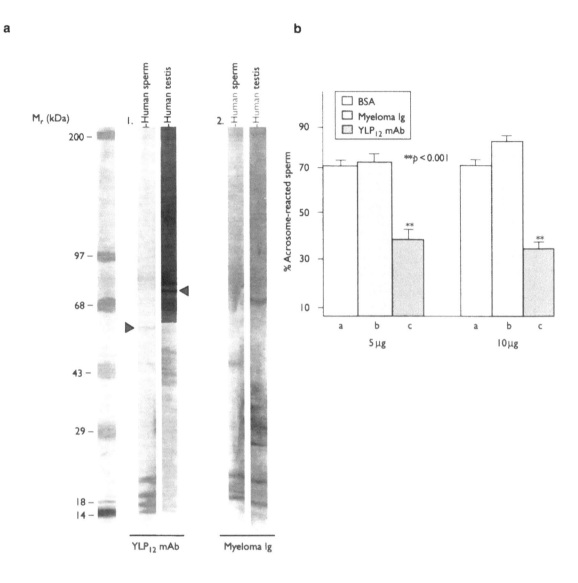

Figure 17.4 (a) Immunoreactivity of YLP$_{12}$ monoclonal antibody (mAb) in the Western blot procedure. The YLP$_{12}$ mAb recognized a specific protein band of about 50 ± 5 kDa in a human sperm extract and about 72 ± 5 kDa in a human testis extract (arrowhead) (panel 1). Myeloma immunoglobulin did not recognize these specific protein bands (panel 2). (b) Effect of YLP$_{12}$ mAb on human sperm acrosome reaction. YLP$_{12}$ mAb significantly inhibited the capacitation/acrosome reaction at both 5 µg and 10 µg/100 µl concentrations. Myeloma Ig did not affect capacitation/acrosome reaction at either concentration. (Reproduced with permission from Naz *et al.* 2002, *Arch Androl*, 48:169–75. www.tandf.co.uk/journals)

vas, but would simply interfere with its chemistry or physiology over a prolonged period.

Vas valve

The aim here was to develop a method for introducing a valve into an intravas device, which would allow the sperm to pass through or not, according to the wishes of the male.

Experimental designs to consider are the following:

(1) Long-term effectiveness of occluding the vas (preventing recanalization or spontaneous reanastomosis);

(2) The size of the lumen of the vas and distensibility of the vas walls, which vary among men;

(3) How much the vas wall is distended or compressed before scarring occurs;

(4) Whether the supply can repair itself following insertion;

(5) Peristalsis, which may prevent tissue growth from the vas wall into the device;

(6) Clotting or coagulation of sperm in epididymal fluid, which may clog a valve or other prosthetic device;

(7) The extent to which the length of the device affects peristaltic activity. Would peristalsis or pressure at the point of vasocclusion cause sperm leakage, granuloma formation, or recanalization?

(8) Any significant difference between a longitudinal and a transverse incision in the vas.

CHAPTER 18

Future research directions

SEMEN EVALUATION

The need to isolate human sperm of acceptable quality is of no less importance in the advanced reproductive technologies than ovulation induction or oocyte aspiration. Particularly given the broad clinical applications for intracytoplasmic sperm injection (ICSI) in current practice, laboratory and operator selection of individual sperm for oocyte injection is critical. Preparation techniques can influence the quantity and quality of the sperm available for use. While several human sperm preparations have been described, most are variants either of density gradient centrifugation or of non-centrifugation-based swim-up methods. While either might be useful in certain clinical circumstances, there is no consensus on the best approach towards processing and selecting human spermatozoa in a particular clinical setting (Sills *et al.* 2000).

There is a need for accurate assessment of membrane permeability, spermatozoal nucleus swelling, sperm–egg fusion, chromatin condensation, cell viability, embryonic viability and metabolism. To this end, the search for fluorescent dyes might solve such a requirement in a quick and easy way (Green, 1992; El-Danasouri *et al.* 1993).

ERECTILE DYSFUNCTION

The introduction of the oral erectogenic agent Viagra® (sildenafil citrate) has revolutionized the therapy of erectile dysfunction (ED). Viagra, a selective phosphodiesterase inhibitor, has become the first-line therapeutic agent of choice for the treatment of ED. Although the efficacy of Viagra in overall use has been claimed to be

60%, a modest 41% satisfaction rate has been documented (Jarow *et al.* 1999) in patients with severe ED (due to organic causes). New derivatives are needed for patients with severe forms ED who fail to show a response to Viagra. Successful therapy with phosphodiesterase inhibitors depends on the preservation of nerve endings to facilitate nitric oxide (NO)-cGMP-mediated neurogenic erection. Research is needed to prevent the onset of ED as well as agents that operate through NO-independent mechanisms (Monga and Rajasekaran, 2002). Currently available treatments for ED induce a temporary erectile response at the time of administration. These therapeutic approaches do not cure the basic vascular cavernosal pathology causing the ED, however. Future research is necessary to evaluate factors that induce new vascular structure formation (vasculogenesis).

THE PROSTATE IN HEALTH AND DISEASE

Further studies are awaited to elucidate each paracrine or autocrine growth factor pathway system to provide precise information on prostate growth and function, as well as a detailed characterization of the interaction between androgen and the signaling pathway of growth factors.

There is a need to develop biomarkers to identify patients with biologically significant prostate cancer who have cancer that can be cured by therapeutic intervention and in whom cure is necessary. Current established treatment options in these patients include radical prostatectomy, radiation therapy – either by external beam or by radioactive seed implantation (brachytherapy) – and cryosurgical ablation of the prostate (freezing). Our view is that currently radical prostatectomy is the treatment of choice in the younger patient who is likely to live 15 years or more, whereas in the older patient with reasonable life expectancy, radiation therapy by external beam or by radioactive seeds, or cryosurgery are appropriate. Patients with advanced disease are currently not curable. They are managed with hormonal manipulation, i.e. androgen deprivation. The major source of androgen in men is the testes. Another source that contributes a small fraction of circulating androgens is the adrenal glands. Our preference for testicular androgen deprivation is simple scrotal orchidectomy (surgical removal of testicles via a small scrotal incision). Compared to medical castration by gonadotropin releasing hormone (GnRH) agonists, orchidectomy is simple, quick and much more economical (the cost orchidectomy is equivalent to the cost of a few months of medical therapy). In addition, patients who have a surgical orchidectomy need anti-androgens. These have additional side-effects and costs.

BIOCHEMISTRY OF SPERMATOGENESIS

Methods need to be developed to separate different cells comprising the seminiferous tubules. Effects need to be evaluated of exogenous androgens administered acutely and chronically on cellular dynamics within the testes, on the circulating levels of endogenous androgens and other hormones, and on the relationship of these factors to libido.

FUNCTIONS OF THE MALE DUCTAL SYSTEM AND ACCESSORY GLANDS

The origin of the constituents of non-human primate semen and their relation to the functional capacity of sperm need to be clarified. Studies are needed on epididymal function as related to sperm transport and fertilizing capacity. The effects of exogenous hormones (androgens) on accessory gland structure and function remain to be identified.

REVERSIBILITY OF VASECTOMY

Research on the reversibility of vasocclusion may be divided into three major approaches:

(1) Surgical reversal of vasectomy;

(2) Preservation of fertility of the vasectomy patient in the form of frozen sperm;

(3) Use of mechanical devices for reversible vasocclusion.

IMMUNE SYSTEM AND SEMINAL CYTOKINES

Further studies are needed to verify the controversial findings that interleukin-10 acts as a suppressor cytokine of the immune system (Huleihel *et al.* 1999; Kelly and Critchley, 1997). The importance of immune balance in semen for human fertility can be evaluated by conducting further research on the nature of pro-inflammatory as well as anti-inflammatory substances.

Further studies will permit a better clarification of the relevance of the androgen receptor gene abnormalities to the development of isolated cryptorchidism, hypospadias, micropenis and impaired spermatogenesis.

References

A

Abbas AK, et al. (1997). *Cellular and Molecular Immunology*, 3rd edn. Philadelphia: WB Saunders

Abdel-Hamid I, et al. (2002). Flow-through immunoassay system for rapid clinical diagnostics. Personal communication

Abou-Haila A, et al. (1996). Androgen regulation of molecular forms of beta-D-glucuronidase in the mouse epididymis: comparison with liver and kidney. *J Androl*, 17:194–207

Abrams PH, et al. (1979a). The results of prostatectomy: a symptomatic and urodynamic analysis of 152 patients. *J Urol*, 121:640–2

Abrams PH (1979b). Perfusion urethral profilometry. *Urol Clin North Am*, 6:103–10

Adami H, et al. (1994). Testicular cancer in nine Northern European countries. *Int J Cancer*, 59:33–8

Adams ML, et al. (1992). Inhibition of the morphine withdrawal syndrome by a nitric oxide synthase inhibitor, N G-nitro-L-arginine methylester. *Life Sci*, 50:35–40

Adams ML, et al. (1994). Effects of nitric oxide-related agents on rat testicular function. *J Pharmacol Exp Ther*, 269:230–7

Ahmadi A, Ng SC (1999). Influence of sperm plasma membrane destruction on human sperm head decondensation and pronuclear formation. *Arch Androl*, 42:1–7

Aiman J, Griffin JE (1982). The frequency of androgen receptor deficiency in infertile men. *J Clin Endocrinol Metab*, 54:725–32

Aitken J (1994). The biochemistry and physiology of human spermatozoa: Consequences for fertility and sterility. In Van Blerkom J, ed. *The Biological Basis of Early Human Reproductive Failure: Application to Medically Assisted Conception and the Treatment of Infertility*, 1994:252–82

Aitken RJ (1983). Clinical assessment of human sperm function. *J Obstet Gynecol*, 3:48

Aitken RJ (2002). Active oxygen in spermatozoa during epididymal transit. Personal communication

Aitken RJ, Baker HWG (1995). Seminal leukocytes: passengers, terrorists or good Samaritans? *Hum Reprod*, 10:1736–9

Aitken RJ, Clarkson JS (1987). Cellular basis of defective sperm function and its association with the genesis of reactive oxygen species by human spermatozoa. *J Reprod Fertil*, 81:459–69

Aitken RJ, et al. (1989). Generation of reactive oxygen species, lipid peroxidation and human sperm function. *Biol Reprod* 40:183–97

Aitken RJ, et al. (1991). Prospective analysis of sperm–oocyte fusion and reactive oxygen species generation as criteria for the diagnosis of infertility. *Am J Obstet Gynecol*, 164:542–51

Akin JW, et al. (1991). Evidence for a partial deletion in the androgen receptor gene in a phenotypic male with azoospermia. *Am J Obstet Gynecol*, 165:1891–4

Alberti I, et al. (1996). Differential nuclear matrix–intermediate filament expression in human prostate cancer in respect to benign prostatic hyperplasia. *Cancer Lett*, 109:193–8

Alexander NJ, Anderson DJ (1987). Immunology of semen. *Fertil Steril*, 47:192–205

Allen JF (1996). Separate sexes and the mitochondrial theory of aging. *J Theor Biol*, 180:135–40

Allera RC, et al. (1995). Mutations of the androgen receptor coding sequence are infrequent in patients with isolated hypospadias. *J Clin Endocrinol Metab*, 80:2697–9

Altura BM, Altura BT (1981). Magnesium ions and contraction of vascular smooth muscle. Relationship to some vascular diseases. *Fed Proc*, 40:2672

Anawalt BD, et al. (1996). Serum inhibin B levels reflect Sertoli cell function in normal men and men with testicular dysfunction. *J Clin Endcrinol Metab*, 81:3341–5

Andrews JC, Bavister BD (1989). Capacitation of hamster spermatozoa with the divalent cation chelators D-penicillamine, L-histidine, and L-cystine in a protein-free culture medium. *Gamete Res*, 23:159–70

Ansbacher R (1973). Vasectomy: sperm antibodies. *Fertil Steril*, 24:788

Ansbacher R, et al. (1971). Sperm antibodies in infertile couples. *Fertil Steril*, 22:298

Aragona F, Glazel GP (1998). Prepubertal varicoceles. *Urology*, 52:348–9

Aragona F, et al. (1994). Correlation of testicular volume, histology and LHRH test in adolescents with idiopathic varicocele. *Eur Urol*, 26:61–6

Araujo AB, et al. (1998). The relationship between depressive symptoms and male erectile dysfunction: cross sectional results from the Massachusetts Male Aging Study. *Psychosom Med*, 60:458–65

Arun P, et al. (1998a). Endogenous alkaloids in the brain of rats loaded with tyrosine/tryptophan in the serum of patients of neurodegenerative and psychiatric disorders. *Ind J Med Res*, 107:231–8

Arun P, et al. (1998b). Identification and estimation of endogenous digoxin in biological fluids and tissues by TLC and HPLC. *Ind J Biochem Biophys*, 35:308–12

Arver S, et al. (1996). Improvement of sexual function in testosterone deficient men treated for 1 year with a permeation-enhanced testosterone transdermal system. *J Urol*, 155:1604–8

Asherson RA, et al. (2001). *Vascular Manifestations of Systemic Autoimmune Diseases*. Boca Raton, FL: CRC Press

Ashkenazi A, Dixit VM (1998). Death receptors signaling and modulation. *Science*, 281:1305

Auger J, et al. (1990). Aniline blue staining as a marker of sperm chromatin defects associated with different semen characteristics discriminates between proven fertile and suspected infertile men. *Int J Androl*, 13:452–62

Avery S, et al. (1990). An evaluation of the hypoosmotic sperm swelling test as a predictor of fertilizing capacity *in vitro*. *Int J Androl*, 13:93–9

B

Bacetti B, et al. (1993). Notulae seminologicae. 2 The 'Short tail' and 'Stump' defect in human spermatozoa. *Andrologica*, 25:331–5

Badran HH, Hermo LS (2002). Expression and regulation of aquaporins 1, 8, and 9 in the testis efferent ducts, and epididymis of adult rats and during postnatal development. *J Androl*, 23:358–73

Bains R, et al. (2002). Human sperm cells express CD44. *Fertil Steril*, 78:307–12

Bajpai M, et al. (2003). Effect of tyrosine kinase inhibitors on tyrosine phosphorylatin and motility parameters in human sperm. *Arch Androl*, 49:229–46

Ball CR (1966). Estimation and identification of thiols in rat spleen after cysteine or glutathione treatment: relevance to protection against nitrogen mustards. *Biochem Pharmacol*, 15:809–16

Bandivdekar AH, Moodbidri SB (2002). Spermicidal activity of seed oil of *Pongamia glabra*. *Arch Androl*, 48:9–13

Bandivdekar AH, et al. (1991). Antifertility effects of human sperm antigen in female rats. *Contraception*, 44:559–89

Bandivdekar AH, et al. (1992). Antifertility effects in rats actively immunized with 80 kDa human semen glycoprotein. *Ind J Exp Biol*, 30:1017–23

Bandivdekar AH, et al. (2001). Characterization of 80 kDa human sperm antigen responsible for immunoinfertility. *Am J Reprod Immunol*, 45:28–34

Bandyopadhyay N. (2002). *Biochemical Studies on Sperm Nuclear Chromatin*. PhD Thesis, University of Calcutta, Calcutta, India

Bangma CH, et al. (1996). Transrectal ultrasonic volumetry of the prostate. *In vivo* comparison of different methods. *Prostate*, 28:107–10

Bartsch W, et al. (1990). Enzymes of androgen formation and degradation in the human prostate. *Acad Sci*, 595:53–66

Basrur PK (1999). *Veterinary Medical Genetics*. Guelph: University of Guelph Press

Batch JA, et al. (1993). Mutations of the androgen receptor gene identified in perineal hypospadias. *J Med Genet*, 30:198–201

Battmann T, et al. (1991). *In vitro* inhibition of the preovulatory LH surge by substance P and *in vitro* modulation of gonadotropin-releasing hormone-induced LH release by substance P, oestradiol and progesterone in the female rat. *J Endocrinol*, 130:169–75

Behre HM, et al. (1997). Diseases of the hypothalamus and the pituitary gland. *Andrology*, 115–29

Behrmen SJ, Menge AC (1979). Immunological aspects of infertility in human reproduction. In Hafez ESE, Evans TN, eds. *Conception and Contraception*. Hagerstown, MD: Harper and Row

Belker AM, et al. (1991). Results of 1469 microsurgical vasectomy reversals by the Vasectomy Study Group. *J Urol*, 145:505–11

Belloli G, et al. (1993). Varicocele in childhood and adolescence and other testicular anomalies. An epidemiological study. *Pediatr Med Chir*, 15:159–62

Belmonte SA, et al. (2002). Compartmentalization of lysosomal enzymes in cauda epididymis of normal and castrated rats. *Arch Androl*, 48:193–201

Belmonte SA, et al. (2002). Mannose-6-phosphate receptors as a molecular indicator of maturation of epididymal sperm. *Arch Androl*, 48:65–72

Bergmeyer HV (1978). *Methods of Enzymatic Analysis.* New York: Academic Press

Berthelsen JG, Skakkeboek NE (1983). Gonadal function in men with testis cancer. *Fertil Steril,* 39:68–71

Besedovsky HO, del Rey A (1996). Immune–neuroendocrine interactions: facts and hypotheses. *Endocr Rev,* 17:64–102

Beutler E, et al. (1963). Modified procedure for the estimation of reduced glutathione. *J Lab Clin Med,* 61:882

Bidwell J, et al. (1997). Tissue matrix protein expression in human osteoblasts, osteosarcoma tumors, and osteosarcoma cell lines. *Mol Biol Rep,* 24:271–82

Biggers JD, et al. (1971). The culture of mouse embryos 'in vitro.' *Methods Mammalian Embryol,* 24:86–116

Bissada N (2001). Prostate cancer: current status and future directions. *Adv Reprod,* 5,91–8

Bloxam LD, Warren WH (1974). Error in the determination of tryptophan by the method of Denkala and Dewey. A revised procedure. *Anal Biochem,* 60:621–5

Boettcher B, et al. (1970). Sperm agglutinating activity in some human sera. *Int J Fertil,* 15:143

Bolander FF (1994). *Mol Endocrinol,* 24:103–240

Bolander FF Jr (2000). Hormone receptors: the basics and recent advances. *Adv Reprod,* 4:1–15

Bornstein SR, Ehrhart-Bornstein M (1999). Interactions of the stress system. In *The Adrenal: Basic and Clinical Aspects, Stress and Adaptation: from Selye's Concept to Application of Modern Formulations.* New York: Marcel Dekker, 89–108

Bornstein SR, Chrousos GP (1999). Clinical review 104: adrenocorticotropin (ACTH)-and non-ACTH-medicated regulation of the adrenal cortex – neural and immune inputs. *J Clin Endocrinol Metab,* 84:1729–36

Bos JD (1997). Skin immune system (SIS). In *Cutaneous Immunology and Clinical Immunodermatology.* Boca Raton, FL: CRC Press

Bostwick et al. (1999). *Prostate Cancer.* New York: American Cancer Society, Villard

Bott SRT, Kirby RS (2001). Benign prostatic hyperplasia. In Lunenfeld B, Gooren L. *Textbook of Men's Health.* London: Parthenon Publishing, 53–68

Bravo PW, et al. (1997a). Semen collection and artificial insemination in alpacas. *Theriogenology,* 47:619–26

Bravo PW, et al. (1997b). Effect of repeated collection on semen characteristics of alpacas. *Biol Reprod,* 57:520–4

Bravo PW, et al. (2002). The ejaculatory process and semen characteristics associated with it of llamas and alpacas. *Arch Androl,* 48:65–72

Breitbart H, Spungin B (1997). The biochemistry of the acrosome reaction. *Mol Hum Reprod,* 3:195–202

Brennemann W, et al. (1997). Gonadal function of patients treated with cisplatin based chemotherapy for germ cancer. *J Urol,* 158:844–50

Brinster RL (1993). Stem cells and transgenic mice in the study of development. *Int J Dev Biol,* 3:89–99

Brinster RL, et al. (1980). Translation of globin messenger RNA by the mouse ovum. *Nature,* 283:499–501

Bucy RP, Golpfert P (2002). Some basic cellular immunology principles applied to the pathogenesis of infectious diseases. In *Immunotherapy for Infectious Diseases.* Totowa, NJ: Humana Press

Burgaud JL, Baserga R (1996). Intracellular transactivation of the insulin-like growth factor I receptor by an epidermal growth factor receptor. *Exp Cell Res,* 233:412–19

Burger HG, Igarashi M (1988). Inhibin: definition and nomenclature, including related substances. *J Clin Endocrinol Metab,* 78:433–9

Bunce PO (1969). *Urologic Survey.* New York: Harper and Row

C

Calkins JH, et al. (1988). Interleukin-1 inhibits Leydig cell steroidogenesis in primary culture. *Endocrinology,* 123:1605–10

Calvin HI (1976). Comparative analysis of the nuclear basic proteins in rat, human, guinea pig, mouse and rabbit spermatozoa. *Biochim Biophys Acta,* 434:377–89

Calzada L, Martinez JM (2002). Induction of nuclear matrix–estradiol receptor complex during capacitation process in human spermatozoa. *Arch Androl,* 48:221–4

Calzada L, et al. (1998). Different affinities of tamoxifen binding sites in the estrogen receptor of breast cancer. *Med Sci Res,* 26:829–30

Calzada L, et al. (2001a). Hormone-related factors associated with hormone receptors levels in breast cancer. *Gynecol Obstet Invest,* 52:264–8

Calzada L, et al. (2001b). Measurement of androgen and estrogen receptors in breast tissue from subjects with anabolic steroid-dependent gynecomastia. *Life Sci,* 69:1465–9

Camejo MI (2003). Relation between immunosuppressive PGE$_2$ and IL-10 to proinflammatory IL-6 in seminal plasma of infertile and fertile men. *Arch Androl,* 49:111–16

Camejo MI, et al. (2001). Interleukin-6 (IL-6) in seminal plasma of infertile men, and lipid peroxidation of their sperm. *Arch Androl,* 47:97–101

Canadian Networking Tox Centre (1998). *Manual of Immunological Methods.* Boca Raton, FL: CRC Press

Capen CC, Martin SL (1989). The pituitary gland. In McDonald LE, Pineda MH, eds. *Veterinary Endocrinology and Reproduction.* Philadelphia: Lea & Febiger

Cappechi MR (1989). Altering the genome by homologous recombination. *Science,* 244:1288–92

Carani C, et al. (1997). Effect of testosterone and estradiol in a man with aromatase deficiency. N Engl J Med, 337:91–5

Carlsen E, et al. (1992). Evidence for decreasing quality of semen during past 50 years. Br Med J, 305:609–13

Carpenter WT Jr, Buchnan RW (1994). Medical progress in schizophrenia. N Engl J Med, 30:681

Carranco A, et al. (1983). Heparin induced nuclei decondensation of mammalian epididymal spermatozoa. Arch Androl, 10:213–18

Carreau S, et al. (1994). La cellule de Sertoli: aspects fonctionnels compares chez le rat, le porc et l'homme. Ann Endocrinol, 55:203–20

Carrell DT, Liu L (2002). Sperm DNA fragmentation is increased in couples with unexplained recurrent pregnancy loss. Arch Androl, 48:147–54

Carroll PR, et al. (1987). Fertility status of patients with clinical stage I testis tumors on a surveillance protocol. J Urol 138:70–2

Casper RF, et al. (1996). The hypo-osmotic swelling test for selection of viable sperm for intracytoplasmic sperm injection in men with complete asthenozoospermia. Fertil Steril, 65:972–6

Catalona WJ, et al. (1991). Measurement of prostate-specific antigen in serum as a screening test for prostate cancer. N Engl J Med, 324:1156–61

Chamberlain NL, et al. (1994). The length and location of CAG trinucleotide repeats in the androgen receptor N-terminal domain affect transactivation function. Nucleic Acids Res, 22:3181–6

Chamness SL, et al. (1995). The effect of androgen on nitric oxide synthase in the male reproductive tract of the rat. Fertil Steril, 63:1101–7

Chan PJ, et al. (2002). A simple DNA disc chip in a microarray design based on modified comparative genomic hybridization for sperm DNA analysis. Fertil Steril, 77:1056–9

Chan PTK, Schlegel PN (2002). Epididymitis and other inflammatory conditions of the male excurrent ductal system. Hum Reprod, 17:121–29

Chan SYW, et al. (1990). Differential evaluation of human sperm hypoosmotic swelling test and its relationship with the outcome of in-vitro fertilization of human oocytes. Hum Reprod, 5:84–8

Check JH, et al. (1995). A comparative prospective study using matched samples to determine the influence of subnormal hypoosmotic test scores of spermatozoa on subsequent fertilization and pregnancy rates following in vitro fertilization. Hum Reprod, 10:1197–200

Check ML, et al. (2001). Pregnancy/implantation rates as related to age following transfer of frozen embryos produced by ICSI. Arch Androl, 47:161–5

Chemes HE, et al. (1987). Dysplasia of the fibrous sheath. An ultrastructural defect of human spermatozoa associated with sperm immotility and primary sterility. Fertil Steril, 48:664–9

Chemes HE, et al. (1990). Extreme asthenozoospermia and chronic respiratory disease. A new variant of the immotile cilia syndrome. Int J Androl, 13:216–22

Chemes HE, et al. (1998). Ultrastructural pathology of the sperm flagellum: association between flagellar pathology and fertility prognosis in severly asthenozoospermic men. Hum Reprod, 13:2521–6

Chen SU, et al. (1995). Comparison between a two-layer discontinuous Percoll gradient and swim-up for sperm preparation on normal and abnormal semen samples. J Assist Reprod Genet, 12:698–703

Chiappelli F, Liu QN (2000). Immunity. In Encyclopedia of Stress. New York: Academic Press.

Chomczynski P, Sacchi N (1987). Single-step method of RNA isolation: scidguanidium thiocynate–phenol–chloroform extraction. Anal Biochem, 162:156–9

Chrousos GP (1998). Stressors, stress, and neuroendocrine integration of the adaptive response. The 1997 Hans Selye Memorial Lecture. Acad Sci, 851:311–35

Chrousos GP (2000a). Disease, stress-induced, overview. In Fink G, ed. Encyclopedia of Stress. New York: Academic Press

Chrousos GP (2000b). Adrenal insufficiency. In Fink G, ed. Encyclopedia of Stress. New York: Academic Press

Ciejek EM, et al. (1982). Ribonucleic acid precursors are associated with the chick oviduct nuclear matrix. Biochemistry, 21:4945–53

Coburn M, Wheeler T (1991). Testicular biopsy in male evaluation. Infertil Male, 17:225–53

Comporti M (1989). Three models of free radical induced cell injury. Chem Biol Interact, 72:1–56

Coombs RRA, et al. (1973). Immunoglobulin classes reactive with spermatozoa in the serum and seminal plasma of vasectomized and infertile men. Immunol Reprod, 45:354–9

Costabile RA, et al. (1992). Testicular volume assessment in the adolescent with a varicocele. J Urol, 147:1348–50

Coutts AS, et al. (1996). Estrogen regulation of nuclear matrix-intermediate filament proteins in human breast cancer cells. J Cell Biochem, 63:174–84

Curzon G, Green AR (1970). Rapid method for the determination of 5-hydroxy tryptophan and 5-hydroxy indoleacetic acid in certain regions of rat brain. Br J Pharmacol, 39:653–5

Cyr DG et al. (2003). Cellular interactions and the blood–epididymal barrier. Arch Androl, 49, in press

D

Davis PJ, Davis FB (1996). Nongenomic actions of thyroid hormone. Thyroid, 6:497–504

de Kretser DM, et al. (1989). Serum inhibin levels in normal men and men with testicular disorders. J Endocrinol, 120:517–23

Delgado NM, et al. (1980). A species-specific decondensation of human spermatozoa nuclei by heparin. Arch Androl, 4:305–13

Delgado NM, et al. (1982). Heparin binding sites in the human spermatozoa membrane. Arch Androl, 8:87–95

Delgado NM, et al. (1999). Nucleons, I: a model for studying the mechanism of sperm nucleus swelling in vitro. Arch Androl, 43:85–95

Delgado NM, et al. (2001). Heparin and glutathione II: correlation between decondensation of bull sperm cells and its nucleons. Arch Androl, 47:47–58

DePaolo LV, et al. (2000). Male contraception: views to the 21st century. Trends Endocrinol Metab, 11:66–9

DeSantis M, et al. (1999). Impact of cytotoxic treatment on long-term fertility in patients with germ-cell cancer. Int J Cancer, 83:864–5

Devi KU, et al. (1997). A maturation-related differential phosphorylation of the plasma membrane proteins of the epididymal spermatozoa of the hamster by endogenous protein kinases. Mol Reprod Dev, 47:341–50

de Wit R, et al. (1995). Four cycles of BEP versus an alternating regime of PVB and BEP in patients with poor-prognosis metastatic testicular non-seminoma: a randomized study of the EORTC Genitourinary Tract Cancer Cooperative Group. Br J Cancer, 71:1311–14

Dickey RA, et al. (2002). Relationship of follicle numbers/estradiol levels in multiple implantation after intrauterine insemination. Adv Reprod, 6:abstr 64

Dickey RP, et al. (2002). Effect of diagnosis, age, sperm quality and number of preovulatory follicles on the outcome of multiple cycles of clomiphene citrate – intrauterine insemination. Fertil Steril, 78:1088–95

Dickmann AB, Herr JC (1997). Sperm antigens and their use in the development of immunocontraceptive. Am J Reprod Immunol, 37:111–17

Dobashi M, et al. (2001). Inhibition of sterodigenesis in Leydig cells by exogenous nitric oxide occurs independently of sterodigenic acute regulatory protein (StAR) mRNA. Arch Androl, 47:203–9

Donovan JF, Winfield HN. (1992). Laparoscopic varix ligation. J Urol, 147:77–81

Dowsing AT, et al. (1999). Linkage between male infertility and trinucleotide repeat expansion in the androgen-receptor gene. Lancet, 354:640–3

Dozortsev D, et al. (1994). Behaviour of spermatozoa in human oocytes displaying one pronucleus after intracytoplasmic sperm injection. Hum Reprod, 9:2139–44

Dozortzev D, et al. (1995). Sperm plasma membrane damage prior to intercytoplasmic sperm injection: a necessary condition for sperm nucleus decondensation. Hum Reprod, 10:2960–4

Duncan AE, Fraser LR (1993). Cyclic AMP-dependent phosphorylation of epididymical mouse sperm proteins during capacitation in vitro: identification of an M, 95000 phosphotyrosine-containing protein. J Reprod Fertil, 97:287–99

E

Eisenbach M, Ralt D (1992). Precontact mammalian sperm–egg communication and role in fertilisation. Am J Physiol, 162:C1095–101

Eisenbach M, Tur-Kaspa I (1994). Human sperm chemotaxis is not enigmatic anymore. Fertil Steril, 62:233–5

El-Danasouri I, et al. (1993). Fluorescence staining of nuclear deoxyribonucleic acid allows for on accurate assessment of the hamster on egg penetration assay. Fertil Steril, 59:470–2

Elliot OJ, et al. (1996). An RMB homologue maps to the mouse Y chromosome and is expressed in germ cells. Hum Mol Genet, 5:869–74

Englebienne P (2000). Immune and Receptor Assays in Theory and Practice. Boca Raton, FL: CRC Press

Evirgen O, et al. (2003). Ultrastructural analysis of TESE and semen sperm tails from patients exhibiting absolute immotility on the day of ICSI. Arch Androl, 49:57–67

Ezner N, Robaire B (2002). Androgenic regulation of the structure and functions of the epididymis. Personal communication

F

Fahmy WE, Bissada N (2003). Cryosurgery for prostate cancer. Arch Androl, 49, in press

Falkenstein E, et al. (1996). Full-length cDNA sequence of a progesterone membrane-binding protein from porcine vascular smooth muscle cells. Biochem Biophys Res Commun, 229:86–9

Farrar DJ (1994). Urodynamics in the elderly. In Urodynamics: Principles, Practice and Application. New York: Marcel Dekker

Fawcett DW (1974). In Maucini RE, Martini L, eds. Male Fertility and Sterility. London: Academic Press

Fehder WP, et al. (2000). Macrophages. In Fink G, ed. Encyclopedia of Stress. New York: Academic Press

Feingold M, Pashaya H (1983). The Chromosome, Genetics and Birth Defects in Clinical Practice. Boston: Little Brown

Felberbaum RE, et al. (2001). GnRH antagonists in assisted reproduction. In GnRH Analogues. New York: Parthenon Publishing

Feng HL (2003). Molecular biology of male infertility. Arch Androl, 49:19–28

Ferin M (2000). Effects of stress on gonadotropin secretion. In Fink G, ed. Encyclopedia of Stress. New York: Academic Press

Fernandez-Botran R, Vetvicka V (2001). *Methods in Cellular Immunology*, 2nd edn. New York: CRC Press

Fey KG, et al. (1984a). Epithelial cytoskeletal framework and nuclear matrix–intermediate filament scaffold: three-dimensional organization and protein composition. *J Cell Biol*, 98:1973–84

Fey KG, et al. (1984b). Epithelial structure revealed by chemical dissection and unembedded electron microscopy. *J Cell Biol*, 99:203s–8s

Fierro R, et al. (2002). Expression of IL-2α and IL-2β receptors on the membrane surface of human sperm. *Arch Androl*, 48:397–404

Fink G (2000). *Encyclopedia of Stress*. New York: Academic Press

Fjallbrant B (1968). Sperm antibodies and sterility in men. *Acta Obstet Gynecol Scand*, 47 (Suppl 4)

Foreman D, et al. (1973). A modification of the Roe procedure for the determination of fructose in tissues. *Anal Biochem*, 56:584–90

Fraioli F, et al. (1984). β-Endorphin, metenkefalin, and calcitonin in human semen: evidence for possible role in human sperm motility. *Acad Sci*, 483:365–70

Franklin RR, Dukes CD (1964). Antispermatozoal antibody and unexplained infertility. *Am J Obstet Gynecol*, 89:6

Friberg J (1974). Clinical and immunological studies on spermagglutinating antibodies in serum and seminal fluid. *Acta Obstet Gynecol Scand*, (Suppl) 36:47

Friedler S, et al. (1997). Intracytoplasmic injection of fresh and cryopreserved testicular spermatozoa in patients with nonobstructive azoospermia: a comparative study. *Fertil Steril*, 68:892–7

Frungieri MB, et al. (2002). Number, distribution pattern, and identification of macrophages in the testes of infertile men. *Fertil Steril*, 78:298–306

Fujisawa M, et al. (2002). Evaluation of health-related quality of life in patients treated for erectile dysfunction with Viagra (Sildenafil citrate) using SF-36 score. *Arch Androl*, 48:15–22

G

Gabor G, Allon N (1994). Spectrofluorometric method for NO determination. *Anal Biochem*, 220:16

Gamett DC, et al. (1997). Secondary dimerization between members of the epidermal growth factor family. *J Biol Chem*, 272:12052–6

Garban H, et al. (1995). Restoration of normal adult penile erectile response on aged rats by long-term treatment with androgen. *Biol Reprod*, 53:1365–72

Garnier PE, et al. (1974). Effect of synthetic luteinizing hormone-releasing hormone (LH-RH) on the release of gonadotrophins in children and adolescents. VI: relations to age, sex and puberty. *Acta Endocrinol*, 77:422–34

Gatewood JM, et al. (1987). Sequence-specific packing of DNA in human sperm chromatin. *Science*, 236:962–4

Gatz M, et al. (1996). Aging and mental disorders. In *Handbook of the Psychology of Aging*. New York: Marcel Dekker, 365–82

Gerdes MG, et al. (1994). Dynamic changes in the higher-level chromatin organization of specific sequences revealed by *in situ* hybridization to nuclear halos. *J Cell Biol*, 126:289–304

Giguere A, et al. (1996). Modulation of microtubule polymerization by thyroid hormones presented at the 78th Annual Meeting of the Endocrine Society; Abstr: 652

Glimelius B, et al. (1978). Binding of heparin to the surface of cultured human endothelial cells. *Thromb Res*, 12:773–82

Golberger L, Breznitz S (1993). *Handbook of Stress: Theoretical and Clinical Aspects*, 2nd edn. New York: Free Press

Gold ER, Fundenberg HH (1967). Chromic chloride: a coupling reagent for passive hemagglutination reactions. *J Immunol*, 99:859–62

Goldberg E (1990). Lactate dehydrogenase C4 as an immuno-contraceptive model. In *Gamete Interaction: Prospects for Immunocontraception*, 6:63–73

Goldstein DS (1995). *Stress Catecholamines and Cardiovascular Disease*. New York: Oxford University Press

Goldstein JL, Brown MS (1990). Regulation of the mevalonate pathway. *Nature*, 343:425–30

Gonzalez-Unzaga M, et al. (2003). Clinical significance of nuclear matrix–estradiol receptor complex in human sperm. *Arch Androl*, 49:77–81

Green DPL (1992). Comparison of Hoechst 33342 and propidium iodide as fluorescent markers for sperm fusion with harmster oocytes. *J Reprod Fertil*, 96:581–91

Green DR, Reed JC (1998). Mitochondria and apoptosis. *Science* 281:1309

Green LC, et al. (1982). Analysis of nitrate, nitrite, and [^{15}N]nitrate in biological fluids. *Anal Biochem*, 126:131–8

Griffiths J, Abrams PA (1990). The Stamey endoscopic bladder neck suspension in the elderly. *Br J Urol*, 65:170–2

Griveau JF, et al. (1995). Reactive oxygen species, lipid peroxidation and enzymatic defense systems in human spermatozoa. *J Reprod Fertil*, 103:17–26

Groux H, et al. (1966). Interleukin-10 induces a long term antigen-specific anergic state in human CD4+ T cells. *J Exp Med*, 184:19–29

Gruschwitz MS, et al. (1996). Cytokine levels in the seminal fluid of infertile men. *J Androl*, 17:158–63

Guillemette C, et al. (1995). Specificity of glucuronosyltransferase activity in the human cancer cell line LNCaP, evidence for the presence of a least two glucuronosyltransferase enzymes. *J Steroid Biochem Mol Biol*, 55:355–62

Gündogan M (2003). Effect of diluents on motility of ram sperm during storage at 5°C. *Arch Androl* 49: 69–75

Gurland BJ (1983). *The Mind and Mood of Aging*. New York: Haworth

Gusse M, et al. (1986). Purification and characterization of nuclear basic proteins of human sperm. *Biochim Biophys Acta*, 884:124–34

H

Habib AA, et al. (1998). The epidermal growth factor receptor associates with and recruits phosphatidylinositol 3-kinase to the platelet-derived growth factor β receptor. *J Biol Chem*, 273:6885–91

Habig WH, et al. (1974). Glutathione-S-transferases. The first enzymatic step in mercapturic acid formation. *J Biol Chem*, 249:7130–9

Hacker GW, Gu J (2002). *Gold and Silver Staining: Techniques in Molecular Morphology*. New York: CRC Press

Hafez ESE, Kanagawa H (1973). Scanning electron microscopy of human monkey and rabbit spermatozoa. *Fertil Steril*, 24:776–87

Haga H (1992). Effects of dietary magnesium supplementation on diurnal variation of BP and plasma Na^+-K^+ ATPase activity in essential hypertension. *Jpn Heart J*, 33:785

Hammadeh ME, et al. (1996). The effect of chromatin condensation and morphology of human spermatozoa on fertilization, cleavage and pregnancy rates in an intracytoplasmatic sperm injection programme. *Hum Reprod*, 11:2468–71

Hammadeh ME, et al. (2001). Predictive value of sperm chromatin condensation (aniline blue staining) in the assessment of male fertility. *Arch Androl*, 46:99–104

Hammadeh ME, et al. (2002). Chromatin decondensation of human spermatozoa *in vitro* and its relation to fertilization rate after intracytoplasmic sperm injection (ICSI). *Arch Androl*, 48:201–10

Hammerstedt RH, Parks JE (1987). Changes in sperm surfaces associated with epididymal transit. *J Reprod Fertil Suppl*, 34:133–49

Hanash KA, Mostofi KF (1992). Androgen effect on prostate specific antigen secretion. *J Surg Oncol*, 49:202–4

Handrow RR, et al. (1984). Specific binding of the glycosaminogly-can ^{3}H-heparin to bull, monkey and rabbit spermatozoa *in vitro*. *J Androl*, 5:51–63

Hansen PJ (2000). Immunology of reproduction. In Hafez B, Hafez ESE, eds. *Reproduction in Farm Animals*, 7th edn. Philadelphia: Lippincott/Willams & Wilkins

Harada Y, et al. (1999). WT1 gene expression in human testicular germ-cell tumors. *Mol Urol*, 3:357–63

Haupert GT (1989). Sodium pump regulation by endogenous inhibition. *Top Membr Transport*, 34:345

Hermo L, et al. (1997). Beta-hexosaminidase immunolocalization and alpha- and beta-subunit gene expression in the rat testis and epididymis. *Mol Reprod Dev*, 46:227–42

Hernandez O, et al. (1977). The human spermatozoa genome analysis by DNA reassociation kinetics. *Biochim Biophys Acta*, 521:557–65

Herr JC, et al. (1990). Biochemical and morphological characterization of the intra-acrosomal antigen SP-10 from human sperm. *Biol Reprod*, 42:181–93

Hess RA, et al. (2002). The role of estrogens in the endocrine and paracrine regulation of the efferent ductules, epididymis and vas deferens. *Arch Androl*, 48:32–41

Hibi H, et al. (2002). Treatment of oligoasthenozoospermia with tranilast, a mast cell blocker: the results of long-term administration. *Arch Androl*, 48:451–60

Hidiroglou M, Knipfel JE (1984). Zinc in mammalian sperm: a review. *J Dairy Sci*, 67:1147–56

Hill JA (1991). Implications of cytokines in male and female sterility. *Cellular and Molecular Biology of the Materno-Fetal Relationship*, New York: Marcel Dekker, 212:123–9

Hill JA. (1989). The effects of lymphokines and monokines on human sperm fertilizing ability in the zona-free hamster egg penetration test. *Am J Obstet Gynecol*, 160:1154–9

Hinton BT, et al. (1998). Testicular regulation of epididymal gene expression. *J Reprod Fertil Suppl*, 53:47–57

Hjort T, Hansen KB (1971). Immunofluorescent studies on human spermatozoa. *Clin Exp Immunol*, 8:9

Hogan B, et al. (1994). *Manipulating the Mouse Embryo: a Laboratory Manual*. Maine: Cold Spring Harbor Laboratory

Horan MA (2000). Immune system, aging. In *Encyclopedia of Stress*. New York: Academic Press

Horan MA, Little RA (1998). *Injury in the Aging*. Cambridge: Cambridge University Press

Horan MA, et al. (2000). Biology of aging and stress. In *Encyclopedia of Stress*. New York: Academic Press

Houdebine LM (1997). *Transgenic Animals: Generation and Use*. Amsterdam: Harwood Academic Publishers

Howard GC, Bethell DR, eds. (2001). *Basic Methods in Antibody Production and Characterization*. New York: Marcel Dekker

Hu Y, et al. (1999). Clinical application of intracytoplasmic sperm injection using *in vitro* cultured testicular spermatozoa obtained the day before egg retrieval. *Fertil Steril*, 72:666–9

Hughes CM, et al. (1996). A comparison of baseline and induced DNA damage in human spermatozoa from fertile men, using a modified comet assay. *Mol Hum Reprod*, 2:613–19

Huleihel M, et al. (1999). Expression of IL-12, IL-10, PGE2, sIL-2R, sIL-6R in seminal plasma of fertile and infertile men. *Andrologia*, 31:283–8

Huleihel M, et al. (2000). Production of interleukin-1-like molecules by human sperm cells. *Fertil Steril*, 73:1132–7

Hulka, Davis (1973). Sterilization in men. In Hafez, Evens, eds. *Human Reproduction*. Hagerstown, MD: Harper and Row

Hunnicutt GR, et al. (1997). Analysis of the process of localization of fertilin to the sperm posterior head plasma membrane domain during sperm maturation in the epididymis. *Dev Biol*, 191:146–59

Husted S (1975). Sperm antibodies in men from infertile couples. *Int J Fertil*, 20:113

Husted S, Hjort T (1975). Microtechnique for simultaneous determination of immobilizing and cytotoxic sperm antibodies. *Clin Exp Immunol*, 22:256

Huston JM (1986). Testicular feminization. A model for testicular descent in mice and men. *J Pediatr Surg*, 21:195–8

Hurt RJ, et al. (1985). The use of vital dyes to assess embryonic viability in the hamster *Mesocricetus auratus*. *Stain Technol*, 60:163–7

Hayat MA (1995). *Immunogold–Silver Staining: Principles, Methods and Applications*. New York: CRC Press

I

Ibahim ME, et al. (1988). Sperm chromatin heterogeneity as an infertility factor. *Arch Androl*, 21:129–33

Ichiyanagi O, et al. (2003). Successful treatment of retrograde ejaculation with amezinium. *Arch Androl*, 49:215–218

Iglesias J, et al. (1999). Albumin is a major serum survival factor for renal tubular cells and macrophages through scavenging of ROS. *Am J Physiol*, 277:F711–22

Iida H, et al. (1999). Identification of Rab3A GTPase as an acrosome-associated small GTP-binding protein in rat sperm. *Dev Biol*, 211:144–55

Illingworth PJ, et al. (1996) Inhibin-B: a likely candidate for the physiologically important form of inhibin in men. *J Clin Endocrinol Metab*, 81:1321–5

Ing NH, et al. (1992). Members of the steroid hormone receptor super family interact with TFIIB (S300-II). *J Biol Chem*, 267:17617–23

Ing NH, et al. (1996). Estrogen enhances endometrial estrogen receptor gene expression by a posttranscriptional mechanism in the ovariectomized ewe. *Biol Reprod*, 54:591–9

Inkster S, et al. (1995). Human testicular aromatase: immunocytochemical and biochemical studies. *J Clin Endocrinol Metab*, 80:1941–7

Irwin MH, et al. (2001). Construction of a mutated mtDNA genome and transfection into isolated mitochondria by electroporation. *Adv Reprod*, 5:57–61

Ishihara K, et al. (2002). *Biocompatible Phospholipid Polymers for Prevention of Unfavorable Bioreactions on the Surface of Medical Devices*. New York: Marcel Dekker

Ishii T, et al. (2001). Micropenis and the AR gene: mutation and CAG repeat-length analysis. *J Clin Endocrinol Metab*, 86:5372–8

Isojima S, et al. (1968). Problem of ABO blood group incompatibility and sterility: the effect of blood group antibody on spermatozoa. *Am J Obstet Gynecol*, 102:304–6

Itoh K, et al. (2003). Results and complications of laparoscopic palomo varicocelectomy. *Arch Androl*, 49: in press

Iwasaki A, Cagnon C (1992). Formation of reactive oxygen species in spermatozoa of infertile patients. *Fertil Steril* 57:409–16

J

Jackson JA, et al. (1989). Prostatic complications of testosterone replacement therapy. *Arch Intern Med*, 149:2365–6

James PS, et al. (1999). Lipid diffusion in the plasma membrane of ram and boar spermatozoa during maturation in the epididymis measured by fluorescence recovery after photobleaching. *Mol Reprod Dev*, 52:207–15

Jarow JP, et al. (1999). Clinical efficacy of slidenafil citrate based on etiology and response to prior treatment. *J Urol*, 162:722–5

Jaya P, Kurup PA (1986). Effect of magnesium deficiency on the metabolism of glycosaminoglycans in rats. *J Biosci*, 10:487

Johnson L, et al. (1978). Scanning electrons and light microscopy of the equine seminiferous tubule. *Fertil Steril*, 29:208–15

Jeyendran R (2003). *Sperm Collection and Processing Methods. A Practical Guide*. New York: Cambridge University Press

Jones KH, Senft JA (1985). An improved method to determine cell viability by simultaneous staining with fluorescein diacetate–propidium iodide. *J Histochem Cytochem*, 33:77–9

Jones R (1998). Plasma membrane structure and remodeling during sperm maturation in the epididymis. *J Reprod Fertil*, 53:73–84

Jones R (2002). *Plasma Membrane Composition and Organisation During Maturation of Spermatozoa in the Epididymis*. New York: Marcel Dekker

Jones R, et al. (1980). Hormonal regulation of protein synthesis in the rat epididymis. *Biochem J*, 188:667–76

Jönsson et al. (1988). *Surfactants and Polymers in Aqueous Solution*. New York: Wiley

Junginger (1994). In Kreuter J, ed. *Colloidal Drug Delivery Systems*. Series volume 66. New York: Marcel Decker

Johns Hopkins University (1992). *Vasectomy: New Opportunities*. Baltimore, MD: Johns Hopkins University School of Medicine and Public Health

K

Kass EJ, Marcol B (1992). Results of varicocele surgery in adolescents. A comparison of techniques. *J Urol*, 148:694–6

Katsoff D, et al. (2000). Evidence that sperm with low hypoosmotic swelling scores cause embryo implantation defects. *Arch Androl*, 44:227–30

Katten S (1998). Incidence and pattern of varicocele recurrence after laparoscopic ligation of the internal spermatic vein with preservation of the testicular artery. *Scand J Urol Nephrol*, 32:335–40

Kelly RW, Critchely HOD (1997). Immunomodulation by human seminal plasma: a benefit for spermatozoon and pathogen. *Hum Reprod*, 12:2200–7

Keyhani E, Storey BT (1973). Energy conservation capacity and morphological integrity of mitochondria in hypotonically treated rabbit epididymal spermatozoa. *Biochim Biophys Acta*, 305:557–69

Khudyakov YE, Fields HA, eds. (2002). *Artificial DNA: Methods/ Applications*. New York: CRC Press

Kibrich S, et al. (1952). Methods for detection of antibodies against mammalian spermatozoa. II A gelatin agglutination test. *Fertil Steril*, 3:430–8

Klocker H, et al. (1992). Point mutation in the DNA binding domain of the androgen receptor in two families with Reifenstein syndrome. *Am J Hum Genet*, 50:1318–27

Knoke I, et al. (1999). A new point mutation of the androgen receptor gene in a patient with partial androgen resistance and severe oligozoospermia. *Androlgia*, 31:199–201

Koehler JK, et al. (1982). Spermaphagy. In Hafez ESE, Kenemans P, eds. *Atlas of Human Reproduction–Scanning Electron Microscopy*. Lancaster, UK: MTP Press

Koh EJ, et al. (2001). Adrenal steroids in human prostatic cancer cell lines. *Arch Androl*, 46:117–25

Kohler G, Milstein C (1976). Derivation of specific antibody-producing tissue culture and tumor lines by cell fusion. *Eur J Immunol*, 6:511–19

Kolk AHJ, et al. (1974). Autoantigens of human spermatozoa. Solubilization of a new auto-antigen detected on swollen sperm heads. *Clin Exp Immunol*, 16:63

Kramer JA, Krawetz SA (1996). Nuclear matrix interactions within the sperm genome. *J Biol Chem*, 271:11619–22

Kremer J (1995). A simple sperm penetration test. *Int J Fertil*, 10:209

Kremer J, Jager S (1976). The sperm–cervical mucus contact test. A preliminary report. *Fertil Steril*, 27:335

Kunert R, Katinger H (2002). Production of immunoglobulins and monoclonal antibodies targeting infectious diseases. In Jacobson JM, ed. *Immunotherapy for infectious Diseases*. Totowa, NJ: Humana Press

Kurup RK, Kurup PA (2003). Isoprenoid pathway dysfunction in human male infertility. *Arch Androl*, 49:117–27

L

Labrie F, et al. (1993). Intracrinology: the basis for the rational design of endocrine therapy at all stages of prostate cancer. *Eur Urol*, 24(Suppl 2):94–105

Labrie F, et al. (1998). DHEA and the intracrine formation of androgens and estrogens in peripheral target tissues: its role during aging. *Steroids*, 63:322–8

Lan ZJ, et al. (1998). Regulation of gamma-glutamyl transpeptidase catalytic activity and protein level in the initial segment of the rat epididymis by testicular factors: role of the basic fibroblast growth factor. *Biol Reprod*, 58:197–206

Lancaster MV, Fields RD (1996). Antibiotic and cytotoxic drug susceptibility assays using resazurin and poisoning agents. U.S. Patent No. 5,501,959

La Spada AR, et al. (1991). Androgen receptor gene mutations in X–linked spinal and bulbar muscular atrophy. *Nature*, 352: 77–9

Law WT, et al., eds. (2002). *Biomedical Diagnostic Science and Technology*. New York: Marcel Dekker

Lee JD, et al. (1996). Analysis of chromosome constitution of human spermatozoa with normal and aberrant head morphologies after injection into mouse oocytes. *Hum Reprod*, 11:1942–6

Lee PA, et al. (1980). Micropenis. I. Criteria, etiologies and classification. *Johns Hopkins Med J*, 146:156–63

Lejeune H, et al. (1996). Regulation paracrine et autocrine des fonctions testiculaires. In *Endocrinologie sexuelle de l'homme*, 77–103

Leung PC, Steele GL (1992). Intracellular signaling in the gonads. *Endocr Rev*, 13:476–98

Levin HS (1979). Testicular biopsy in the study of male infertility: its current usefulness, histologic techniques and prospects for the future. *Hum Pathol*, 10:569–84

Levy JB, Husmann DA (1995). The hormonal control of testicular descent. *J Androl*, 16:459–63

Leyton L, Saling P (1989). Evidence that aggregation of the mouse sperm receptor triggers the acrosome reaction. *J Cell Biol*, 108:2163–8

Lim HN, et al. (2000). Longer polyglutamine tracts in the androgen receptor are associated with moderate to severe undermasculinized genitalia in XY males. *Hum Mol Genet*, 9:829–34

Lin CY, et al. (2002). Intrascrotal hemangioma. *Arch Androl*, 48:259–65

Lin TP (1966). Microinjection of mouse eggs. *Science*, 151: 333–7

Lin T, et al. (1998). Interleukin-1 inhibits Leydig cells steroidogenesis without affecting steroidogenic acute regulatory protein messenger ribonucleic acid or protein levels. *J Endocrinol*, 156:461–7

Lindman B, et al. (1999). In Kumar P, Mittal K, et al., eds. *Handbook of Microemulsion Science and Technology*. New York: Marcel Dekker

Lithgow GJ (1996). Invertebrate gerontology: the age mutations of *Caenorhabditis elegans*. *Bioessays*, 18:809–15

Liu HW, et al. (2000). GP-83 and GP-39, two glycoproteins secreted by human epididymis are conjugated to spermatozoa during maturation. *Mol Hum Reprod*, 6:422–8

Liu J, et al. (1997). High fertilization rate obtained after intracytoplasmic sperm injection with 100% nonmotile spermatozoa selected by using a simple modified hypo-osmotic swelling test. *Fertil Steril*, 68:373–5

Liu M-Y, et al. (2003). Inhibitory mechanisms of lead on steroidogenesis in MA-10 mouse Leydig tumor cells. *Arch Androl*, 49:29–38

Lovell-Badger R, Hacker A (1995). The molecular genetics of SRY and its role in mammalian sex determination. *Phil Trans R Soc Lond B*, 350:205–14

Lowenstein JM (1969). *Methods in Enzymology*. New York: Academic Press

Lowry LJ, et al. (1999). Evaluation of semen and sperm chromosome aneuploidy rates in couples with unexplained recurrent pregnancy loss, Abstract number O-133. *Abstracts of the Conjoint Annual Meeting of the American Society for Reproductive Medicine and Canadian Fertility and Andrology Society*, S53

Lubahn DB, et al. (1988). Cloning of human androgen receptor complementary DNA and localization to the X chromosome. *Science*, 40:327–30

Lunenfeld B, ed. (2001). *GnRH Analogues, The State of the Art 2001*. London: Parthenon Publishing

Lunenfeld B, Gooren L, eds (2002). Aging men – challenges ahead. In *Textbook of Men's Health*. London: Parthenon Publishing

Lyon RP, et al. (1982). Varicocele in childhood and adolescence: implication in adulthood infertility? *Urology*, 19:641–4

M

Maeda K, et al. (1997). Possible different mechanism between amyloid-B and substance vP induced chemotaxis of murine microglia. *Gerontology*, 43(Suppl 1):11–15

Maehly AC, Chance B (1954). The assay of catalase and peroxidase. *Methods Biochem Anal*, 2:357

Majorino M, et al. (1998). Testosterone mediates expression of the selenoprotein PHGPx by induction of spermatogenesis and not by direct transcriptional gene activation. *FASEB J*, 12:1359–70

Malmsten M (2002). *Surfactants and Polymers in Drug Delivery*. New York: Marcel Dekker

Manjunath P, et al. (2002). Seminal plasma phospholipid-binding proteins in farm animals. *Adv Reprod*, 6, abstr 72

Marcelli M, et al. (1991). Androgen resistance associated with a mutation of the androgen receptor at amino acid 772 (Arg-Cys) results from a combination of decreased messenger ribonucleic acid levels and impairment of receptor function. *J Clin Endocrinol Metab*, 73:318–25

Marie E, et al. (2001). Increased testicular steroid concentrations in patients with idiopathic infertility and normal FSH levels. *Arch Androl*, 47:177–84

Markova MD (2001). Electron microscopic observations of mouse sperm whole mounts after extraction for nuclear matrix and intermediate filaments. *Arch Androl*, 47:37–46

Marks S (1999). *Prostate Cancer. A Family Guide to Diagnosis, Treatment and Survival*, Revised edition. Tucson, AZ: Fisher Books

Martikainen H, et al. (1982). Rapid and slow response of human testicular steroidogenesis to hCG by measurements of steroids in spermatic and peripheral vein blood. *J Steroid Biochem*, 16:287–91

Martinez O, Goud B (1998). Rab proteins. *Biochim Biophys Acta*, 1404:101–12

Mason J (1995). Psychological influences on the pituitary–adrenal cortical system. *Recent Prog Horm Res*, 345–89

Mathews C, et al. (1992). Motility and fertilizing capacity of epididymal spermatozoa in normal and pathological cases. *Fertil Steril*, 57:871–6

Matsuda T (2000). Diagnosis and treatment of post-herniorraphy vas deferens obstruction. *Int J Urol*, 7:S35–8

Matsuda T, et al. (1992). Laparoscopic varicocelectomy. A simple technique for clip ligation of the spermatic vessels. *J Urol*, 147:636–8

Matsuda T, et al. (1998). Seminal tract obstruction caused by childhood inguinal herniorrhaphy: results of microsurgical reanastomosis. *J Urol*, 159:837–40

Matsui Y, et al. (1992) Derivation of pluripotential embryonic stem cells from murine primordial germ cells in culture. *Cell*, 70: 841–7

Matthews GJ, et al. (1995). Patency following microsurgical vaso-epididymostomy and vasovasostomy: temporal considerations. *J Urol*, 154:2070–3

Mayorga LS, Bertini F (1985). The origin of some acid hydrolases of the fluid of the cauda epididymis. *J Androl*, 6:243–7

Mbizvo MT, et al. (1990). Human follicular fluid stimulates hyperactivated motility of human sperm. *Fertil Steril*, 54:708–712

McCann SM (2000). Nitric oxide. In *Encyclopedia of Stress*. New York: Academic Press

McCann SM, et al. (1994). Induction by cytokines of the pattern of pituitary hormone secretion in infection. *Neuroimmunomodulation*, 1:2–13

McCann SM, et al. (1998). The nitric oxide hypothesis of aging. *Exp Gerontol*, 33:813–26

McEwen BS (2000). Definitions and concepts of stress. In *Encyclopedia of Stress*. New York: Academic Press

McGrady AV (1984). Effects of psychological stress on male reproduction. *Arch Androl*, 13:1–7

McKenzie SJ, Halsey JF (1984). Cholera toxin B subunit as a carrier protein to stimulate a mucosal immune response. *J Immunol*, 133:1818–24

McLachlan RI, et al. (1995). Hormonal control of spermatogeneis. *Trans Electr Micros*, 6:95–101

McLare (1980). In Hafez ESE, ed. *Reproduction in Farm Animals*, 4th edn. Philadelphia: Lea & Febiger, p. 229

McLaren A (1970). In *Ciba Foundation Symposium on the Family and its Future*. London: Churchill

McLaren A (1980). Ferilization, cleavage and implantation. In Hafez ESE, ed. *Reproduction in Farm Animals*, 4th edn. Philadelphia: Lea & Febiger

McMahon CG, et al. (2000). Efficacy, safety and patient acceptance of sildenafil citrate as treatment for erectile dysfunction. *J Urol*, 164:1192–6

Mendis-Handagama C, Ariyaratne S (2001). Differentiation of the adult Leydig cell population in the postnatal testis. *Biol Reprod*, 65:660–71

Michaut M, et al. (2000). Calcium-triggered acrosomal exocytosis in human spermatozoa requires the coordinated activation of Rab3A and N-ethylmaleimide-sensitive factor. *Proc Natl Acad Sci USA*, 97:9996–10001

Monastersky GM, Robl JM (1995). *Strategies in Transgenic Animal Science*. American Society for Microbiology Press.

Moncada S, et al. (1991). Nitric oxide: physiology, pathophysiology, and pharmacology. *Pharmacol Rev*, 43:109–42

Monga M, Rajasekaran M (2003). Erectile dysfunction, current concepts and future directions. *Arch Androl*, 49:7–18

Monga M, et al. (2002). Patient satisfaction with testosterone supplementation for the treatment of erectile dysfunction. *Arch Androl*, 48: 433–442

Monia BP, et al. (1990). Ubiquitination enzymes. *Biotechnology* 8:209

Montiel EE, et al. (2003). Glutathione related enzymes in cell cultures from different regions of human epididymis. *Arch Androl*, 49:95–105

Morishima A, et al. (1995). Aromatase deficiency in male and female siblings caused by a normal mutation and the physiological role of estrogens. *J Clin Endocrinol Metab*, 80: 3689–98

Morley JE (1986). Impotence. *Am J Med*, 80:897–905

Morley JE (2000). Nutrition. In Fink G, ed. *Encyclopedia of Stress*. New York: Academic Press

Morley JE (2001). Testosterone, depression and cognitive function. In *Textbook of Men's Health*. New York: Parthenon Publishing, 401–407

Moschos S, et al. (2002). Leptin and reproduction: a review. In *Encyclopedia of Stress*. New York: Academic Press

Muroya K, et al. (2001). Hypospadias and the androgen receptor gene: mutation screening and CAG repeat length analysis. *Mol Hum Reprod*, 7:409–13

Musa FR, et al. (2000). Effects of luteinizing hormone, follicle-stimulating hormone, and epidermal growth factor on expression and kinase activity of cyclin-dependent kinase 5 in Leydig TM3 and Sertoli TM4 cell lines. *J Androl*, 21:392–402

Mutlu S, et al. (2002). *Glow-Discharge-Treated Quartz Crystal Microbalance as Immunosensor*. New York: Marcel Dekker

N

Nadel B, et al. (1995). Cell-specific organization of the 5s ribosomal RNA gene cluster DNA loop domains in spermatozoa and somatic cells. *Biol Reprod*, 53:1222–8

Nagy L, Freeman DA (1990). Effect of cholesterol transport inhibitors on steroidogenesis and plasma membrane cholesterol transport in cultured MA-10 Leydig tumor cells. *Endocrinology*, 126:2267–76

Nakhla AM, et al. (1999). Sex hormone-binding globulin receptor signal transduction proceeds via a G protein. *Steroids*, 64:213–16

Naz RK (2000). Fertilization-related sperm antigens and their immunocontraceptive potentials. *Am J Reprod Immunol*, 44:41–6

Naz RK, Chauhan SC (2001). Presence of antibodies to sperm YLP_{12} synthetic peptide in sera and seminal plasma of immunoinfertile men. *Mol Hum Reprod*, 7:21–6

Naz RK, Evans L (1998). Presence and modulation of Interleukin-12 in seminal plasma of infertile and fertile men. *J Androl*, 19:302–7

Naz RK, Packianathan JLR (2000). Antibodies to human sperm YLP_{12} peptide that is involved in egg binding inhibit human sperm capacitation/acrosome reaction. *Arch Androl*, 45:227–32

Naz RK, et al. (1984). Monoclonal antibody to a human germ cell membrane glycoprotein that inhibits fertilization. *Science*, 225:342–4

Naz RK, et al. (1995). Levels of interferon-gamma and tumor necrosis factor-alpha in sera and cervical mucus of fertile and infertile women: implication of infertility. *J Reprod Immunol*, 29:105–17

Naz RK, et al. (2002). Monoclonal antibody against human sperm-specific YLP_{12} peptide sequence involved in oocyte binding. *Arch Androl*, 48:169–75

Netter FH (1992). The Ciba Collection of Medical Illustrations. Volume 2: Reproductive system. © Icon Learning Systems, LLC

Nicola NA (1994). An introduction to the cytokines. In *Guidebook to Cytokines and their Receptors*. Oxford: Oxford University Press, 1–7

Niederberger C, Ross LS (1993). Microsurgical epididymovasostomy: predictors of success. *J Urol*, 149:1364–7

Nieman DC, Pedersen BK, eds. (2000). *Nutrition and Exercise Immunology*. New York: CRC Press

Nishimura K, et al. (2001). Association of selenoprotein P with testosterone production in cultured Leydig cells. *Arch Androl* 47:85–94

Noboris T, et al. (1997). Nitric oxide production by cultured rat Leydig cells. *Endocrinology*, 138:994–8

Nussbaum RL, et al. (2002). *Thompson and Thompson Genetics in Medicine*, 6th edn. Philadelphia, PA: WB Saunders

O

Obinata M (1997). Conditionally immortalized cell lines with differentiated functions established from temperature-sensitive T-antigen transgenic mice. *Genes Cells*, 2:235–44

O'Brien DA, et al. (1991). Mannose 6-phosphate receptors: potential mediators of germ cell-Sertoli cell interactions. *Ann NY Acad Sci*, 637:327–39

Odeblad E. (1969). Cervical mucus characteristics based on nuclear magnetic resonance (NMR). *Acta Eur Fertil*, 1:99

Odgen PR, et al. (1996). Phylogenetic occurrence of coiled coil proteins: implications for tissue structure in Metazoa via a coiled coil tissue matrix. *Prot Struct Funct Genet*, 24:467–84

O'Donnell L, et al. (2001). Estrogen and spermatogenesis. *Endocr Rev*, 22:289–313

O'Hern PA, et al. (1995). Reversible contraception in female baboons immunized with a synthetic epitope of sperm specific lactate dehydrogenase. *Biol Reprod*, 52:331–9

Ohninger SC, et al. (1991). Recurrent failure of *in vitro* fertilization: role of the hemizona assay in the sequential diagnosis of specific sperm–oocyte defects. *Am J Obstet Gynecol*, 164:1210–15

Ohta S, et al. (2002a). Establishment of a Leydig cell line, TTE1, from transgenic mice harboring temperature-sensitive simian virus 40 large T-antigen gene. *Arch Androl*, 48:43–51

Ohta S, et al. (2002b). DNA microarray analysis of genes involved in the process of differentiation in mouse Leydig cell line TTE1. *Arch Androl*, 48:203–8

Olanow WC, Arendash GW (1994). Metals and free radicals in neurodegenerative disorders. *Curr Opin Neurol*, 7:548

Olson GE, et al. (2003). Structural differentiation of spermatozoa during post-testicular maturation. *Arch Androl*, 49: in press

Orlowsky M, Meister A (1963). Gamma-glutamyl-*p*-nitoanilide: a new convenient substrate for determination of L- and D-gamma-glutamyl transpeptidase activities. *Biochim Biophys Acta*, 73:679–81

Orne MT, Whitehouse WG (2000). Relaxation techniques. In *Encyclopedia of Stress*. New York: Academic Press

O'Rourke L, et al. (1997). Co-receptors of B-lymphocytes. *Curr Opin Immunol*, 9:324–9

Oster J (1971). Varicocele in children and adolescents. An investigation of the incidence among Danish children. *Scand J Urol Nephrol*, 5:27–32

Osuna CJ, et al. (2001). GnRH and hCG tests in healthy adolescents and adults. *Arch Androl*, 47:9–14

Ozbek E, et al. (2001). Depressed total antioxidant enzyme activity in the seminal plasma of patients with varicocele. *Adv Reprod*, 5:17–24

P

Paduch DA, Neidzielski J (1997). Repair versus observation in adolescent varicocele: a prospective study. *J Urol*, 158:1128–32

Paglia DE, Valentine WN (1967). Studies on quantitative and qualitative characterization of erythrocyte glutathione peroxidase. *J Lab Clin Med*, 70:158

Palermo GD, et al. (1996). Intracytoplasmic sperm injection: a powerful tool to overcome fertilization failure. *Fertil Steril*, 65:899–908

Palladino MA, Hinton BT (1994). Expression of multiple gamma-glutamyl transpeptidase messenger ribonucleic acid transcripts in the adult rat epididymis is differentially regulated by androgens and testicular factors in a region-specific manner. *Endrocrinology*, 135:146–56

Palmer DN, et al. (1984). Separation of some neutral lipids by normal phase high performance liquid chromatography on cyanopropyl column. *Anal Chem*, 140:315–19

Palmiter RD, et al. (1982). Dramatic growth of mice that develop from eggs microinjected with metallothionein-growth hormone fusion genes. *Nature*, 300:611–15

Palomo A (1949). Radical cure of varicocele by new technique. Preliminary report. *J Urol*, 61:604–6

Paoletti LC, McInnes PM, eds. (1998). *Vaccines from Concept to Clinic: a Guide to the Development and Clinical Testing of Vaccines for Human Use*. New York: CRC Press

Papanicolaou DA (1997). Cytokines and adrenal insufficiency. *Curr Opin Endocrinol Diabetes*, 4:194–8

Papanicolaou A, et al. (2001). Can maturation arrest occur at the stage of spermiogenesis? *Arch Androl*, 46:105–7

Parkin DM, et al. (1993). Estimates of the world-wide incidence of eighteen major cancers in 1985. *Int J Cancer*, 54:594–606

Parnet P, et al. (1990). Estrous cycle variations in gonadotropin-releasing hormone, substance P and β-endorphin contents in median eminence, the arcuate nucleus and the median pre-optic nucleus in the rat; a detailed analysis of proestrus changes. *J Neuroendocrinol*, 2:291–6

Parrish JJ, et al. (1993). Increases in bovine sperm intracellular calcium (Ca_i) and pH (pH_i) during capacitation. *Biol Reprod*, 48(Suppl 1): 192 (abstract)

Parvinen M, Soderstrom KL (1977). Microanalytical techniques of living testis cells. In Hafez ESE, ed. *Techniques of Human Andrology*. Amsterdam: Elsevier/North Holland Biomedical Press

Patrizio P, Amin A-H (2003). Infertility, ICSI, and the epididymis. *Arch Androl*, 49: in press

Pavlovich CP, Schlegel PN (1997). Fertility options after vasectomy – a cost-effectiveness analysis. *Fertil Steril*, 67:133–41

Penninx BWJH, Deeg DJH (2000). Aging and psychological stress. In *Encyclopedia of Stress*. New York: Academic Press

Penson DF, et al. (1996). Androgen and pituitary control of penile nitric oxide synthase and erectile function in the rat. *Biol Reprod*, 55:567–74

Pentikainen V, et al. (2000). Estradiol acts as germ cell survival factor in human testis *in vitro*. *J Clin Endocrinol Metab*, 85: 2057–67

Perey B, et al. (1961). The wave of the seminiferous epithelium in the rat. *Am J Anat*, 108:47–77

Peters KE, Comings DE (1980). Two-dimensional gel electrophoresis of rat liver nuclear washes, nuclear matrix and hnRNA proteins. *J Cell Biol*, 86:135–55

Pfeffer SR (1988). Mannose-6-phosphate receptors and their role in targeting proteins to lysosomes. *Membrane Biol*, 103: 7–16

Pfeffer SR (1999). Transport-vesicle targeting: tethers before SNAREs. *Nature Cell Biol*, 1:E17–22

Picket CB, Lu AY (1989). Glutathione S-transferases: gene structure, regulation and biological function. *Ann Rev Biochem*, 58:743–64

Pinkert CA (1994a). *Transgenic Animal Technology. A Laboratory Handbook*. New York: Academic Press

Pinkert CA (1994b). Transgenic swine models for xenotransplantation. *Xeno*, 2:10–15

Pinkert CA (1997). The history and theory of transgenic animals. *Lab Anim*, 26:29–34

Pinkert CA (2000). Genetic engineering of farm mammals. In Hafez B, Hafez ESE, eds. *Reproduction in Farm Animals*, 7th edn. Philadelphia: Lippincott Williams and Wilkins

Pinkert CA, Murray JD (1998). Transgenic farm animals. In *Transgenic Animals in Agriculture*. Wallingford, UK: CAB International

Pinkert CA, et al. (1997). Transgenic animal modeling. In *Encyclopedia of Molecular Biology and Molecular Medicine*. New York: VCH, 6:63–74

Politch JA, et al. (1993). Comparison of methods to enumerate white blood cells in semen. *Fertil Steril*, 60:372–5

Posinocec J (1976). The necessity for bilateral biopsy in oligo and azoospermia. *Intern J Fertil*, 21:189

Potts RJ, et al. (1999). Antioxidant capacity of the epididymis. *Hum Reprod*, 14:2513–16

Prasad S, et al. (1998). Expression of cytokine-19 as a marker of neoplastic progression of human prostate epithelial cells. *Prostate*, 35:203–11

Primakoff P, et al. (1997). Reversible contraceptive effect of PH-20 immunization in male guinea pigs. *Biol Reprod*, 56:1142–6

Purvis K, Christinsen E (1996). The impact of infection on sperm quality. *Hum Reprod*, 11:31–41

Q

Qungley CA, et al. (1995). Androgen receptor defects: historical, clinical and molecular perspectives. *Endocr Rev*, 16:271–321

R

Rajasekaran M, et al. (1995). Oxidative stress and interleukins in seminal plasma during leukocytospermia. *Fertil Steril*, 64:166–71

Ramalho-Santos J, Schatten G (2003). Presence of N-ethyl maleimide sensitive factor (NSF) on the acrosome of mammalian sperm. *Arch Androl*, 49: in press

Ramauge M, et al. (1996). Evidence that type III iodothyronine deiodinase in rat astrocyte is a selenoprotein. *Endocrinology*, 137:3021–5

Rao CV (2002). *An Introduction to Immunology*. New York: CRC Press

Ratcliffe SG, Paul N, eds. *Prospective Studies on Children with Sex Chromosome Aneuploidy*. March of Dimes Birth Defects Foundation, Birth Defects Original Article Series 22(3). New York: Alan R. Liss, 1986

Ravikumar KA, et al. (2001): ^{14}C-acetate incorporation into digoxin in rat brain and effect of digoxin administration. *Ind J Exp Biol*, 3:420–6

Rawe YV, et al. (2001). Incidence of tail structure distortions associated with dysplasia of the fibrous sheat in human spermatozoa. *Hum Reprod*, 16:879–86

Razandi M, et al. (1999). Cell membrane and nuclear estrogen receptors (Ers) originate from a single transcript: studies of $Er\alpha$ and $Er\beta$ expressed in Chinese hamster ovary cells. *Mol Endocrinol*, 13:307–19

Rexroad CE Jr, Hawk HW (1994). Production of transgenic ruminants. In *Transgenic Animal Technology: A Laboratory Handbook*. New York: Academic Press, 339–55

Reyes R (1989). Heparin and glutathione physiological decondensing agents of human sperm nuclei. *Gamete Res*, 23:39–47

Reyes A, et al. (1978). Calcium ion requirement for rabbit spermatozoa capacitation and enhancement of fertilizing ability by ionophore A23187 and cyclic adenosine 3'5' monophosphate. *Fertil Steril*, 29:451–5

Reyes R, et al. (2002). Heparin–glutathione III. Study with fluorescent probes as indicators of membrane status of bull sperm. *Arch Androl*, 48:209–19

Rhodes ME (2000). Adrenocorticotropic hormone (ACTH). In *Encyclopedia of Stress*. New York: Academic Press

Rimini R, et al. (1995). Interaction of normal and mutant SRY proteins with DNA. *Phil Trans R Soc Lond B*, 350:215–20

River C (1998). Role of NO and carbon monoxide in modulating the ACTH response to immune and nonimmune signals. *Neuroimmunomodulation*, 5:203–13

Robaire B. (2002) Aging of the epididymis: In Robaire B, Hinton BT, eds. *The Epididymis From Molecules to Clinical Practice. A Comprehensive Survey of the Efferent Ducts, the Epididymis and the Vas Deferens*. New York: Kluwer Academic/Plenum Publishers

Roberts JL (2001). Geriatric hair and scalp disorders. In Norman RA, ed. *Geriatric Dermatology*. London, UK: Parthenon Publishing, 35–64

Roberts JT, Essenhigh DM (1986). Adenocarcinoma of prostate in 40-year-old body-builder. *Lancet*, 2:742

Rosnina Y, et al. (2000). Genetics of reproductive failure. In Hafez B, Hafez ESE, eds. *Reproduction of Farm Animals*, 7th edn. Philadelphia: Lippincott Williams & Wilkins

Roth JC, et al. (1972). FSH and LH response to luteinizing hormone-releasing factor in prepubertal and pubertal children, adult males and patients with hypogonadotropic and hypergonadotropic hypogonadism. *J Clin Endocrinol Metab*, 35:926–30

Rothman JE (1994). Mechanisms of intracellular protein transport. *Nature*, 372:55–63

Rotman B, Papermaster BW (1966). Membrane properties of living mammalian cells as studied by enzymatic hydrolysis of fluorogenic esters. *Proc Natl Acad Sci USA*, 55:134–13

Roveri A, et al. (1992). Phospholipid hydroperoxide glutathione peroxidase of rat testis. *J Biol Chem*, 267:6142–6

Rovert J, et al. Intelligence and achievement in children with extra X aneuploidy: a longitudinal perspective. *Am J Med Genet* 1986; 60: 356–63

Rubio C, et al. (1999). Implications of sperm chromosome abnormalities in recurrent miscarriage. *J Assist Reprod Genet*, 16:253–8

Rubio C, et al. (2001). Incidence of sperm chromosomal abnormalities in a risk population: relationship with sperm quality and ICSI outcome. *Hum Reprod*, 16:2084–92

Rumke P, Hellinga G (1959). Antibodies against spermatozoa in sterile men. *Am J Clin Pathol*, 32:357

Rupprecht R, Holsboer F (1999). Neuroactive steroids: mechanisms of action and neuropsychopharmacological perspectives. *Trends Neurosci*, 22:410–16

S

Sakaki SY, et al. (2002). *Water-Soluble Phospholipid Polymers as a Novel Synthetic Blocking Agent in an Imunoassay System*. New York: Marcel Dekker

Sakin-Kaindl F, et al. (2001). Decreased suppression of antibody-dependent cellular cytotoxicity by seminal plasma in unexplained infertility. *Fertil Steril*, 75:581–7

Salzman C, Leibowitz BD (1991). *Anxiety in the Elderly: Treatment and Research*. New York: Springer-Verlag

Sanchez-Vazquez ML, et al. (1996). Differential decondensation of class I (rat) and class II (mouse) spermatozoa nuclei by physiological concentrations of herapin–glutathione. *Arch Androl*, 36:161–76

Saremi A, et al. (2002). The first successful pregnancy following injection of testicular round spermatid in Iran. *Arch Androl*, 48:315–19

Sasagawa I, Nakada T (2003). Epidemiology of prostatic cancer in East Asia. *Arch Androl*, 49: in press

Sasagawa I, et al. (2000a). CAG repeat length of the androgen receptor gene in Japanese males with cryptorchidism. *Mol Hum Reprod*, 6:973–5

Sasagawa I, et al. (2000b). Laparoscopic varicocelectomy in adolescents using an ultrasonically activated scalpel. *Arch Androl*, 45:91–4

Sasagawa I, et al. (2001). CAG repeat length analysis and mutation screening of the androgen receptor gene in Japanese men with idiopathic azoospermia. *J Androl*, 22:804–8

Sasagawa I, et al. (2002). Androgen receptor gene and male genital anomaly. *Arch Androl*, 48: 467–74

Scanlan JM, et al. (1988). CD4 and CD8 counts are associated with interactions of gender and psychosocial stress. *Psychosom Med*, 60:644–53

Schiavi RC, et al. (1993). Hormones and nocturnal tumesence in healthy aging men. *Arch Sex Behav*, 22:207–15

Schlegel PN (1999). Testicular sperm extraction: microdissection improves sperm yield with minimal tissue excision. *Hum Reprod*, 14:131–5

Schlegel PN, Su LM (1997). Physiological consequences of testicular sperm extraction. *Hum Reprod*, 12:1688–92

Schneyer AL, et al. (1991). Precursors of a-inhibin modulate follicle-stimulating hormone receptor binding and biological activity. *Endocrinology*, 129:1987–99

Seeman MV (2000). Sex steroids, response to stress/susceptibility to depression. In *Encyclopedia of Stress*. New York: Academic Press

Selva J, et al. (1993). Cytogenetic analysis of human oocytes after subzonal insemination. *Pren Diagn*, 13:311–21

Selye H (1936). A syndrome produced by diverse nocuous agents. *Nature*, 138:32

Selye H (1955). Stress and disease. *Science*, 122:625–31

Serrano H, et al. (2001). Pig sperm membrane integrity evaluated by lectin labeling. *Arch Androl*, 47:59–65

Setchell BP (1977). In Cole HH, Cupps PT, eds. *Reproduction in Domestic Animals*, 3rd edn. New York: Academic Press

Sharlip ID, et al. (2002). Best practice policies for male infertility. *Fertil Steril*, 77:873–82

Sharma RK, Agarwal A (1996). Role of reactive oxygen species in male infertility. *Urology*, 48:835–50

Sharma RK, *et al.* (1999). The reactive oxygen species – total antioxidant capacity score is a new measure of oxidative stress to predict male infertility. *Hum Reprod*, 14:2801–7

Sharpe RM (1994). Regulation of spermatogenesis. In *The Physiology of Reproduction*, 1363–434

Sherwood A, Carels RA (2000). Blood pressure. In *Encyclopedia of Stress*. New York: Academic Press

Shibasaki T, *et al.* (2001). Effect of testosterone replacement therapy on serum prostate specific antigen in patients with Klinefelter's syndrome. *Arch Androl*, 47:173–6

Shiraishi K, *et al.* (2003). Activation of endothelial nitric oxide synthase in the contralateral testis during unilateral testicular torsion in rat. *Arch Androl*, 49:179–90

Shively CA (2000). Reproduction, effects of social stress. In *Encyclopedia of Stress*. New York: Academic Press

Sikka SC, *et al.* (1995). Role of oxidative stress and antioxidants in male infertility. *J Androl*, 16:464–8

Sills ES, *et al.* (2000). Comparison of centrifugation and non-centrifugation based techniques for recovery of motile human sperm. *Arch Androl*, 47:110–20

Sliwa L (1992). Effect of heparin on human spermatozoa migration *in vitro*. *Arch Androl*, 30:199–203

Sliwa L (1993). Heparin as a chemo-attractant for mouse spermatozoa. *Arch Androl*, 31:75–8

Sliwa L (1994). Chemotatic effect of hormones in mouse spermatozoa. *Arch Androl*, 32:83–8

Sliwa L (1995a). Chemotaction of mouse spermatozoa induced by certain hormones. *Arch Androl*, 35:105–10

Sliwa L (1995b). Effect of some sex steroid hormones on human spermatozoa migration *in vitro*. *Eur J Obstet Gynecol Reprod Biol*, 58:173–5

Silwa L (2001). Substance P and β-endorphin act as possible chemoattractants of mouse sperm. *Arch Androl*, 46:135–40

Simmen RC, *et al.* (1984). Estrogen modulation of nuclear matrix-associated steroid hormone binding. *Endocrinology*, 115:1197–202

Simoni M, *et al.* (1997). Screening for deletions of the Y-chromosome involving the DAZ (deleted in azoospermia) gene in azoospermia and severe oligozoospermia. *Fertil Steril*, 67:542–7

Skudlarek MD, Orgebin-Crist MC (1986). Glycosidases in cultured rat epididymal cells: enzyme activity, synthesis and secretion. *Biol Reprod*, 35:167–78

Sofikitis NV, *et al.* (1994). Reproductive capacity of the nucleus of the male gamete after completion of meiosis. *J Assist Reprod Genet*, 11:335–41

Sosa A, *et al.* (1974). Capacidad metabolica de nucleos aislados de espermatozoides humanos. *Gaceta Med Mexico*, 108:385–91

Sosa MA, *et al.* (1991). Binding of β-galactosidase from rat epididymal fluid to the sperm surface by high affinity sites different from phosphomannosyl receptors. *J Reprod Fertil*, 93:279–85

Sprat DI, *et al.* (1985). Pituitary luteinizing hormone responses to intravenous and subcutaneous administration of gonadotropin-releasing hormone in men. *J Clin Endocrinol Metab*, 61:890–5

Stalf T, *et al.* (1995). Pregnancy and birth after intracytoplasmic sperm injection with spermatozoa from a patient with tail stump syndrome. *Hum Reprod*, 10:2112–14

Staney TA, *et al.* (1989). Prostate specific antigen in the diagnosis and treatment of adenocarcinoma of the prostate. II. Radical prostatectomy treated patients. *J Urol*, 141:1076–83

Stavropoulos NE, *et al.* (2002). Varicocele in school boys. *Arch Androl*, 48:187–97

Stearns T, Kirschner M (1994). *In vitro* recondensation of centrosome assembly and function: the central role of gamma tubulin. *Cell*, 76: 623–37

Steiner MS (1993). Role of peptide growth factors in the prostate: a review. *Urology*, 42:99–110

Stillman RJ (1982). *In utero* exposure to diethylstilbestrol: adverse effects on reproductive tract and reproductive performance in male and female offspring. *Am J Obstet Gynecol*, 142:905–41

St John DC, *et al.* (1997). Mitochondrial mutations and male infertility. *Nature Med*, 3:124–5

Stocco DM, Clark BJ (1996). Regulation of the acute production of steroids in steroidogenic cells. *Endocr Rev*, 17:221–44

Stoney CM, *et al.* (1987). Sex differences in physiological responses to stress and in coronary heart disease: a casual link? *Psychophysiology*, 24:127–31

Sutherland RW, *et al.* (1996). Androgen receptor gene mutations are rarely associated with isolated penile hypospadias. *J Urol*, 156:828–31

Suzuki Y, *et al.* (2001). Screening for mutations of the androgen receptor gene in patients with isolated cryptorchidism. *Fertil Steril*, 76:834–6

Suzuki Y, *et al.* (2002). 5α-reductase type 2 genes in Japanese males do not appear to be associated with cryptorchidism. *Fertil Steril*, 78:330–4

Swan SH, *et al.* (2000). The question of declining sperm density revisited: an analysis of 101 studies published 1934–1996. *Environ Health Perspect*, 108:961–6

T

Talbot P, Chacon RS (1980). A new procedure for rapidly scoring acrosome reactions of human sperm. *Gamete Res*, 3:211–16

Talbot P, Chacon RS (1981). A triple-stain technique for evaluating normal acrosomal reactions of human sperm. *J Exp Zool*, 215:201–8

Tamlinson MJ, et al. (1992). Preliminary communication: possible role of reactive nitrogen intermediates in leucocyte-mediated sperm dysfunction. *Am J Reprod Immunol*, 127:89–92

Tan R (1997). Pathological fracture due to testosterone deficiency in an elderly man. Abstract. Presented at the *Annual Scientific Meeting of the American Geriatric Society*, San Francisco

Tan RS, Bransgrove LB (1997). Andropause: is there a role for hormone replacement therapy? *Clin Geriatr*, 5:46–58

Tan RS, Bransgrove L (1998). Testosterone replacement therapy. What is its potential in elderly men? *Postgrad Med*, 103:247–56

Tanji N, et al. (2001). Growth factors: roles in andrology. *Arch Androl*, 47:1–7

Tejada RI, et al. (1984). A test for the practical evaluation of male fertility by acridine orange (AO) fluorescence. *Fertil Steril*, 42:87–91

Tenniswood M (1986). Role of epithelial-stromal interactions in the control of gene expression in the prostate: an hypothesis. *Prostate*, 9:375–85

Tenover JS (1992). Effects of testosterone supplementation in the aging male. *J Clin Endocrinol Metab*, 75:1092–8

Terquem A, Dadoune JP (1983). Aniline blue staining of human sperm chromatin: evaluation of nuclear maturation. *Cell*, 34:249–52

Tomlinson MJ, et al. (1993). Prospective study of leukocytes and leukocyte sub-populations in semen suggests they are not a cause of male infertility. *Fertil Steril*, 60:1069–75

Tomomasa H, et al. (2002). Gonadal function in patients with testicular germ cell tumors. *Arch Androl*, 48:405–16

Tsafriri A, et al. (1983). Control of the development of meiotic competence and of oocyte maturation in mammals. In *Fertilization of the Human Egg In Vitro*. Berlin: Springer-Verlag

Tsujimura A, et al. (2002). Outcome of surgical treatment for obstructive azoospermia. *Arch Androl*, 48:29–36

Tsukada T, et al. (1994). An androgen receptor mutation causing androgen resistance in undervirilized male syndrome. *J Clin Endocrinol Metab*, 79:1202–7

Tung KSK, et al. (1997). Mechanism of infertility in male guinea pigs immunized with sperm PH-20. *Biol Reprod*, 56: 1133–41

Tuohimaa P, et al. (1993). Change in location and processing of inhibin a-subunit precursors during sexual maturation of the Djungarian hamster testis. *Endocrinology*, 132:629–33

Turner TT, et al. (1995). Protein synthesis and secretion by the rat caput epididymis *in vivo*: influence of the luminal environment. *Biol Reprod*, 52:1012–9

Tut TG, et al. (1997). Long polyglutamine tracts in the androgen receptor are associated with reduced transactivation, impaired sperm production, and male infertility. *J Clin Endocrinol Metab*, 82:3777–82

U

Urner F, et al. (1993). Evidence of sperm entry into assumed unfertilized human oocyte after subzonal sperm micro-injection. *Hum Reprod*, 8:2167–73

Ursini F, et al. (1999). Dual function of the selenoprotein PHGPx during sperm maturation. *Science*, 285:1393–6

V

Vale W, Bilezikjian LM, River C (1994). Reproductive and other roles of inhibins and activins. In Knobil E, Neill JD, eds. *Reproductive Physiology*, 2nd edn, vol. 1. New York: Raven Press, p. 34

Van den Berg TL, Hellstrom WJ (1997). Individualizing androgen replacement therapy. *Contemp Urol*, 9:25–40

Van den Ham R, et al. (2002). Identification of candidate genes involved in gonocyte development. *J Androl*, 23:410–18

Van der Kolk BA, et al. (1996). *Traumatic Stress: the Effects of Overwhelming Experience on the Mind, Body and Society*. New York: Guilford Press

Vazama F, et al. (1988). The fine structure of the blood-testis barrier in the boar. *Jap J Vet Sci*, 50:1259

Vermeulen A (1991). Clinical review 24: androgens in the aging male. *J Clin Endocrinol Metab*, 73:221–4

Vermeulen A (1993). The male climacterium. *Ann Med*, 25:531–4

Vermeulen A, et al. (1986). Prognosis of subfertility in men with corrected or uncorrected varicocele. *J Androl*, 7:147–55

Vigier B, et al. (1983). Use of monoclonal antibody techniques to study the ontogeny of bovine anti-Mullerian hormone. *J Reprod Fertil*, 69:207

Vingerhoets AJ, Van Heck GL (1990). Gender coping and psychosomatic symptoms. *Psychol Med*, 20:125–135

W

Wallach DFH, Kamath VB (1966). *Methods in Enzymology*. New York: Academic Press

Walther N, et al. (1996). Sertoli cell lines established from H-2K^b-tsA58 transgenic mice differentially regulate the expression of cell-specific antigen. *Exp Cell Res*, 225:411–21

Wang C, et al. (2000). Transdermal testosterone gel improves sexual function, mood, muscle strength and body composition parameters in hypogonadal men. *J Clin Endocrinol Metab*, 85:2839–53

Ward CR, Kopf GS (1993). Molecular events mediating sperm activation. *Dev Biol*, 158:9–34

Ward CR, et al. (1999). The monomeric GTP binding protein, rab3a, is associated with the acrosome in mouse sperm. *Mol Reprod Dev*, 53:413–21

Weber T, et al. (1998). SNAREpins: minimal machinery for membrane fusion. *Cell*, 92:759–72

Weighardt F, et al. (1996). The roles of heterogeneous nuclear ribonucleoproteins (hnRNP) in RNA metabolism. *Bioassays*, 18:747–56

Weinberger JB, et al. (1995). Nitric oxide inhibition of human sperm motility. *Fertil Steril*, 64:408–13

Weissenberg R, et al. (2001). Procarbazine effects on spermatogenesis in the golden hamster (*Mesocricetus auratus*): a flow cytometric evaluation

Weiss-Messer E, et al. (1996). Prolactin and MA-10 Leydig cell steroidogenesis: biphasic effects of prolactin and signal transduction. *Endocrinology*, 137:5509–18

Well-Malherbe (1971). *Methods of Biochemical Analysis*. New York: Inter Science

Wiener JS, et al. (1998). Androgen receptor gene alternations are not associated with isolated cryptorchidism. *J Urol*, 160:863–5

Willenberg HS, et al. (2000a). Disease, stress-induced, overview. In *Encyclopedia of Stress*. New York: Academic Press

Willenberg HS, et al. (2000b). Adrenal insufficiency. In *Encyclopedia of Stress*. New York: Academic Press

Wilmut I, et al. (1997). Viable offspring derived from fetal and adult mammalian cells. *Nature*, 385:810–13

Wolff H, Anderson DJ (1988). Immunohistologic characterization and quantification of leukocyte subpopulation in human semen. *Fertil Steril*, 49:497–504

Wolff H, et al. (1990). Leukocytospermia is associated with poor semen quality. *Fertil Steril*, 53:528–36

Wong ML, et al. (1996). Inducible nitric oxide synthase gene expression in the brain during systemic inflammation. *Nature Med*, 2:581–4

Wong PWK, et al. (1964). Fluorimetric method for tyrosine. *Clin Chem*, 10:1098–100

Wong TW, et al. (1973). Testicular biopsy in the study of male infertility, I: testicular causes of infertility. *Arch Pathol*, 95:151–9

Wood SA, et al. (1993). Non-injection methods for the production of embryonic stem cell–embryo chimaeras. *Nature*, 365:87–9

World Health Organization (WHO) (1992). *Laboratory Manual for the Examination of Human Semen and Semen Cervical Muscus Interaction*. Cambridge, UK: Cambridge University Press, 6–50

Wu H, et al. (1997). Functional interaction of erythropoietin and stem cell factor receptors is essential for erythroid colony formation. *Proc Natl Acad Sci USA*, 94:1806–10

Wu SH, et al. (1973). Effects of selenium, vitamin E and antioxidants on testicular function in rats. *Biol Reprod*, 8:625–9

Wyllie GG (1985). Varicocele and puberty. The critical factor? *Br J Urol*, 57:194–6

Y

Yamauchi T, et al. (1997). Tyrosine phosphorylation of the EGF receptor by the kinase Jak2 is induced by growth hormone. *Nature*, 390:91–6

Yan W, et al. (2000). Stem cell factor functions as a survival factor for mature Leydig cells and a growth factor for precursor Leydig cells after ethylene dimethane sulfonate treatment: implication of a role of the stem cell factor/c-Kit system in Leydig cell development. *Dev Biol*, 227:169–82

Yanagamachi R (1994). Mammalian fertilization. In *The Physiology of Reproduction*, 189–317

Yanushpolsky EH, et al. (1996). Is leukocytospermia clinically relevant? *Fertil Steril*, 66:822–5

Yong EL, et al. (1994). Pregnancy after hormonal correction of severe spermatogenic defect due to mutation in androgen receptor gene. *Lancet*, 344:826–7

Yong EL, et al. (1998). Androgen receptor transactivation domain and control of spermatogenesis. *Rev Reprod*, 3:141–4

Young EA (1995). The role of gonadal steroids in hypothalamic–pituitary–adrenal axis regulation. *Crit Rev Neurobiol*, 9:371–81

Z

Zamboni L (1992). Sperm structure and its relevance to infertility. *Arch Pathol Lab Med*, 116:325–44

Zamboni L (1994). Detection of human sperm pathology by fine structure analysis. In *The Biological Basis of Early Human Reproductive Failure: Application to Medically Assisted Conception and the Treatment of Infertility*. New York: Academic Press, 327–44

Zaneveld LJD, Polakoski P (1979). Collection and physical examination of the ejaculate. In Hafez ESE, ed. *Techniques of Human Andrology*. MTP Press, 142

Zhu X, Naz RK (1997). Fertilization antigen-1: cDNA cloning, testis-specific expression, and immunocontraceptive effects. *Proc Natl Acad Sci USA*, 94:4704–9

Zini A, et al. (1993). Reactive oxygen species in semen of infertile patients: levels of superoxide dismutase and catalase-like activities in seminal plasma and spermatozoa. *Int J Androl*, 16:183–8

Zini A, *et al.* (1995). Low level of nitric oxide promotes human sperm capacitation *in vitro. J Androl*, 16:424–31

Zini A, *et al.* (2001a). Correlations between two markers of sperm DNA integrity, DNA denaturation and DNA fragmentation, in fertile and infertile men. *Fertil Steril*, 75:674–7

Zini A, *et al.* (2001b). Biologic variability of sperm DNA denaturation in infertile men. *Urology*, 581:258–61

Zlotta AR (2001). GnRH analogues in prostate cancer. In *Lunenfeld B, ed.* GnRH Analogues. New York: Parthenon Publishing

Appendix

GLOSSARY OF COMMON ABBREVIATIONS

ACTH	Adrenocorticotropic hormone
ADH	Antidiuretic hormone
AFP	α-Fetoprotein
AI	Artificial insemination
AIDS	Acquired immune deficiency syndrome
AMP	Adenosine monophosphate
ARC	AIDS-related complex
ATP	Adenosine triphosphate
BBB	Blood–brain barrier
BBT	Basal body temperature
bFGF	Basic fibroblast growth factor
BP	Blood pressure
BSA	Bovine serum albumin
cAMP	Cyclic AMP
cDNA	DNA complementary to RNA
CDP	Cytidine 5′-phosphate
CIC	Circulating immune complexes
CL	Corpus luteum
CRH	Corticotropin releasing hormone
CSF	Colony-stimulating factor
CT	Computed tomography
D&C	Dilatation and curettage
D&E	Dilatation and evacuation
DES	Diethylstilbestrol
DHEA	Dehydroepiandrosterone
DHT	Dihydrotestosterone
DMSO	Dimethyl sulfoxide (Me_2SO)
DNA	Deoxyribonucleic acid
EF	Elongation factor
EGF	Epidermal growth factor

ELISA	Enzyme-linked immunosorbent assay
FCS	Fetal calf serum
FGF	Fibroblast growth factor
FSH	Follicle stimulating hormone
GnRH	Gonadotropin releasing hormone
GHRH	Growth hormone releasing hormone
GLC	Gas–liquid chromatography
GM-CSF	Granulocyte–macrophage colony-stimulating factor
GTT	Glucose tolerance test
hCB	Human cord blood
hCG	Human chorionic gonadotropin
hMG	Human menopausal gonadotropin
hMT	Human mammary tumor
HPLC	High-pressure liquid chromatography
HSV	Herpes simplex virus
ICM	Inner cell mass
IF	Immunofluorescence
IFN	Interferon
Ig	Immunoglobulin
IGF	Insulin-like growth factor
IL	Interleukin
IM	Intramuscular
IUGR	Intrauterine growth restriction
IV	Intravenous
IVF	*In vitro* fertilization
kDa	Kilodalton
LBW	Low birth weight
LH	Luteinizing hormone
LHRH	Luteinizing hormone releasing hormone
LHRF	Luteinizing hormone releasing factor
LI	Luteinizing inhibitor

LPS	Lipopolysaccharide
NGF	Nerve growth factor
NK	Natural killer
PAF	Platelet-activating factor
PAGE	Polyacrylamide gel electrophoresis
PBL	Peripheral blood lymphocytes
PBS	Phosphate-buffered saline
PDGF	Platelet-derived growth factor
PG	Prostaglandin
PGE_2	Prostaglandin E_2
PGF_2	Prostaglandin F_2
PIF	Prolactin inhibiting factor
PVS	Perivitelline space
RNA	Ribonucleic acid
rRNA	Ribosomal RNA
SMC	Somatomedin-C
STH	Somatotropic hormone
TBG	Thyroxine-binding globulin
TDF	Testis-determining factor
TGF	Transforming growth factor
TNF	Tumor necrosis factor
VIP	Vasoactive intestinal peptide

UNITS OF MEASURE

mg	Milligram (10^{-3} g)
μg	Microgram (10^{-6} g)
ng	Nanogram (10^{-9} g)
pg	Picogram (10^{-12} g)
IU	International unit

FURTHER INFORMATION AND USEFUL ADDRESSES

Eisenhower Army Medical Center

Website: http://www.ddeamc.amedd.army.mil/info_pat/takingcare/health_info/testicular.htm

MenWeb

Website: http://www.vix.com/menmag/testican.htm

Sex education

USA

The Sex Education Coalition
PO Box 341 751, Bethesda, MD 20827-1751, USA
E-mail: Webmaster@SexEdCoalition.org

UK

Sex Education Forum
National Children's Bureau, 8 Wakley Street, London ECIV 7QE, UK
E-mail: sexedforum@ncb.org.uk
Web: http://www.ncb.org.uk/sexed.htm

Brook Centres
Web: http://www.brook.org.uk
E-Mail: information@brookcentres.org.uk

Contraception

USA

Engender Health
440 Ninth Avenue, New York, New York 10001, 212-561-8067, USA
Web: http://www.engenderhealth.org

The World Health Organization has a online booklet called *Vasectomy:*
http://www.who.int/rht/documents/FPP94-3/fpp943.htm
They also offer a film called *No Scalpel Vasectomy* for $10.

JAMA Women's Health
Contraception Information Center
Web: www.ama-assn.org/special/contra/support/ppfa/vasecto4.htm

UK

International Planned Parenthood Federation
Regent College, Regent's Park, London NW1 4NS, UK
Phone: 020 7486 0741

Infertility

Resolve
The National Infertility Association
1310 Broadway, Somerville, MA 02144, USA
E-mail: resolveinc.@aol.com
Web: http://www.resolve.org

InterNational Council on Infertility Information Dissemination (INCIID)
PO Box 6386, Arlington, Virginia 22206, USA
Phone: 703-379-9178
Fax: 703-379-1593
E-mail: INCIIDinfo@inciid.org
Web: http://www.inciid.org

The American Infertility Association
666 Fifth Avenue, Suite 278, New York, NY 10103, USA
Phone: 718-621-5083
E-mail: 718-621-5083
Web: http://www.americaninfertility.org

http://www.infertility-info.com
A website with information about *in vitro* fertilization.
Sponsored by Zander

Ferti.Net
Web: http://www.ferti.net

International Federation of Infertility Patient Associations
Charter House, Suite 8, 43 St. Leonards Road, Bexhill-on-Sea, East Sussex, TN40 1JA, UK
Phone: 01424 732361
Fax: 01424 7311858
E-mail: office@child.org.uk
Web: http://www.repromed.org.uk

The National Fertility Association (ISSUE)
114 Lichfield Street, Walsall WSI ISZ, UK
Phone: 01922 722 888
Web: http://www.issue.co.uk
E-mail: info@issue.co.uk

National Infertility Support and Information Group
P.O. Box 131, Eglinton Street, Cork, Republic of Ireland
E-Mail: nisig@indigo.ie

International Program on Chemical Safety (WHO/UNEP/ILO)
Global State of the Science Assessment of endocrine disruptors
Web: http://endocrine.ei.jrc.it/gaed.html

Rachel's Environment & Health weekly
Web: http://www.rachel.org/bulletin
Published by
Environmental Research Foundation, P.O. Box 5036, Annapolis, MD 21403, USA
Fax: 410-263-8944
E-mail: info@rachel.org

Occupational health

USA

National Institute for Occupational Safety and Health
Web: www.cdc.gov/niosh/homepage.html
NIOSH Publication No. 96-132
Phone: 1-800-356 4674

UK

Directory of Sites in Occupational and Environmental Health
Web: http://www.agius.com/hew/links

British Occupational Health Strategy
Web: http://www.ohstrategy.net/strategy/strat_intro.htm

Prostate health and disease

USA

American Cancer Society
Web: http://www.cancer.org

Centers for Disease Control and Prevention (CDC)
Cancer Prevention and Control
4770 Buford Hwy., NE MS K64, Atlanta, GA 30341
Phone: 1-888-842-6355
Web: http://www.cdc.gov

National Cancer Institute
Web: http://cancernet.nci.nih.gov/Cancer_Types/Prostrate_Cancer.shtml
Phone: 1-800-4-CANCER

MedlinePlus
Web: http://www.nlm.nih.gov/medlineplus/prostatecancer.html
This service of the National Library of Medicine has a website listing news from various publications – popular press and governmental agencies – on prostate cancer.

http://www.prostate.com
A site dedicated to prostate cancer, with special sections about treatment options, and a 'what to ask your doctor' section. Affiliated with pharmaceutical company TAP, the company that produces a drug used in the treatment of advanced prostate cancer.

http://www.prostatehealth.com
Informative site with general and specific information, about the prostate in general and about infections and diseases and their treatment.

UK

CancerBACUP
Web: http://cancerbacup.org.uk/info/prostate.htm

CancerHelp UK
Web: http://www.cancerhelp.org.uk

Some organizations of interest

CaP Cure (The Association for the Cure of Cancer of
    the Prostate)
1250 4th Street, Santa Monica, CA 90401, USA
Phone: 1-800-757-CURE or 310-458-2873
Web: http://www.capcure.org

National Prostate Cancer Coalition
1156 15th Street, NW, Washington, DC 20005, USA
Phone: 202-463-9455
Web: http://www.4npcc.org

Index

Note to index: page numbers of tables (where not already covered by the reference) are shown in bold

T - #1058 - 101024 - C260 - 285/214/12 [14] - CB - 9781842142356 - Gloss Lamination